Problem-based Approach to Gastroenterology and Hepatology

Problem-based Approach to Gastroenterology and Hepatology

Edited by

John N. Plevris MD, PhD, FRCPE, FEBGH
Consultant and Reader in Gastroenterology
Centre for Liver and Digestive Disorders
The Royal Infirmary of Edinburgh
Edinburgh, Scotland
UK

Colin W. Howden MD, FRCP (Glasg.), FACP, AGAF, FACG
Professor of Medicine
Division of Gastroenterology and Hepatology,
Northwestern University Feinberg School of Medicine
Chicago
Illinois
USA

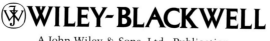

A John Wiley & Sons, Ltd., Publication

This edition first published 2012 © 2012 by Blackwell Publishing Ltd

Blackwell Publishing was acquired by John Wiley & Sons in February 2007. Blackwell's publishing program has been merged with Wiley's global Scientific, Technical and Medical business to form Wiley-Blackwell.

Registered office: John Wiley & Sons, Ltd, The Atrium, Southern Gate, Chichester, West Sussex, PO19 8SQ, UK

Editorial offices: 9600 Garsington Road, Oxford, OX4 2DQ, UK
The Atrium, Southern Gate, Chichester, West Sussex, PO19 8SQ, UK
111 River Street, Hoboken, NJ 07030-5774, USA

For details of our global editorial offices, for customer services and for information about how to apply for permission to reuse the copyright material in this book please see our website at www.wiley.com/wiley-blackwell

Library of Congress Cataloging-in-Publication Data

Problem-based approach to gastroenterology and hepatology / edited by John N. Plevris, Colin W. Howden.
    p. ; cm.
  Includes bibliographical references and index.
  ISBN-13: 978-1-4051-8227-0 (pbk. : alk. paper)
  ISBN-10: 1-4051-8227-X (pbk. : alk. paper)
  1. Gastrointestinal system–Diseases xDiagnosis–Case studies. 2. Liver–Diseases–Diagnosis–Case studies. I. Plevris, John N. II. Howden, Colin W.
  [DNLM: 1. Gastrointestinal Diseases–diagnosis–Case Reports. 2. Gastrointestinal Diseases–therapy–Case Reports. 3. Liver Diseases–diagnosis–Case Reports. 4. Liver Diseases–therapy–Case Reports. WI 140]
  RC808.P76 2012
  616.3'3–dc23

        2011015322

A catalogue record for this book is available from the British Library.

Wiley also publishes its books in a variety of electronic formats. Some content that appears in print may not be available in electronic books.

Set in 9 on 11.5 pt Sabon by Toppan Best-set Premedia Limited
Printed and bound in Singapore by Markono Print Media Pte Ltd

1 2012

Contents

Preface

Problem-based approaches are commonly used in Medicine as effective learning tools; the problem drives knowledge, thus promoting critical thinking and making the whole educational process interesting and relevant. We hope that this book, based on the above principles, will be of value to physicians who are training in Gastroenterology and Hepatology and who may be preparing to take a specialty postgraduate examination. Given its size, this book is clearly not intended to be a major treatise on digestive disorders. Furthermore, we do not claim that reading it will guarantee success in a relevant postgraduate examination in Gastroenterology/Hepatology. Rather, we hope that it will stimulate further reading, will supplement other preparations for those examinations and provide valuable insight into how some of the experts – from both sides of the Atlantic – approach common, important clinical issues in these specialties. Each chapter contains a number of case scenarios that raise questions of diagnosis and management. Our expert authors then present valuable discussion and important learning points about each case.

We have been fortunate to be able to draw on the expertise of friends and colleagues from both sides of the Atlantic (and beyond). We therefore expect that this book will be of value to a broad, multinational readership. It has been said that the UK and the USA are *"two countries separated by a common language"*. (The derivation of that is uncertain having been variously attributed to Winston Churchill, Oscar Wilde and George Bernard Shaw – any of whom could have prepared a more entertaining preface than this). We hope that this is not the perception of this book. Authors based in the USA have used American spelling and units of measurement; those based in the UK have used their own frames of reference. Hopefully, both are clear and readers will learn from both.

We would like to take this opportunity to thank all of our invited authors for their contributions to this book and their commitment to this project. We are also grateful to the editorial team at Wiley-Blackwell for all the support and effective co-ordination.

John N. Plevris
Colin W. Howden
January 2012

Contributors

Michael P. Angarone DO
Clinical Instructor
Northwestern University, Division of Infectious
  Disease
Northwestern University Feinberg School of
  Medicine
Chicago, IL, USA

Malcolm B. Barnes MBBS(Hons), FRACP
Consultant Gastroenterologist
Monash Medical Centre
Victoria, Australia

Andrew J. Bathgate MB.CHB, MD, FRCPE
Consultant Hepatologist
Scottish Liver Transplant Unit
The Royal Infirmary of Edinburgh
Edinburgh, Scotland, UK

Paul Beck PhD, MD, FRCPC
Associate Professor of Medicine
Division of Gastroenterology
University of Calgary
Calgary, Alberta, Canada

Tiffany J. Campbell BSC(Hons), MB ChB,
  MRCP, FRCR
Consultant Radiologist
Forth Valley Royal Hospital
Larbert, UK

Lotte Dinesen MD
Specialist Registrar
Gastroenterology Section, Division of Medicine
Imperial College London
Hammersmith Hospital
London, UK

Joanna K. Dowman MBChB(Hons), MRCP
Clinical Research Fellow and Specialist Registrar in
  Gastroenterology
Queen Elizabeth Hospital Birmingham, and NIHR
  Biomedical Research Unit and Centre for Liver
  Research
University of Birmingham, UK

Mary Farid MD
Fellow in Gastroentrology
UCLA Affiliated Training Program in Digestive
  Diseases
University of California
Los Angeles, USA

Ronnie Fass MD
Professor of Medicine
University of Arizona and Chief of Gastroenterology
Southern Arizona VA Health Care System
Tucson, AZ, USA

John P. Flaherty MD
Professor of Medicine
Division of Infectious Diseases
Northwestern University Feinberg School of
  Medicine
Chicago, IL, USA

O. James Garden BSc, MBChB, MD, FRCS(Glas),
  FRCS(Ed), FRCP(Ed), FRACS(Hon), FRCSC(Hon)
Regius Professor of Clinical Surgery
Clinical Surgery
The Royal Infirmary of Edinburgh
Edinburgh, Scotland, UK

Subrata Ghosh MBBS, MD(Edin.), FRCP, FRCPE,
  FRCPC
Professor of Medicine
Chairman of Department of Medicine
University of Calgary
Calgary, Alberta, Canada

Simon Glance MDBBS(Hons)
Consultant Gastroenterologist
The Northern Hospital
Melbourne, Australia

Nirmala Gonsalves MD
Assistant Professor of Medicine
Division of Gastroenterology
Northwestern University – The Feinberg School of
  Medicine
Chicago, IL, USA

Timothy T. Gordon-Walker MBChB, BSc
Specialist Registrar in Gastroenterology
The Royal Infirmary of Edinburgh
and
MRC Centre for Inflammation Research
Queen's Medical Research Institute
Edinburgh, Scotland, UK

Peter C. Hayes MD, PhD, FRCPE
Professor of Hepatology
Centre for Liver and Digestive Disorders
The Royal Infirmary of Edinburgh
Edinburgh, Scotland UK

Neil C. Henderson BMSc(Hons), MBChB(Hons),
  MSc, PhD, MD, FRCP(Ed)
Senior Clinical Scientist and Consultant
  Hepatologist
Centre for Liver and Digestive Disorders
The Royal Infirmary of Edinburgh
Edinburgh, Scotland, UK

Tiberiu Hershcovici MD
Research Fellow
Southern Arizona VA Health Care System
Tucson, AZ, USA

Ikuo Hirano MD
Professor of Medicine
Division of Gastroenterology
Northwestern University Feinberg School of
  Medicine
Chicago, IL, USA

John P. Iredale DM, FRCP, FMedSci
Professor of Medicine
Tissue Injury and Regeneration Group
MRC Centre for Inflammation Research
Queen's Medical Research Institute
Edinburgh, Scotland, UK

Brian E. Lacy MD, PhD
Associate Professor of Medicine
Dartmouth Medical School
and
Director
Gastrointestinal Motility Laboratory
Dartmouth-Hitchcock Medical Center
Lebanon, NH, USA

Anne-Marie Lennon MB, PhD, MRCP(UK)
Assistant Professor of Medicine
Department of Gastroenterology and Hepatology
Johns Hopkins Hospital
Baltimore, MA, USA

Grigorios I. Leontiadis MD, PhD
Assistant Professor
McMaster University Department of Medicine
Division of Gastroenterology
Health Sciences Centre
Hamilton, ON, Canada

Norma C. McAvoy MBChB, MRCP(UK)
Clinical Lecturer
Centre for Liver and Digestive Disorders
The Royal Infirmary of Edinburgh
Edinburgh, Scotland, UK

Lisa J. Massie MBChB
Specialist Surgical Registrar
Clinical Surgery
The Royal Infirmary of Edinburgh
Edinburgh, Scotland, UK

Lynne A. Meekison MBChB
Associate Specialist
Centre for Liver and Digestive Disorders
The Royal Infirmary of Edinburgh
Edinburgh, Scotland, UK

Phil N. Newsome PhD, FRCP
Senior Lecturer in Hepatology and Honorary
  Consultant Physician
Queen Elizabeth Hospital Birmingham, and NIHR
  Biomedical Research Unit and Centre for Liver
  Research
University of Birmingham, UK

Remo Panaccione MD, FRCPC
Associate Professor of Medicine
Division of Gastroenterology
University of Calgary
Calgary, Alberta, Canada

Dilip Patel BMedSci (Hons), MB BS, FRCP(Ed),
  FRCR
Consultant Radiologist and Honorary Clinical
  Senior Lecturer
The Royal Infirmary of Edinburgh
University of Edinburgh
Edinburgh, Scotland, UK

Prakash Ramachandran BSc, MBChB, PhD,
  MRCP(UK)
Specialist Registrar in Gastroenterology and
  Hepatology
Scottish Liver Transplant Unit
The Royal Infirmary of Edinburgh
Edinburgh, Scotland UK

Erica J. Revie BSc, MBChB, MRCS
Specialist Surgical Registrar
Clinical Surgery
The Royal Infirmary of Edinburgh
Edinburgh, Scotland, UK

Veerendra Sandur MBBS, MD, DNM,
  DM(Gastro)
Liver Transplantation Fellow
Multiorgan Transplant Program
Toronto General Hospital
Toronto, Ontario, Canada

Matthew Shale MRCP
Academic Clinical Fellow
Gastroenterology Section
Division of Medicine
Imperial College London, Hammersmith Hospital
London, UK

Virender K. Sharma FASGE, FACG, AGAF
Professor of Medicine and Director
Arizona Center for Digestive Health
Gilbert, AZ, USA

Kenneth J. Simpson MBChB, MD, PhD, FRCPE
Senior Lecturer in Hepatology
Centre for Liver and Digestive Disorders
The Royal Infirmary of Edinburgh
Edinburgh, Scotland, UK

Chad C. Spangler MD
Instructor in Medicine
Division of Gastroenterology and Hepatology
Dartmouth-Hitchcock Medical Center
Lebanon NH, USA

Brennan Spiegel MD, MSHS
Associate Professor of Medicine
VA Greater Los Angeles Healthcare System David
  Geffen School of Medicine at UCLA
and
Director
UCLA/VA Center for Outcomes Research and
  Education
Los Angeles, CA, USA

George Therapondos MBChB(Hons), PhD,
  MD, FRCP(Ed)
Assistant Professor of Medicine
Multiorgan Transplant Program
Toronto General Hospital
University Health Network
Toronto, Ontario, Canada

PART ONE
Gastroenterology

1

Dysphagia

Nirmala Gonsalves[1], Ikuo Hirano[1], and John N. Plevris[2]

[1]Division of Gastroenterology, Northwestern University Feinberg School of Medicine, Chicago, USA
[2]Centre for Liver & Digestive Disorders, The Royal Infirmary, University of Edinburgh, Edinburgh, UK

Dysphagia refers to difficulty or inability in swallowing food or liquids. Most dysphagia patients are candidates for urgent upper digestive endoscopy, to exclude the presence of esophageal cancer. The annual incidence of upper gastrointestinal malignancy, particularly esophageal adenocarcinoma, is steadily increasing in the western world, being the 5th most common primary site in Scotland [1].

Traditionally, dysphagia has been classified as oropharyngeal or esophageal. Oropharyngeal dysphagia is due to impaired food bolus formation or propagation into hypopharynx. Causes include neuromuscular disorders, cerebrovascular events, mechanical obstruction in the oral cavity or hypophanynx, decreased salivation, Parkinson's and Alzheimer's disease or depression. Esophageal dysphagia can be due to mechanical obstruction, (benign or malignant stricture), dysmotility disorders or secondary to gastro-esophageal reflux. Significant dysphagia is often associated with aspiration pneumonia.

A detailed history is important to elicit a possible etiology. In younger patients dysmotility is more common. The presence of chest pain during swallowing strongly suggests esophageal spasm; dysphagia for both liquids and solids is common is achalasia. In young patients with food impaction eosinophilic esophagitis should always be considered. In the elderly, neurological causes should be considered if the dysphagia is high, while esophageal cancer usually presents with short duration progressive dysphagia for solids with regurgitation and weight loss. New onset hoarse voice and dysphagia, point towards malignant infiltration of the recurrent laryngeal nerve. High dysphagia associated with regurgitation of undigested food from previous days, is strongly suggestive of a pharyngeal pouch.

Despite the different presenting features associated with different causes of dysphagia, there is no reliable way to predict at presentation those patients likely to have a malignant cause. Recently, a scoring system based on 6 parameters (advanced age, male gender, weight loss of >3 kg, new onset dysphagia, localisation to the chest and absence of acid reflux at presentation) could strongly predict malignancy [2]. In this chapter, three selected cases will illustrate the different etiologies of this important alarm symptom.

Case 1: dysphagia for liquids and solids

Case presentation

A 52-year-old man reports a 9-month history of difficulty swallowing both liquids and solids with meals and localizes the problem to upper sternum. He gets frequent episodes of coughing and choking when lying flat at night after meals. More recently, he has noticed spontaneous regurgitation of clear, foamy liquid and undigested food into his mouth, especially when bending over after dinner. He has lost over 15 lb (6.8 kg) since his symptoms began. Heartburn, which had been a problem in the past, has notably improved

---

since his dysphagia began. Additional complaints include episodes of squeezing pain lasting for several minutes to 1 hour without radiation that can occur at any time and are unrelated to physical activity or meals. Drinking cold water sometimes alleviates the pain.

Past medical history: hypertension

Medications: lisinopril

Social history: employed as a businessman. Moved to the USA from Bolivia 20 years ago. Smokes 20 cigarettes per day. Drinks 3–4 glasses of wine per week

Family history: no family history of cancer or swallowing disorders

Physical examination: unremarkable

In particular, oral cavity without mucosal abnormalities, intact dentition, with no neck masses, lymphadenopathy or goiter. No evidence of sclerodactyly or telangiectasia.

Upper endoscopy revealed a dilated esophagus with approximately 200 mL of retained, semisolid debris despite a 36-hour liquid diet (Figure 1.1a). The underlying mucosa appeared with scattered superficial erosions and mild, diffuse nodularity. Constriction of the esophagogastric junction was noted with minimal resistance to passage of the endoscope into the stomach (Figure 1.1b). Pylorus was patent and the duodenum was normal.

Esophageal manometry was performed using a high-resolution, solid-state catheter assembly with contour pressure topography (Figure 1.2) showed panesophageal pressurization or common cavity phenomenon in response to a water swallow. Failed deglutitive relaxation of the lower esophageal sphincter was evident. The presence of an esophagogastric pressure gradient is seen in the esophagus before the swallow suggestive of achalasia.

Questions

• What are the diagnostic considerations in this patient?
• What are the clinical symptoms of achalasia?
• What diagnostic tests are useful in achalasia?
• What is the pathophysiology of achalasia?
• What are the benefits and risks of different treatment options that should be discussed with this patient?
• What are the complications of achalasia?

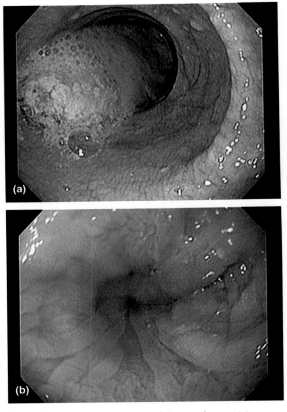

Figure 1.1 Endoscopic images of the esophagus: (a) a moderately dilated esophageal body with retained food and secretions in spite of a 12-hour fast; (b) a constriction at the level of the esophagogastric junction in the same patient.

Differential diagnosis

Esophageal dysmotility should be considered in any patient presenting with dysphagia for both liquids and solids. A few caveats to this rule exist:

• First, patients with oropharyngeal dysphagia may present with liquid and solid dysphagia and, in fact, may have greater difficulty with liquids than solids. However, the fact that this patient localizes his dysphagia to the sternal area excludes an oropharyngeal etiology.

• Second, patients with esophageal food impaction typically have difficulty swallowing liquids and even their own saliva. However, the history was not consistent with repeated food impactions in this case.

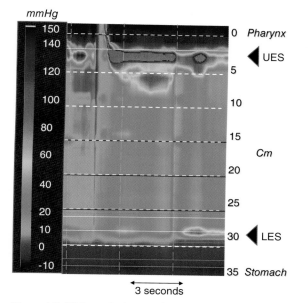

mmHg

0 *Pharynx*
◄ UES
5
10
15
Cm
20
25
30 ◄ LES
35 *Stomach*

← 3 seconds →

Figure 1.2 High-resolution esophageal manometry pressure contour plot depicting a water swallow. Panesophageal pressurization above intragastric pressure is seen and failed lower esophageal sphincter relaxation is evident.

• Third, the dysphagia that accompanies an advanced esophageal malignancy produces progressive obstruction. Although a consideration here, such patients present with a more rapid transition from solid to semisolid to liquid dysphagia over time.

The three major esophageal motor disorders are achalasia, scleroderma, and diffuse esophageal spasm (DES). Patients with scleroderma have typically mild dysphagia and in most cases is accompanied with cutaneous manifestations. Although both DES and achalasia are possible diagnoses in this patient, dysphagia in DES is generally less severe and more intermittent than in achalasia.

Clinical presentation of achalasia

Achalasia is an uncommon but important disease. The clinical manifestations as well as treatment center on the integrity of the lower esophageal sphincter (LES). Dysphagia and regurgitation are the most commonly reported symptoms. Nocturnal regurgitation can lead to night cough and aspiration. With progres-

sive disease weight loss can occur. Chest pain is well recognized in achalasia and has been reported in 17–63% of patients but its mechanism is unclear although proposed etiologies include secondary or tertiary esophageal contractions, esophageal distension by retained food, gastro-esophageal reflux, esophageal irritation by retained medications, food, and bacterial or fungal overgrowth. Paroxysmal pain may be neuropathic in origin. Inflammation within the esophageal myenteric plexus could also be a contributory factor. More than one mechanism is likely operative in an individual patient.

A prospective study found no association between the occurrence of chest pain and either manometric or radiographic abnormalities [3]. Patients with chest pain were younger and had a shorter duration of symptoms compared with patients with no pain, but treatment of achalasia had little impact on the chest pain, in spite of adequate relief of dysphagia. Counter to this, a recent surgical series reported adequate relief of chest pain after a Heller myotomy [4]. Importantly, chest pain is not a universal feature in achalasia. In fact, many patients appear unaware of either esophageal distension or the prolonged the prolonged esophageal retention of food. Recent studies using esophageal barostat stimulation have demonstrated that some patients with achalasia have diminished mechanical and chemosensitivity of the esophagus [5]. Such differences may explain the heterogeneity of visceral sensitivity in the achalasia population.

Diagnostic evaluation

Upper endoscopy is the first line investigation in suspected achalasia. Findings include esophageal dilation with retained saliva or food and annular constriction of the gastroesophageal junction. Intubation of the stomach is achieved with minor resistance due to raised LES pressure. Significant difficulty passing an endoscope through the gastroesophageal junction should raise the index of suspicion for pseudoachalasia due to neoplastic infiltration of the distal esophagus or gastric cardia. In spite of these recognized endoscopic features, upper endoscopy was reported as normal in 44% of a series of newly diagnosed achalasia patients [6]. A barium esophagogram (swallow) can be highly suggestive of achalasia, particularly when there is the combination of esophageal dilation with retained food and barium, and a smooth, tapered constriction of the gastroesophageal junction. However, the diagnosis of achalasia was suggested in only 64% of barium examinations in the previous study [6].

Esophageal manometry has the highest diagnostic sensitivity for achalasia and should be performed when the etiology of dysphagia is not evident by endoscopy alone. Findings include distal esophageal aperistalsis and incomplete or absent LES relaxation. Additional supportive features include a hypertensive LES and low-amplitude esophageal body contractions. by endoscopic or radiographic examination.

Although manometry is regarded as the "gold standard" for the diagnosis of achalasia, heterogeneity exists in the manometric presentation. The most commonly recognized variant is known as "vigorous achalasia," variably defined by the presence of normal to high amplitude esophageal body contractions in the presence of a non-relaxing LES. Such contractions are generally simultaneous and can be difficult to distinguish from common cavity phenomena. Although vigorous achalasia may represent an early stage of achalasia, studies have failed to demonstrate differences in terms of clinical presentation, although botulinum toxin has been reported to be more effective in patients with vigorous achalasia. Additional manometric variants of achalasia include rare individuals with intact peristalsis through most of the esophageal body and with preservation of either deglutitive or transient LES relaxation [7]. The significance in defining these variants lies in the recognition that these sometimes confusing manometric findings are still consistent with achalasia when combined with clinical data supportive of the diagnosis.

High-resolution esophageal manometry (HRM) combined with contour plot topographic analyses can significantly improve the accuracy of esophageal manometry. HRM allows for automated analysis of more detailed quantitative data. An example of the utility of this methodology is the interpretation of impaired LES deglutitive relaxation in the setting of exaggerated respiratory contractions of the crural diaphragm. Intrabolus pressure elevations are more readily apparent and quantified using HRM. A recent retrospective study subclassified 99 achalasia patients into those with classic achalasia with minimal esophageal pressurization, achalasia with esophageal compression (panesophageal pressurization in excess of 30 mmHg), and achalasia with spasm [8]. Panesophageal pressurization was a positive predictor whereas esophageal spasm was a negative predictor of treatment response.

Secondary forms of achalasia

The most concerning secondary etiology is cancer, which can present as achalasia by one of three mechanisms. The first and most common occurs through direct mechanical obstruction of the gastroesophageal junction. This is referred to as pseudoachalasia, and has been most commonly described with distal esophageal and proximal gastric adenocarcinomas. Cancer can also infiltrate the submucosa and muscularis of the LES and disrupt the myenteric neurons, resulting in achalasia without an endoscopically visible mucosal abnormality. Finally, achalasia can be a manifestation of paraneoplastic syndrome with circulating autoantibodies that are directed at the myenteric neurons. This syndrome is a rare but important complication of small cell lung cancer.

Chagas' disease, a parasitic infection caused by *Trypanosoma cruzi*, is endemic to areas of Central and South America. The esophagus is most commonly involved, and manifests itself as secondary achalasia in 7–10% of chronically infected individuals. Chagas' disease should be a consideration in the evaluation of achalasia patients in the USA, given that the gastrointestinal sequelae can manifest years or decades after the acute infection. Our patient had positive serological testing for antibodies to *T. cruzi*, consistent with chronic infection. The management of his achalasia does not change but evaluation for other cardiac and visceral manifestations of the parasite are indicated.

Pathogenesis

While the etiology of primary achalasia remains unknown, several hypotheses have been proposed. Several studies have implicated viral agents. A study using DNA hybridization techniques found evidence of varicella-zoster virus in three of nine myotomy specimens from patients with achalasia [9]. The herpes virus family was specifically targeted in this study, given their neurotropic nature. The predilection of the herpesviruses for squamous epithelium as opposed to columnar epithelium makes this an attractive hypothesis and could explain why achalasia involves only the esophagus, while sparing the remainder of the gastrointestinal tract. More recent studies however, failed to detect the presence of measles, herpes, or human papillomaviruses in myotomy specimens of 13 patients with achalasia. This negative study does not exclude the possibility of either an alternate viral species or past viral infection with clearance of the inciting pathogen from the host tissue. Supporting the viral hypothesis is a recent study demonstrating immunoreactivity of lymphocytes from the LES of patients with achalasia in response to herpes simplex virus HSV-1 antigens. In this study, analysis of oligoclonal expansion of T cells provided evidence for immune activation thus resulting in autoimmune destruction of enteric neurons [10].

An autoimmune etiology of achalasia is supported by the presence of circulating autoantibodies against the myenteric plexus. These have been shown in a few studies to be more prevalent in achalasia patients than in controls. However, a recent study detected significantly higher immunostaining of the esophageal myenteric plexus neurons using serum from both achalasia and gastroesophageal reflux disease (GERD) patients than controls, suggesting that such antibodies represent an epiphenomenon rather than a causative factor [11]. The presence of a lymphocytic infiltrate consisting of CD3+ and CD8+ T cells in the myenteric plexus not found in controls, also supports an autoimmune etiology [11,12].

Treatment

Treatment options for idiopathic achalasia include medical therapy, endoscopic botulinum toxin injection, endoscopic pneumatic dilation, and surgical myotomy [13–15]. All forms of therapy seek to reduce the LES pressure to allow for improved esophageal clearance by gravity because the esophageal peristalsis is impaired.

Medical therapy with calcium channel antagonists or nitrates has demonstrated limited efficacy. Medical therapy is generally restricted to patients awaiting more definitive therapy or patients who are not candidates for more invasive therapies and who have not responded to treatment with botulinum toxin.

Botulinum toxin is both easy and safe to administer [16]. To date, there have been over 15 prospective studies involving over 450 patients from around the world that have examined its efficacy. Response rates at 1 month after administration average 78% (range 63–90%). By 6 months, the clinical response drops to 58% (range 25–78%), and to 49% (range 15–64%) at 12 months. Moreover, improvement in objective measures of esophageal function are significantly lower after botulinum toxin than other more definitive therapies for achalasia [17]. Given the limitations to the efficacy and durability of response, botulinum toxin is generally reserved for patients who are not candidates for pneumatic dilation or Heller myotomy.

Dilation of the esophagus is the oldest form of therapy for achalasia. Currently, the Rigiflex pneumatic dilator (Boston Scientific Corp, Boston, MA) is the most widely used dilating system. A non-compliant polythylene balloon that comes in three sizes designed to inflate to fixed diameters of 3, 3.5, or 4 cm is used. The overall success rates defined by good to excellent relief of symptoms averages 85% (range 70–92%) with a mean follow-up period of 20 months. Age, balloon diameter, post-dilation LES pressure, clearance of barium on an esophagogram, and prior dilation have been identified as predictors of success. Similar to the botulinum toxin experience, several studies have reported that older patients respond better. Eckardt found a 2-year remission rate of 29% in patients under 40 compared with 67% for those over 40 [18]. Long-term follow-up studies of the effectiveness of pneumatic dilation have reported a substantially lower response rate of 30–40% – approximately half that reported in the short-term studies. Thus, repeated dilations are to be expected when using pneumatic dilation as primary therapy. The main complication of pneumatic dilation is esophageal perforation. Published series have reported perforation rates of 0–8% with a mean rate of 2.6%.

Laparoscopic Heller myotomy has greatly advanced the surgical approach to achalasia. It allows for shorter hospital stays and less recovery time than open cardiomyotomy. Furthermore, the laparoscopic approach has substantially challenged the use of dilation as primary therapy since perforation from pneumatic dilation generally necessitates repair via open thoracotomy. Success rates reported in large series approximate 90%, with mean follow-up approaching 2 years. Perioperative complications of perforation, hemorrhage, or pneumothorax are uncommon and readily managed intraoperatively. Reflux is a not infrequent complication of both endoscopic and surgical therapies in the setting of an aperistaltic esophagus. In one of the larger surgical series, reflux was documented by pH testing in 17% of patients after laparoscopic myotomy with most of these patients not reporting heartburn [19]. Barrett's esophagus and peptic stricture have been documented in several reported series after a Heller myotomy. Surgical approaches to the problem have included creation of a loose Nissen, partial posterior Toupet, or partial anterior Dor fundoplication. Similar to the experience with pneumatic dilation, the reported remission rates after Heller myotomy for achalasia reflect a gradual deterioration over time. Malthaner reported a 95% success rate at 1 year, 77% at 5 years, 68% at 10 years, and 67% at 20 years [20]. Thus, the effectiveness of what is considered the most definitive therapy for achalasia appears to wane with time.

Several studies have reported superior success rates for surgery compared with pneumatic dilation. A recent, retrospective, longitudinal study using an administrative database in Ontario, Canada compared outcomes of 1181 patients treated with pneumatic dilation with 280 patients treated with Heller myotomy as initial therapy [13]. Although the risk of subsequent therapeutic intervention at 10 years was significantly higher with dilation (64%) than with surgery (38%), this outcome is expected and attributed to repeated dilations that did not lead to a significantly higher risk of surgical intervention in the dilation group. On the other hand, the 38% risk of therapeutic intervention after surgery stresses that recurrent dysphagia occurs in a significant proportion of surgical patients. Currently, the choice of therapy remains an individualized decision that weighs factors including available expertise, patient's acceptance of possible risks, and patient factors such as age and comorbidity.

Complications

The main complications of untreated achalasia include progressive malnutrition and aspiration; in particular postprandial and nocturnal coughing. Uncommon but important secondary complications include the formation of epiphrenic diverticula and esophageal cancer. Epiphrenic diverticula presumably form as a result of increased intraluminal pressures, and are most commonly detected in the distal esopha-

gus immediately proximal to the LES. Squamous esophageal cancer is seen with an increased frequency in idiopathic achalasia although adenocarcinomas are also reported. A large cohort study from Sweden found a 16-fold increased risk of esophageal cancer during years 1 through 24 after initial diagnosis. Cancers detected in the first year after diagnosis of achalasia were excluded to eliminate primary cancers that may have presented as pseudoachalasia [21]. The overall prevalence of esophageal cancer in achalasia is approximately 3% with an incidence of approximately 197/100 000 per year [22]. The incidence significantly increases after 15 years of achalasia-related symptoms. However, routine endoscopic screening of patients with achalasia is not generally recommended due to low overall incidence of esophageal cancer. Nevertheless, some experts still advocate surveillance in long-standing achalasia patients who would be candidates for esophageal resection were a cancer to be detected [22]. Treatment of achalasia does not reduce cancer risk, and several cases of cancer have been reported after therapy with pneumatic dilation or surgical myotomy.

Case 2: dysphagia with food impactions

Case presentation

A 46-year-old white man has had difficulty swallowing for the past 20 years. He first noticed symptoms in high school with meat and bread. He has had multiple food impactions and has needed repeated dilations but has no problems with liquids. His symptoms are intermittent and localize to his lower chest. He denies any coughing with eating and does not have any difficulty initiating a swallow. His weight has been stable, he denies arthralgia or myalgia, fevers, chills, or sweats (or the american term swets is preferable?).

Past medical history: allergic rhinitis, which is exacerbated in the spring and fall.

Medications: loratidine, esomeprazole intermittently

Allergies: beer (wheezing and hives), seasonal allergies to pollen and grass. During high school he went through immunotherapy for seasonal allergies

Social history: he is married with two children, Works in finance. Denies any smoking or alcohol

Physical exam: normal

Questions

- What is the differential diagnosis?
- What would be the next step in the workup of this patient?
- What treatment options are available?

Differential diagnosis for dysphagia

The differential diagnosis includes gastro-esophageal reflux, esophageal dysmotility, eosinophilic esophagitis, Schatzki's ring or a peptic stricture.

Diagnostic findings

The patient underwent an upper endoscopy; findings are presented in Figure 1.3. The concentric mucosal rings and linear furrows are typical endoscopic features of eosinophilic esophagitis (EoE). Diagnosis was confirmed on biopsy. Figure 1.4 shows the characteristic histological features of EoE, including intraepithelial eosinophils, superficial layering of eosinophils, and epithelial hyperplasia.

Epidemiology

Over the last few years, EoE has become a topic of increasing attention by gastroenterologists, pathologists, and allergists. EoE may occur in isolation or in conjunction with eosinophilic gastroenteritis. Previously considered a rare condition, there has been a dramatic increase in reports of EoE worldwide [23]. The cause for this rise is probably a combination of an increasing incidence of EoE and a growing awareness of the condition. The incidence of EoE has been rising in a population of children residing in Hamilton County in Ohio. In 2000, Noel et al. estimated the incidence to be 0.91 per 10 000 with a prevalence of 1 per 10 000, compared with 1.3 in 10 000 and a prevalence of 4.3 in 10 000 in 2003 [24]. Straumann and colleagues studied a population of adults in Olten County, Switzerland and found a similar trend [25]. These studies are likely to underestimate the true incidence and prevalence of EoE in the general population because these data are based on patients with symptoms sufficient to warrant endoscopy.

A population-based study in Sweden randomly surveyed 3000 adult members of the population and 1000 healthy adults underwent endoscopy with esophageal biopsies. Probable EoE was present in 1% of the population [26].

EoE tends to have a male predilection. Among 323 adult patients from 13 studies, 76% were male with a mean age of 38 (range 14–89). Among 754 children from 16 studies, 66% were boys with a mean age of 8.6 (range 0.5–21.1) [27]. One pediatric review suggested that there was a racial predilection, with 94.4% of the patients being white [28]. Wang and

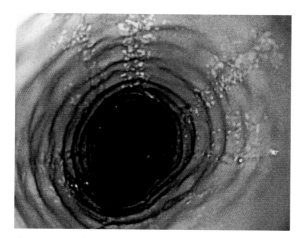

Figure 1.3 Endoscopic image of the esophagus in a patient with eosinophilic esophagitis. Findings present include concentric mucosal rings, linear furrows, and white exudates. (Image courtesy of Dr Gonsalves and Dr Hirano.)

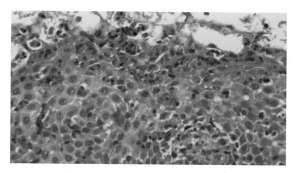

Figure 1.4 Histomicrograph of esophageal biopsy with H&E staining in a patient with eosinophilic esophagitis. Characteristic histopathological changes are present which include intramucosal eosinophils, superficial layering of eosinophils, eosinophilic microabcesses, epithelial hyperplasia, and spongiosis. (Image courtesy of Dr Gonsalves and Dr Hirano.)

colleagues found a seasonal variation of EoE presentations in the children; fewer patients presented in winter, a season with low outdoor allergens, compared with spring, summer, or fall [29]. Eosinophilia was also decreased in winter. A familial pattern has been recognized among children with the condition. In a case series of 381 children with EoE, 5% of patients had siblings with EoE and 7% had a parent with either an esophageal stricture or a known diagnosis of EoE [30]. Eotaxin-3, a gene encoding an eosinophil-specific chemoattractant, was found to be the most highly induced gene in children with EoE, suggesting a potential genetic predisposition [31]. Therefore, workup of patients should include a thorough family history.

Clinical features of EoE

Clinical presentation differs in adults from children. Adults usually present with dysphagia, food impaction, heartburn, and chest pain [27]. In one study, 50% of adults presenting with food impaction were ultimately diagnosed with EoE [32]. Younger children, tend to present with vomiting, heartburn, regurgitation, emesis, and abdominal pain [30], while dysphagia and food impaction, are more commonly seen in older children and adolescents [24]. In adults, this diagnosis has often been overlooked and many patients have had endoscopies with alternate diagnoses, including Schatzki's rings or GERD before a diagnosis of EoE. Eosinophils are commonly seen in GERD and in the past many EoE cases were misdiagnosed as GERD. The presence ≥15 eosinophils per high power field is highly suggestive of EoE [27], so eosinophil counts on esophageal biopsies should be specifically requested if there is suspicion of such diagnosis.

Pathophysiology

Studies have shown that the esophageal infiltration of eosinophils may be related to an allergic response to both food and aeroallergens. Mishra et al. have induced eosinophilic esophagitis by exposing mice to an aeroallergen, *Aspergillus fumigatus* [33]. This group further investigated the roles of cytokines in the pathogenesis of this inflammatory response using interleukin-5 (IL5) and eotaxin knockout mice. They demonstrated that, in response to aeroallergen exposure, eotaxin knockout mice showed decreased esophageal eosinophilia whereas IL5 knockout mice did not demonstrate any esophageal eosinophilia. They thus concluded that both IL5 and eotaxin play important roles in eosinophil recruitment and may be potential therapeutic targets [33].

Certain environmental allergens contributing to esophageal eosinophilia has also been suggested in humans. A recent case report, of an adult with allergic rhinoconjunctivitis and asthma demonstrated an increase in symptoms as well as esophageal eosinophilia during the pollen season [34]. Interestingly, biopsies obtained during non-pollen months were normal, suggesting that tissue eosinophilia was triggered by pollen exposure. In addition, numerous clinical studies have shown an association between food allergies and EoE. The most commonly identified food allergens include milk, soy, egg, wheat, peanuts, and shellfish and after elimination of these agents or use of a elemental diet, esophageal eosinophilia resolves [35,36]. Future studies regarding the pathogenesis of this illness are critical to developing appropriate treatments.

Endoscopic findings

Common endoscopic features in adults include linear furrows (80%), mucosal rings (64%), small-caliber esophagus (28%), white plaques/exudates (16%), and strictures (12%). In children, common endoscopic features include linear furrows (41%), normal appearance (32%), esophageal rings (12%), and white plaques (15%) [30]. However, the classic endoscopic features may be subtle or absent during endoscopy. therefore, biopsies should be taken in unexplained dysphagia, refractory heartburn, or chest pain despite such normal in appearances findings [27].

Pathology

EoE is ultimately diagnosed by the presence of increased intramucosal eosinophils in the esophagus, without concomitant eosinophilic infiltration in the stomach or duodenum [27]. Other features include superficial layering of the eosinophils, eosinophilic microabscesses, intercellular edema, and degranulation of eosinophils. Other inflammatory cells such as lymphocytes, polymorphonuclear leukocytes, and mast cells may also be present [37]. Epithelial hyperplasia, defined by papillary height elongation and basal zone proliferation is common [37] similarly to reflux esophagitis. Subepithelial fibrosis is sometimes seen in EoE, suggesting that deeper layers of the esophagus may be involved [38]. This has been confirmed by endoscopic ultrasonography [39]. It is speculated that this mucosal and submucosal fibrosis may lead to esophageal remodeling and decreased compliance of the esophagus, thus explaining the presence of dysphagia even in the absence of an identifiable stricture.

Although a single diagnostic threshold of eosinophil density has not been universally agreed, a recent consensus statement suggests using a threshold value of ≥15 eosinophils per high power field to diagnose EoE [27]. It is also recognized that the eosinophilic infiltration of the esophagus may not be evenly distributed [40]. Therefore, it is suggested that biopsies be obtained from both the proximal and the distal esophagus to obtain a higher diagnostic yield. A retrospective review suggested at least five biopsies to improve diagnostic yield in the adult population [40]. Prospective studies need to be performed to validate this recommendation.

Diagnostic criteria

Recent consensus recommendations based on a systematic review of the literature and expert opinion have led to the following diagnostic criteria to diagnose EoE:
• the presence of symptoms including, but not limited to, dysphagia and food impaction in adults and feeding intolerance, and GERD in children
• ≥15 eosinophils per high power field in the esophageal biopsy
• exclusion of other disorders associated with similar clinical, histologic, or endoscopic features such as GERD, with either the use of high-dose acid suppression before biopsy procurement or normal pH monitoring [27].

Intraesophageal pH testing

There have been 9 adult and 11 pediatric studies reporting data from pH monitoring. Of 228 adult patients, 40% had pH monitoring with normal results in 82% of patients. Of 223 children, 78%

had pH monitoring with normal results in 90% of patients [27].

Radiography

Radiological studies such as barium esophagrams (swallow) are non-diagnostic although occasionally may identify esophageal strictures and esophageal rings thus alerting the endoscopist to use a smaller-caliber endoscope or to proceed more cautiously with passage of the endoscope [27].

Manometry

Esophageal manometry, studied in 77 adults in 7 studies and 14 children in 3 studies [27], was abnormal in 41 of 77 adult patients. In the adults, the LES was normal in 66, hypotensive in 10, and hypertensive in 1 patient. Peristaltic abnormalities were seen in 30 of 77 patients: 28 of 30 patients had nonspecific peristaltic abnormalities and one each had DES and nutcracker esophagus. Compared with these abnormalities in adults, all 14 children had normal esophageal manometry. In a recent study by Chen and colleagues HRM was used in 24 adult patients with EoE [41]. The most common abnormality noted was elevation in peristaltic velocity. Some patients also had failed esophageal peristalsis and impaired relaxation of the LES.

Natural history

Straumann and colleagues followed a cohort of 30 adults with EoE for a mean of 7 years [42]. Although dysphagia persisted in almost every patient, eosinophil levels in the esophagus decreased in the absence of treatment. No patient had concomitant eosinophilic infiltration of the stomach or duodenum on either the index or follow-up endoscopy. Furthermore, none of the patients progressed to hypereosinophilic syndrome or developed a malignancy. Liacouras and colleagues followed 381 children with EoE over a period of 10 years [30] and found that, although medical treatment with either oral corticosteroids or topical fluticasone was effective in obtaining remission, all patients had recurrence of symptoms and esophageal eosinophilia upon discontinuation of treatment. Dietary treatment with either amino acid-based formula or dietary restriction was highly effective in inducing and maintaining remission. Assa'ad and colleagues studied another group of 89 children over a period of 8 years [29]. They found that the disease was chronic and relapsing in this population. For instance, of the 66% of patients who had initial resolution of their EoE, 79% later relapsed. An important question raised is whether children with EoE outgrow the condition or progress to long-term sequelae such as fibrosis and strictures. Additional long-term follow-up studies in both the pediatric and the adult populations are needed to address this concern.

Treatment

Treatment approaches for EoE vary between children and adult patients. In children treatment with an elemental diet for 1 month has been shown to improve both clinical symptoms and histological changes. Spergel et al. used skinprick and patch testing to identify food allergens in a cohort of children [35]. Once food allergens were identified, patients underwent either a food elimination diet or an elemental diet with an amino acid-based formula; 18 of 26 patients had complete resolution of symptoms and 6 of 26 had partial resolution. Overall, after dietary intervention, esophageal eosinophilia significantly improved. Recently Kagalwalla and colleagues showed that a targeted diet eliminating milk, soy, egg, wheat, nuts, and seafood has a remission rate of 74% [36]. This approach was recently tried in adults with a 52% response rate.

Systemic corticosteroids have shown to effectively treat children with EoE. In one study, 20 patients with EoE with symptoms of refractory reflux were treated with methylprednisolone (1.5 mg/kg per day, divided into twice daily dosing) for 4 weeks [43] 65% of patients became asymptomatic while the rest had significant improvement in symptoms within 4 weeks. The average time for clinical improvement was 8 ± 4 days. All patients in this group demonstrated decreased eosinophilia on biopsy, in addition to decreased peripheral eosinophilia and IgE levels. Topical corticosteroids have also demonstrated effectiveness. In a study by Remedios et al., 19 adults were studied after treatment with topical fluticasone (250 μg two puffs twice daily for 4 weeks) [44]. This therapy resulted in complete relief of dysphagia, significant decrease in esophageal eosinophilia and was well tolerated in all patients. Encouraging results have

also been obtained in children with an approximate 50% response rate.

Attwood et al. treated with montelukast eight adult patients with EoE [45]. An initial dose of 10 mg daily was used and increased if needed to a total of 100 mg daily. Maintenance dosages for all patients were between 20 and 40 mg/day for 4 months. Therapy resulted in resolution of dysphagia while continuing the medication. However, 75% of patients had recurrence within 3 weeks of cessation or reduction in the medication. Also, treatment with montelukast for 4 months did not reduce the density of eosinophils on repeat biopsy. Another agent that has been shown to improve symptoms and histology of EoE is anti-IL5 (mepolizumab). This agent is currently being investigated in clinical trials for both EoE and eosinophilic gastroenteritis.

Esophageal dilation has been used to treat patients with strictures. Although dysphagia improves initially, symptoms recurred in all patients 3–8 months after dilation, with most patients requiring repeat dilation, on an average twice a year [23]. Such dilatations are associated with significant esophageal wall disruption with the potential for perforation. This risk might have been over-emphasized and for some patients dilatations are the only means for effective symptom relief if medical therapy fails [15].

Case 3 dysphagia for solids

Case presentation

A 68 year old man complains of a 6 month history of intermittent dysphagia at the lower sternum and nocturnal gastro-esophageal reflux with occasional regurgitation of food. He denies any weight loss and he has a good appetite. Past medical history has been unremarkable apart from progressive 10 kg weight gain since retirement as a hospital porter. He was diagnosed with celiac disease at the age of 35 and he has been on a gluten-free diet although he admits to erratic compliance. At the age of 58, and while at work, he suffered crush fractures of the vertebrae at the level of T12 and L1. A bone DEXA density scan confirmed osteoporosis of the spine and he was started on biphosphonates (alendronate sodium) and calcium/vitamin D supplements. He was also advised to adhere to a strict gluten free diet. He has been on omeprazole 20 mg for the last 3 years; recently increased to 40 mg because of worsening acid reflux.

Social history: Retired hospital porter; smokes 20 cigarettes per day and drinks approximately 24 units of alcohol per week, mainly spirits. Family history: No family history of cancer or swallowing disorders.

Physical examination was unremarkable apart from a BMI of 29.1 and a slightly distended abdomen with epigastric discomfort on palpation, but no organomegaly; bowel sounds were normal.

He had not been keen for an upper endoscopy but reluctantly agreed following the development of dysphagia. Endoscopy showed Barrett's esophagus with the squamous-columnal junction at 36 cm with mild stricturing at 39 cm. Three tongues of Barrett's esophagus were extending within the squamous epithelium. (C3M4 by the Prague classification criteria [46]). Four-quadrant biopsies every 2 cm from Barrett's esophagus [47] confirmed the presence of specialised intestinal metaplasia and goblet cells. Fibrin and neutrophil infiltration were also present suggestive of active inflammation. In addition, focal glandular atypia in keeping with low-grade dysplasia was evident but no high-grade dysplasia.

Questions

• What are the main diagnostic considerations and the most appropriate management?

Diagnostic considerations:

This patient has long-standing acid reflux in a background history of celiac disease. Gaining weight, with alcohol intake above the upper limit exacerbated his acid reflux. He has an established inflamed Barrett's esophagus with a mild benign esophageal stricture and low-grade dysplasia. It is well recognised that in the presence of chronic inflammation, it is difficult to differentiate between reactive changes and true dysplasia. In addition, this patient has been treated with a biphosphonates, which can cause esophageal ulceration and strictures. More recently, long term use of biphosphonates has been associated with higher risk of esophageal cancer. [48]

The principles of management are two fold: (a) to improve dysphagia and acid reflux and (b) to establish whether he has true low-grade dysplasia. If the patient suffers from mild intermittent dysphagia, one may treat him with high dose PPIs alone and observe whether his symptoms improve. If dysphagia

persists, esophageal dilatation may be necessary to improve swallowing. This patient was prescribed add: dispersible lansoprazole (FasTab) 30 mg bd and he reluctantly undertook a second endoscopy 12 weeks later as he had symptomatically improved; the stricture was not present and repeat biopsies demonstrated less inflammation but persistent focal glandular atypia, suggestive of true low-grade dysplasia. The patient was advised to remain on high-dose PPIs and have a repeat endoscopy.

Questions

• How often would you endoscope this patient?
• Would you advise the patient to stop taking the Biphosphonates for osteoporosis?

Answers:

A repeat endoscopy is advised 6 months later with four-quadrant biopsies every 2 cm. If low-grade dysplasia persists, yearly endoscopies thereafter are necessary to detect if there is progression to high-grade dysplasia.

The decision to continue with biphosphonate treatment would be based on the benefit/risk ratio. The patient would be advised to have a further bone DEXA scan and if there is a significant probability of further osteoporotic fractures, he should continue on osteoporosis therapy. Alternative medications, such as risedronate sodium or strontium ranelate, could be considered. Also the patient is now committed to long-term treatment with a PPI, which might further increase the risk of osteoporosis [49]. The importance of strict adherence to a gluten free diet should also be emphasised.

Patient Management

The patient declined further endoscopies as he became asymptomatic on PPIs. He agreed to a bone DEXA scan which showed significant osteoporosis of the spine (cumulative 10-year fracture risk in excess of 15%). Alendronate sodium was changed to risedronate sodium and the patient was advised to return for a follow up endoscopy, but he did not attend despite repeated calls.

Four years later he consulted his general practitioner because of a 3-month history of progressive dysphagia for solids with frequent choking and 4 kg weight loss. Clinical examination was normal.

Questions

What is the differential diagnosis?

Answer:

The differential diagnosis includes development of esophageal adenocarcinoma on Barrett's or development of further esophageal stricture due to acid reflux or due to treatment with biphosphonates. An upper GI endoscopy demonstrated an obstructed esophagus with an irregular exophytic lesion at 36 cm. He had a balloon dilatation of the stricture and biopsies confirmed esophageal adenocarcinoma developing on Barrett's esophagus.

Questions

- How would you investigate this patient further?
- What are the treatment options?

Answer:

This patient will require staging investigations and discussion at the upper GI cancer multidisciplinary case conference. A chest and abdomen CT followed by a PET scan and an endoscopic ultrasound (EUS) would be appropriate staging investigations. CT is mostly of value to exclude any distant metastases, particularly in the liver or lungs, and a PET scan is of value to further assess suspicious areas on CT in other organs or to establish whether some lymph nodes seen on CT are malignant or benign [50]. EUS remains the gold standard of tumour and nodal (TN) staging in esophageal cancer. The 3 tests should be considered complementary rather than being interpreted independently. A recent study highlighted the importance of case conference for those cases as the final staging following a multi disciplinary discussion approached 92% using pathology of surgical specimen as gold standard. [51]

Patient Management:

A chest and abdominal CT was clear of metastases but the tumour radiologically was a T3 (tumour invading into the adventitia) with regional lymphadenopathy (N1). A PET/CT has shown that the regional lymphadenopathy was 18FFDG avid suggestive of malignant lymph nodes. The patient had an endoscopic ultrasound, which confirmed a T3 tumour with 3 peri-tumour nodes. Final staging T3N1.

Therapeutic options for the treatment of a T3N1 esophageal tumour include surgery, preoperative chemotherapy followed by surgery, or chemoradiotherapy. Patient co-morbidity is important in deciding treatment options, as there is significant operative risk (5 to 10% mortality). This has to be balanced against the limited 5-year survival of T3N1 disease (approximately 10–15%), which could be increased to 25 to 30% with preoperative chemotherapy prior to surgery. Preoperative chemotherapy consisting of cisplatin and 5-FU (fluoroucil) can also help to achieve complete surgical clearance of cancer (60% of patients versus 54% if not receiving preoperative chemotherapy) and improvement in the 2-year survival from 34 to 43% [52].

This patient tolerated preoperative chemotherapy well with no side effects, such as leucopenia, cardiotoxicity, thromboembolic events or gastrointestinal upset and undertook surgery. Histology on the excised specimen confirmed a T3N1 tumour with 3 out of 20 nodes excised positive. The patient remains well 18 months later.

Discussion

Despite improvements in the management of esophageal cancer, prognosis remains poor because of the late presentation of the disease. At presentation over 60% of patients are inoperable. In general, patients who are fit for surgery with localised tumour and no nodal involvement will be candidates for surgery alone. The presence of lymph nodes significantly worsens prognosis and such patients will benefit from preoperative chemotherapy. In early T1N0 disease, endoscopic mucosal resection or endoscopic submucosal dissection can be considered, provided there is no satellite lymphadenopathy present. If in doubt, an EUS with sampling of suspicious nodes is recommended. For patients with advanced disease not fit for surgery, palliative measures such as esophageal stent insertion, argon plasma coagulation or Nd-YAG laser are appropriate to establish lumen patency and improve dysphagia, nutritional status and offer better quality of life. Esophageal stent technology has greatly advanced and a variety of covered and uncovered metal self-expandable stents are available depending on the length and the position of the malignant stricture. Such endoprostheses are placed under fluoroscopic control or direct endoscopic view under sedation. They are of value for sealing broncho-esophageal fistulas in advanced (T4) disease and are particularly suitable for elderly patients or those not keen to receive repeated endoscopic treatments. Complications of stenting are generally few with stent migration rate of approximately 5%. Perforations are rare. The most commonly encountered complications are pain following stent insertion, which is usually controlled by simple analgesia; in patients with advanced disease severe pain may herald very poor prognosis and may require use of opiate analgesia. Food bolus obstruction, cleared by endoscopy and tumour in-growth are common complications. Using covered stents reduces tumour in-growth. Patients with esophageal stents should be advised to drink warm or carbonated drinks before and after meals to clear food debris, to have a soft diet and regularly use PPIs particularly for the stents crossing the gastro-esophageal junction.

References

1 Scottish Audit of Gastric & Oesophageal Cancer; report 1997, 2000, 2002; http://www.crag.scot.nhs.uk/committees/CEPS/reports/O prelims.pdf
2 Rattigan E, Tyrmpas I, Murray G, Plevris JN. Scoring system to identify patients at high risk of esophageal cancer. *British J Surgery* 2010;97(12):1831–7.
3 Eckardt VF, Stauf B, Bernhard G. Chest pain in achalasia: patient characteristics and clinical course. *Gastroenterology* 1999;116:1300–4.
4 Perretta S, Fisichella PM, Galvani C, et al. Achalasia and chest pain: effect of laparoscopic Heller myotomy. *J Gastrointest Surg* 2003;7:595–8.
5 Brackbill S, Shi G, Hirano I. Diminished mechano-sensitivity and chemosensitivity in patients with achalasia. *Am J Physiol Gastrointest Liver Physiol* 2003;285:G1198–203.
6 Howard PJ, Maher L, Pryde A, et al. Five year prospective study of the incidence, clinical features, and diagnosis of achalasia in Edinburgh. *Gut* 1992;33:1011–15.
7 Hirano I, Tatum RP, Shi G, Sang Q, Joehl RJ, Kahrilas PJ. Manometric heterogeneity in patients with idiopathic achalasia. *Gastroenterology.* 2001;120:789–98.
8 Pandolfino JE, Kwiatek MA, Nealis T, et al. Achalasia: a new clinically relevant classification by high-resolution manometry. *Gastroenterology* 2008;135:1526–33.
9 Robertson CS, Martin BA, Atkinson M. Varicella-zoster virus DNA in the oesophageal myenteric plexus in achalasia. *Gut* 1993;34:299–302.
10 Facco M, Brun P, Baesso I, et al. T cells in the myenteric plexus of achalasia patients show a skewed TCR repertoire and react to HSV-1 antigens. *Am J Gastroenterol* 2008;103:1598–609.
11 Moses PL, Ellis LM, Anees MR, et al. Antineuronal antibodies in idiopathic achalasia and gastro-oesophageal reflux disease. *Gut* 2003;52:629–36.
12 Clark SB, Rice TW, Tubbs RR, et al. The nature of the myenteric infiltrate in achalasia: an immunohistochemical analysis. *Am J Surg Pathol* 2000;24:1153–8.
13 Lopushinsky SR, Urbach DR. Pneumatic dilatation and surgical myotomy for achalasia. *JAMA* 2006;296:2227–33.
14 Spiess AE, Kahrilas PJ. Treating achalasia: from whalebone to laparoscope. *JAMA* 1998;280:638–42.
15 Walzer N, Hirano I. Achalasia. *Gastroenterol Clin North Am* 2008;37:807–25, viii.
16 Pasricha PJ, Rai R, Ravich WJ, et al. Botulinum toxin for achalasia: long-term outcome and predictors of response. *Gastroenterology* 1996;110:1410–15.
17 Vaezi MF, Richter JE, Wilcox CM, et al. Botulinum toxin versus pneumatic dilatation in the treatment of achalasia: a randomised trial. *Gut* 1999;44:231–9.
18 Eckardt VF, Aignherr C, Bernhard G. Predictors of outcome in patients with achalasia treated by pneumatic dilation. *Gastroenterology* 1992;103:1732–8.
19 Patti MG, Pellegrini CA, Horgan S, et al. Minimally invasive surgery for achalasia: an 8-year experience with 168 patients. *Ann Surg* 1999;230:587–93; discussion 593–84.
20 Malthaner RA, Tood TR, Miller L, Pearson FG. Long-term results in surgically managed esophageal achalasia. *Ann Thorac Surg* 1994;58:1343–6; discussion 1346–7.
21 Sandler RS, Nyren O, Ekbom A, et al. The risk of esophageal cancer in patients with achalasia. A population-based study. *JAMA* 1995;274:1359–62.
22 Dunaway PM, Wong RK. Risk and surveillance intervals for squamous cell carcinoma in achalasia. *Gastrointest Endosc Clin North Am* 2001;11:425–34, ix.
23 Potter J, Saeian K, Staff D, et al. Eosinophilic esophagitis in adults: an emerging problem with unique esophageal features. *Gastrointest Endosc* 2004;59:355–61.
24 Noel R, Putnam P, Rothenberg M. Eosinophilic esophagitis. *N Engl J Med* 2004;351:940–1.
25 Straumann A, Simon H. Eosinophilic esophagitis: escalating epidemiology? *J Allergy Clin Immunol* 2005;115:418–19.

26 Ronkainen J, Talley N, Aro P, et al. Prevalence of oesophageal eosinophils and eosinophilic esophagitis in adults: the population based Kalixanda study. *Gut* 2007;**56**:615–20.

27 Furuta G, Liacouras C, Collins M, et al. Eosinophilic esophagitis in children and adults: A systematic review and consensus recommendations for diagnosis and treatment. *Gastroenterology* 2007;**133**:1342–63.

28 Assa'ad A, Putnam P, Collins M, et al. Pediatric patients with eosinophilic esophagitis: an 8-year follow-up. *J Allergy Clin Immunol* 2007;**119**:731–8.

29 Wang FY, Gupta SK, Fitzgerald JF. Is there a seasonal variation in the incidence of intensity of allergic eosinophilic esophagitis in newly diagnosed children. *J Clin Gastroenterol* 2007;**4**:451–3.

30 Liacouras C, Spergel J, Ruchelli E, et al. Eosinophilic esophagitis: A 10-year experience in 381 children. *Clin Gastroenterol Hepatol* 2005;**3**:1198–206.

31 Blanchard C, Wang N, Stringer K, et al. Eotaxin-3 and a uniquely conserved gene-expression profile in eosinophilic esophagitis. *J Clin Invest* 2006;**116**:536–47.

32 Desai TK, Stecevic V, Chang C, et al. Association of eosinophilic inflammation with esophageal food impaction in adults. *Gastrointest Endosc* 2005;**61**:795–801.

33 Mishra A. Mechanism of eosinophilic esophagitis. *Immunol Allergy Clin North Am* 2009;**29**(1):29–40.

34 Morrow J, Vargo J, Goldblum J, et al. The ringed esophagus: Histologic features of GERD. *Am J Gastroenterol* 2001;**96**:984–9.

35 Spergel J, Beausoleil J, Mascarenhas M, et al. The use of skin prick tests and patch tests to identify causative foods in eosinophilic esophagitis. *J Allergy Clin Immunol* 2002;**109**:363–8.

36 Kagalwalla A, Sentongo T, Ritz S, et al. Effect of six-food elimination diet on clinical and histologic outcomes in eosinophilic esophagitis. *Clin Gastroenterol Hepatol.* 2006;**4**:1097–1102.

37 Parfitt JR, Gregor JC, Suskin NG, et al. Eosinophilic esophgitis in adults: distinguishing features from gastro-esophageal reflux disease: a study of 41 patients. *Mod Pathol* 2006;**19**:90–6.

38 Chehade M, Sampson HA, Morrotti RA. Esophageal subepithelial fibrosis in children with eosinophilic esophagitis. *J Pediatr Gastroenterol Nutr* 2007;**45**:319–28.

39 Stevoff C, Rao S, Parsons W, et al. EUS and histopathologic correlates in eosinophilic esophagitis. *Gastointest Endosc* 2001;**54**:373–7.

40 Gonsalves N, Policarpio-Nicolas M, Zhang Q, et al. Histopathologic variability and endoscopic correlates in adults with eosinophilic esophagitis. *Gastroenterology* 1978;**74**:1298.

41 Chen J, Ghosh S, Pandolfino J, et al. Esophageal dysmotility in eosinophilic esophagitis: analysis using high resolution esophageal manometry. *Gastroenterology* 2007;**132**(suppl):A6.

42 Straumann A, Spichtin H, Grize L, et al. Natural history of primary eosinophilic esophagitis: A follow-up of 30 adult patients for up to 11.5 years. *Gastroenterology* 2003;**125**:1660–9.

43 Liacouras CA, Wenner WJ, Brown K, et al. Primary eosinophilic esophagitis in children: successful treatment with oral corticosteroids. *J Pediatr Gastroenterol Nutr* 1998;**26**:380–5.

44 Remedios M, Campbell C, Jones D, et al. Eosinophilic esophagitis in adults: clinical, endoscopic, histologic findings, and response to treatment with fluticasone propionate. *Gastrointest Endosc* 2006;**63**:3–12.

45 Attwood S, Lewis C, Bronder C, et al. Eosinophilic esophagitis: a novel treatment using montelukast. *Gut* 2003;**52**:181–5.

46 Sharma P, Dent J, Armstrong D, Bergman JJ, et al. The development and validation of an endoscopic grading system for Barrett's esophagus: the Prague C & M criteria. *Gastroenterology* 2006;**131**(5):1392–9.

47 Jo-Etienne Abela, James J. Going, John F. Mackenzie, Margaret McKernan, et al. Systematic Four-Quadrant Biopsy Detects Barrett's Dysplasia in More Patients Than Nonsystematic Biopsy. *Am J Gastroenterol* 2008;**103**(4):850–855.

48 Green J, Czanner G, Reeves G, Watson J, et al. Oral bisphosphonates and risk of cancer of oesophagus, stomach, and colorectum: case-control analysis within a UK primary care cohort. *BMJ* 2010;1;**341**:c4444.

49 Insogna KL. The effect of proton pump-inhibiting drugs on mineral metabolism. *Am J Gastroenterol* 2009 Mar;**104** Suppl 2:S2–4.

50 Jamil LH, Gill KR, Wallace MB. Staging and restaging of advanced esophageal cancer. *Curr Opin Gastroenterol* 2008;**24**(4):530–4.

51 Davies AR, Deans DA, Penman I, Plevris JN, et al. The multidisciplinary team meeting improves staging accuracy and treatment selection for gastro-esophageal cancer. *Dis Esophagus* 2006;**19**(6):496–503.

52 Bancewica J, Clark P, Smith D, et al. Surgical resection with or without preoperative chemotherapy in oesophageal cancer: a randomized controlled trial. *Lancet* 2002;**9319**:1727–1733.

2

The Problem of Heartburn, and Atypical Chest Pain

Ronnie Fass and Tiberiu Hershcovici

University of Arizona, Southern Arizona VA Health Care System, Tucson, AZ, USA

Case 1: patient with heartburn

Case presentation

A 46-year-old woman complains of heartburn that started 6 years ago. Her symptoms occurred up to three times daily during "bad" months and about three times a week during the rest of the year. The patient describes a burning sensation behind the sternum that travels to her neck. Symptoms occasionally waken her from sleep during the night, particularly if she had a heavy meal that evening. She has rarely experienced a sour or bitter taste in the mouth.

She denies dysphagia, odynophagia, chest pain, early satiety, epigastric pain or discomfort, bloating, nausea, or vomiting. Her appetite is good, and she has not lost any weight.

Past medical and surgical history: unremarkable
Current medications: none
Social history: employed as a social worker. She considers her work to be very stressful. She is married and has two toddlers at home. Both of her pregnancies were unremarkable
Family history: unremarkable
Habits: she denies smoking or drinking alcohol. However, she admits to occasional late-night meals
Physical examination: BP 120/70 mmHg; heart rate 88/min; weight 91 kg; height: 180 cm; BMI: 28
General appearance: well appearing woman with mild obesity, sitting comfortably. Oral cavity without mucosal abnormalities

Neck: no masses, lymphadenopathy, or goiter
Heart: regular rhythm, normal heart sounds without murmurs
Lungs: clear to auscultation
Abdomen: soft and not distended. No masses or tenderness. Normal bowel sounds
Extremities: no edema or cyanosis

The patient was initially seen by her primary care physician, who suggested lifestyle modifications, including an attempt to lose weight, and that she consider a less busy work schedule. She was also started on an H_2-receptor antagonist twice daily. The patient stated that she felt no improvement in her symptoms despite 2 months of therapy. In addition, she was unable to lose weight or change her work schedule. Consequently, she was initiated on a standard dose of a proton pump inhibitor (PPI) once daily, taken 30 min before breakfast. She stated that the PPI appeared to help her during the first 2 weeks, but her symptoms then recurred, although with less severity and frequency than before.

Questions

- What are the diagnostic considerations in this patient?
- What is the pathophysiology of this condition?
- What diagnostic tests are useful in this condition?
- What therapeutic options can be offered to this patient?

Problem-based Approach to Gastroenterology and Hepatology, First Edition. Edited by John N. Plevris, Colin W. Howden.
© 2012 Blackwell Publishing Ltd. Published 2012 by Blackwell Publishing Ltd.

The problem

Between 10% and 40% of patients with gastro-esophageal reflux disease (GERD) fail to respond symptomatically, either partially or completely, to a standard dose PPI treatment [1,2]. During a period of only 7 years (1997–2004), there was an increase by almost 50% in the use of at least double-dose PPIs in patients with GERD [3]. In a recent US survey of 617 GERD patients taking PPIs, 71% used PPIs once a day, 22.2% twice a day, and 6.8% more than twice a day or on an "as-needed" basis [4]. Approximately 42.1% of all patients supplemented their prescription PPIs with other antireflux therapies, including over-the-counter antacids and H_2-receptor antagonists. Over 85% of the patients still experienced GERD-related symptoms, but 72.8% were satisfied or very satisfied with their PPI treatment.

In the *2000 Gallup Study of Consumers' Use of Stomach Relief Products*, 36% reported taking non-prescription medication in addition to a prescription medication for GERD [2]. Of those, 56% stated that they used their prescription medication daily but still needed to supplement with non-prescription medication for breakthrough symptoms. Interestingly, 28% stated that only the combination of prescription and non-prescription medications relieved their symptoms, and 24% reported that prescription medication worked better in the long run but that non-prescription medications were faster acting.

Failure of PPI treatment to resolve GERD-related symptoms has become the most common presentation of GERD in gastrointestinal (GI) practice. Although cost analysis of PPI failure has yet to be carried out, it is likely an expensive clinical problem due to repeated utilization of healthcare resources such as clinic visits, diagnostic tests, and prescription medications [5].

Most of the patients with heartburn who are not responsive to PPIs have either non-erosive reflux disease (NERD) or functional heartburn (FH). These patients may comprise up to 70% of the heartburn patient population and often exhibit a low response rate to PPI once daily [3,6]. In contrast, patients with erosive esophagitis (EE), which account for 30–40% of the GERD population, have a symptom response rate that is significantly higher than what has been reported in patients with NERD [3,7].

Underlying mechanisms for refractory GERD

Figure 2.1 depicts the proposed underlying mechanisms for persistent heartburn despite PPI treatment.

Compliance

Compliance should be assessed in all patients with GERD who report lack of response to PPI treatment, particularly before ordering any diagnostic test. Unfortunately, a subset of patients may not disclose that they are poorly compliant during their clinic visit. Physicians should emphasize the need to consume antireflux treatment on a regular, daily basis. It is the role of the treating physician to ensure proper compliance with the prescribed PPI through patient education about the disease and the value of compliance with treatment.

Dosing time

In addition to compliance, patients need to be evaluated for proper consumption of the PPIs because timing and frequency of dosing are critical for their maximum efficacy. PPIs should be taken 30–60 min before a meal. In one study, it was demonstrated that the control of gastric pH was significantly better when omeprazole or lansoprazole was taken before breakfast rather than without breakfast [8].

Patients' preferences and lack of physicians' clear instructions on how to consume PPIs are commonly to blame for inadequate symptom control. In a study of 100 patients with persistent GERD symptoms on PPIs, only 46% dosed their PPI optimally [9]. Of those who dosed suboptimally, 39% consumed their PPI at bedtime and 4% as needed. However, there is no clear evidence thus far that restoring adequate PPI dosing time improves the symptoms of patients with refractory GERD. Despite the latter argument, most authorities emphasize the need to ensure that refractory GERD patients dose their PPIs optimally.

Weakly acidic or alkaline reflux

Studies have suggested that persistent GERD-related symptoms on PPIs might be due to less acidic or non-acidic reflux. The first stationary, postprandial, multichannel, intraluminal impedance pH (MII-pH) study in patients who failed PPI twice daily, at baseline and during therapy, documented a shift from primarily acidic reflux to mostly weakly acidic reflux.

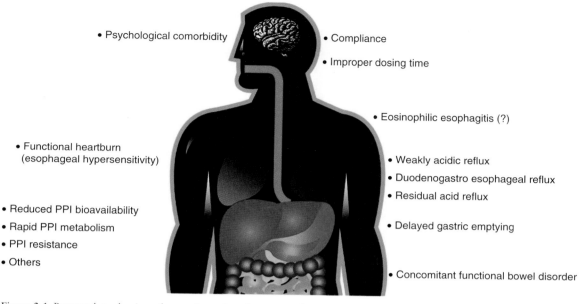

• Psychological comorbidity

• Compliance

• Improper dosing time

• Eosinophilic esophagitis (?)

• Functional heartburn
(esophageal hypersensitivity)

• Weakly acidic reflux

• Duodenogastro esophageal reflux

• Residual acid reflux

• Reduced PPI bioavailability

• Rapid PPI metabolism

• Delayed gastric emptying

• PPI resistance

• Others

• Concomitant functional bowel disorder

Figure 2.1 Proposed mechanisms for persistent heartburn despite proton pump inhibitor (PPI) treatment. (Redrawn with permission after Fass R, Sifrim D. Management of heartburn not responding to proton pump inhibitors. *Gut* 2009;58:295–309.)

Unlike untreated patients, regurgitation became the predominant symptom in patients who failed PPI twice daily [10]. Further studies using ambulatory MII-pH monitoring in patients who failed PPI twice daily demonstrated that acidic reflux was associated with 7–28% of the persistent GERD-related symptoms. In contrast, weakly acidic reflux preceded 30–68% of the symptoms and 30–60% of the symptoms were not preceded by any reflux [11–14].

The mechanism by which weakly acidic reflux causes GERD-related symptoms remains poorly understood. Two possible explanations have been proposed and they include esophageal distension by increased reflux volume and hypersensitivity to weakly acidic refluxate. Thus far, there is no evidence that weakly acidic reflux is more commonly associated with increased volume of the refluxate than acidic reflux. Although this association has been proposed, MII is unable to measure volume and thus to substantiate this claim.

Recently, several studies have demonstrated that proximal extent of weakly acidic reflux (a possible indirect marker of reflux volume) was the most important determinant of symptomatic reflux events in patients who failed PPI treatment [14,15]. However, these studies also showed a considerable overlap in the proximal extent of symptomatic and asymptomatic weakly acidic reflux episodes. In addition to proximal extent, symptomatic reflux episodes in patients who failed PPI twice daily were primarily composed of both gas and liquid [15]. Proximal migration of reflux is more likely to elicit symptoms because the transition zone between the striated and smooth muscle in the esophagus seems to be more sensitive to mechanical stimulus than the distal esophagus, which is composed solely of smooth muscle [16].

Duodeno-gastroesophageal reflux

There is evidence that esophageal exposure to bile acids can result in heartburn. Bile reflux probably accounts for 10–15% of non-acid reflux events. However, most bile reflux events occur concomitantly with acid reflux events. It has been demonstrated that acid rather than bile is the dominant factor responsible for generating GERD-related symptoms.

Tack et al. suggested a possible role for duodenogastroesophageal reflux (DGER) in a subset of patients with difficult to manage symptomatic reflux [17]. In a study that included 65 patients with persistent heartburn and regurgitation while on single- or double-dose PPI therapy, the authors demonstrated that 64% of the patients experienced symptoms that were associated with bile reflux alone or bile reflux together with acid reflux.

The role of the residual reflux

Most studies evaluating patients with refractory GERD tend to compare reflux patterns at baseline and during treatment in the PPI failure group. However, these studies do not address whether residual reflux (acidic, non-acidic, or bile) is a unique PPI failure phenomenon or a general PPI phenomenon, regardless of whether the patient is responsive or non-responsive to treatment. To answer this question, the reflux pattern of responders and non-responders to the same dose of PPI should be compared. Recently, a study evaluated 24 patients who failed PPI once daily and 23 patients who fully responded to PPI once a day with both 24-h esophageal Bilitec and pH monitoring while on treatment [18]. The authors demonstrated that abnormal DGER was documented in 82% of the responders versus 67% of the non-responders. All pH testing and Bilitec parameters were similar between the two groups. GERD symptoms in the PPI failure group were more commonly associated with acid reflux than with DGER. This study demonstrated for the first time that the level of bile and acid exposure is similar among patients who failed and those who were successfully treated with PPI once daily. In addition, in patients who failed to respond to PPI once daily, acidic reflux still plays an important role in symptom generation.

Esophageal hypersensitivity

The role of esophageal hypersensitivity has not been specifically studied in patients who failed PPI treatment. However, most patients who do not respond to PPI therapy have either NERD or FH, conditions in which esophageal hypersensitivity is highly important.

The pH-negative NERD patients have consistently demonstrated lower perception thresholds for pain compared with patients with other GERD phenotypes

when using either esophageal balloon distension or electrical stimulation. A recent study in pH-negative NERD patients demonstrated that perception of reflux events was significantly higher when gas was present in the refluxate [19]. These patients are also more sensitive to less acidic reflux than EE patients. NERD patients form a continuum of esophageal afferent sensitivity with a correlation between the degree of acid exposure and esophageal pain thresholds. Furthermore, objective neurophysiological measures of esophageal-evoked potential latency revealed that pH-negative NERD patients achieve equivalent latency and amplitude esophageal-evoked potential responses with reduced afferent input, suggesting heightened esophageal sensitivity [20].

Most patients in whom reflux symptoms are associated with weakly acidic reflux do not have an increased number of reflux events, suggesting hypersensitivity of the esophagus to less acidic refluxate. Furthermore, none of the studies that assessed the extent and relationship between weakly acidic reflux and GERD-related symptoms using esophageal impedance compared PPI failure with PPI success patients. There is no obvious reason why PPI success patients will demonstrate fewer episodes of weakly acidic reflux than those who failed PPIs. In patients who failed twice daily PPIs Vela et al. showed that acidic reflux almost completely disappeared [21]. Consequently, a similar reflux pattern in PPI success patients would be expected. If the frequency of weakly acidic reflux is similar between PPI success and PPI failure patients, then PPI failure is an esophageal-hypersensitivity phenomenon to weakly acidic reflux.

Differential diagnosis

• Patients with achalasia may develop heartburn as a result of fermentation of retained food in the esophagus.
• Patients who are taking non-steroidal anti-inflammatory drugs (NSAIDs), aspirin, tetracyclines (especially doxycycline), bisphosphonates, potassium chloride, quinidine preparations, and iron compounds can develop pill-induced esophagitis that is unresponsive to PPI treatment.
• In addition to acid, a variety of other causes can lead to esophagitis. Examples include caustic ingestion, infectious esophagitis (e.g. *Candida* sp., Herpes

Simplex), and radiotherapy. These causes should be excluded.

- Impaired gastric emptying – either idiopathic or as a result of medications or comorbidities – can predispose to gastroesophageal reflux.
- Eosinophilic esophagitis in adults is most commonly associated with dysphagia although a third of the patients may also report classic heartburn. However, heartburn alone is uncommon in eosinophilic esophagitis.
- Zollinger–Ellison syndrome, which is characterized by gastric acid hypersecretion, is associated with increased risk of GERD and esophageal mucosal injury.
- Skin disorders such as pemphigus vulgaris, and bullous pemphigoid can involve the esophageal mucosa and present with GERD-like symptoms.

Diagnostic evaluation

Upper gastrointestinal endoscopy

Upper endoscopy is commonly used in clinical practice to evaluate patients with GERD who failed PPI treatment. This clinical strategy has been endorsed by the American Society for Gastrointestinal Endoscopy (ASGE) [22]. The hope is to identify anatomic and histological abnormalities that can explain patients' refractoriness to potent and adequate antireflux treatment. In very rare cases, endoscopy in heartburn patients who failed PPI treatment may reveal non-GERD-related causes, which could explain the symptoms (e.g. ulcers due to Zollinger–Ellison syndrome, pill-induced esophagitis, achalasia, gastroparesis, and skin diseases with esophageal involvement) [23]. In addition, eosinophilic esophagitis or other causes of persistent gastric or duodenal ulcer could be identified.

A recent study evaluated GERD-related endoscopic and histological findings in 105 patients with refractory GERD (failure to respond to once-daily PPI therapy) and 91 GERD patients not receiving antireflux treatment [24]. Refractory GERD patients had a significantly lower prevalence of endoscopic and histological findings compared with the no-treatment group. Refractory GERD was associated with a significantly decreased odds ratio of erosive esophagitis compared with no treatment when adjusted for age, sex, and body mass index (BMI). Eosinophilic esophagitis was extremely rare (only 0.9%) in refractory GERD patients.

In general, the value of endoscopy in discovering GERD-related findings in patients with refractory GERD is very low. This is primarily due to the predominance of NERD and FH among this group of patients and the high efficacy of PPIs in healing erosive esophagitis.

Esophageal pH monitoring

Esophageal pH monitoring is commonly used in the evaluation of patients with refractory GERD. In the assessment of such patients, pH monitoring can be performed off PPI (to assess whether the heartburn was due to acid reflux) or on PPI (to test whether the symptoms are due to residual acid reflux). Inclusion of a symptom–reflux correlation measure such as symptom index (SI) and/or symptom association probability (SAP) helps to determine the relationship between heartburn episodes and acid reflux events, whether the pH test is normal or abnormal.

A positive pH testing on PPI suggests that a patient's persistent heartburn might be related to ongoing acid reflux. If the pH test is normal on PPI treatment but the SI is abnormal, then heartburn induced by physiological levels of acid exposure could be the explanation. A normal pH test on PPI and a negative SI suggests that the patient's heartburn is unlikely to be related to ongoing acid reflux. However, one has to recall that a negative pH test may occur due to poor tolerability of the pH probe which can result in a significant impact on reflux-provoking activities [25].

Residual acid reflux has been documented in GERD patients with persistent heartburn despite treatment with a PPI once or twice daily. In one study, 38.6% of the GERD patients undergoing pH testing for persistent symptoms while on a once-daily PPI, had an abnormal pH test [26]. In another study, 31% and 4% of the GERD patients with refractory symptoms on once- or twice-daily PPI, respectively, had an abnormal pH test [27]. Overall, positive SI was documented in 40% and 7–11% of the patients who remained symptomatic on once- or twice-daily PPI, respectively [12,28,29].

Extending the use of wireless pH monitoring to 4 days may provide a better comparison of esophageal acid exposure and symptom–reflux association between off and on PPI treatment periods [30].

However, studies evaluating this diagnostic strategy in refractory GERD patients are still missing.

Esophageal impedance–pH monitoring

MII–pH monitoring has diagnostic value primarily in patients with refractory GERD. Approximately 10% of refractory GERD patients on PPI treatment have a positive SI to acid reflux, and 37% to non-acid reflux [12]. Adding MII to pH monitoring improves the diagnostic yield by 15–20% and allows better symptom analysis than pH monitoring alone [13]. As MII–pH monitoring is currently the most sensitive method for reflux detection, a negative study (normal number of reflux events and negative symptom analysis) rules out GERD as a cause for persistent symptoms.

Treatment options

Lifestyle modifications

The specific value of lifestyle modifications in patients with refractory GERD has yet to be elucidated. However, in a recent systematic review, only weight loss and elevation of the head of bed were found to be effective in improving GERD symptoms [31]. There were insufficient data to support any of the other commonly practiced lifestyle modifications. Regardless, in patients with refractory GERD, it is reasonable to recommend avoidance of specific lifestyle activities that have been identified by patients or physicians to trigger reflux symptoms.

H_2-receptor antagonists

Early studies have shown that the addition of an H_2-receptor antagonists at bedtime significantly reduced the duration of nocturnal acid breakthrough (NAB) and the number of GERD patients on twice-daily PPI who demonstrated NAB [32]. The effect on NAB was no different between standard-dose and double-dose H_2-receptor antagonists. Despite lack of any clinical correlation between the presence of NAB and nocturnal GERD symptoms, the addition of H_2-receptor antagonists at bedtime has become common practice in GERD patients who failed PPIs regardless of dosing. However, concerns were raised about the rapid development of tolerance (within 1 week) in patients taking an H_2-receptor antagonist daily [33].

In a study that evaluated 100 patients (58 on twice-daily PPI and 42 on twice-daily PPI + H_2-receptor antagonist at bedtime for at least 1 month), the addition of a bedtime H_2-receptor antagonist significantly reduced the percentage time with intragastric pH < 4 [34]. Unfortunately, the authors failed to provide any evidence for similar effects on clinical endpoints. Rackoff et al. evaluated 56 GERD patients on twice-daily PPIs who were receiving H_2-receptor antagonists at bedtime [35]; 72% reported improvement in overall symptoms, 74% in nighttime reflux symptoms, and 67% in GERD-associated sleep disturbances.

These studies, and the vast experience that the authors have accumulated thus far with H_2-receptor antagonist treatment for GERD, suggest that H_2-receptor antagonists improve GERD-related symptoms in the long term in a substantial number of patients. If clinical tolerance has been encountered, then using H_2-receptor antagonists intermittently or on demand could be helpful.

Proton pump inhibitors

In GERD patients who failed on once-daily PPIs, there are two potential therapeutic strategies that could be utilized in clinical practice: switching to another PPI or doubling the PPI dose. However, doubling the PPI dose is by far the most common therapeutic strategy that is used by practicing physicians when managing patients who failed once-daily PPIs, as also acknowledged by the 2008 American Gastroenterological Association technical review on the management of GERD [36]. A Cochrane review suggested that doubling the PPI dose is associated with improved healing of erosive esophagitis with a number needed to treat of 25. However, there is no clear dose–response relationship for heartburn resolution in either erosive esophagitis or NERD [37].

Switching to another PPI is an attractive therapeutic strategy that could be utilized in the management of patients who failed once-daily PPIs. In one study, patients who failed on once-daily 30 mg lansoprazole were randomized to either double-dose lansoprazole or once-daily 40 mg esomeprazole. Single-dose esomeprazole was as effective as double-dose lansoprazole in reducing the percentage of heartburn-free days as well as the symptom score for heartburn, acid regurgitation, and epigastric pain [38].

Although doubling the PPI dose has became the standard of care, there is no evidence to support further dose escalation beyond twice-daily PPI either in symptom control or in healing of erosive esophagitis. When doubling the PPI dose, it should be given twice daily, with the first dose before breakfast and the second before dinner. The support for splitting the dose originates primarily from physiological studies demonstrating an improved control of intragastric pH when one dose was given in the morning and the second dose in the evening compared with giving both doses in the morning before breakfast [39].

In the USA, one other potential strategy would be to use dexlansoprazole MR, the R-enantiomer of lansoprazole in a dual delayed release formulation. However, the effectiveness of this agent in patients who failed treatment with a conventional delayed-release PPI remains to be elucidated [40,41]. Potentially, the two separate releases of dexlansoprazole, separated by 4–5 hours, may be helpful in patients who failed PPI once daily.

Baclofen

A variety of compounds have been shown to reduce the rate of transient lower esophageal sphincter relaxation (TLESR) and thus the number of reflux events. However, only baclofen, a γ-aminobutyric acid B receptor agonist, has been introduced into the clinical arena as a potential add-on treatment for patients who failed PPI treatment (once or twice daily). The drug reduced TLESR rate by 40–60% and reflux episodes by 43%, increased lower esophageal sphincter basal pressure, and accelerated gastric emptying [42]. Baclofen has been shown to significantly reduce weakly acidic reflux and DGER, as well as DGER-related symptoms [43,44]. In patients with persistent heartburn despite PPI treatment, doses up to 20 mg three times daily have been used. As the drug crosses the blood–brain barrier, a variety of central nervous system (CNS)-related side effects may occur. They primarily include somnolence, confusion, dizziness, lightheadedness, drowsiness, weakness, and trembling. The side effects are an important limiting factor in the routine use of baclofen in clinical practice.

Baclofen should be considered in patients with clear evidence of persistent symptoms that are related to weakly acidic reflux, as documented by intraesophageal impedance or in those with regurgitation, or a sour or bitter taste in the mouth as the predominant symptom.

Promotility (prokinetic) drugs

Presently, there are no available data about the value of adding a promotility drug in patients who failed either one or two daily doses of PPI. However, in patients with delayed gastric emptying and persistent GERD symptoms on PPIs, the use of a promotility drug is an attractive option. It is unclear if patients with refractory GERD with normal gastric emptying would also benefit from adding a promotility drug.

Visceral pain modulators

Thus far, there are no studies that specifically evaluated the value of visceral pain modulators in refractory GERD patients. However, given the fact that most of the patients who fail PPI treatment have NERD or FH, and that up to 40% of the patients who fail PPI treatment demonstrate lack of either weakly or acidic reflux, the use of these agents is highly attractive [12,45]. In addition, it could be argued that, even for weakly acidic reflux that has not been shown to be associated with esophageal mucosal damage, visceral pain modulators could be helpful.

Pain modulators such as tricyclic antidepressants, trazodone, and selective serotonin reuptake inhibitors (SSRIs) have all been shown to improve esophageal pain in patients with non-cardiac chest pain [12,46,47]. It is believed that these agents confer their visceral analgesic effect by acting at the CNS and/or esophageal sensory afferent level. The pain modulators are used in non-mood-altering doses, and they currently provide a therapeutic alternative until more novel and esophageal-specific compounds will be available.

Antireflux surgery

A recent surgical study reported that refractory GERD was the most common (88%) indication for antireflux surgery. Interestingly, the most common preoperative symptom under failure of medical antireflux treatment was regurgitation (54%). Overall, 82% of the patients reported that the preoperative reflux symptom completely resolved, and 94% were satisfied with the results of the surgery. In another study that included only 30 participants with refractory GERD who were followed for a period of 12 months, the main preoperative symptoms were regurgitation

(93%) and heartburn (60%). At the end of 1 year post-surgery, all patients were completely relieved of heartburn, but only 86% reported resolution of regurgitation. Patient satisfaction rate with the surgery was 87%.

Thus far, it is believed that antireflux surgery should be considered only in refractory GERD patients who clearly demonstrate that residual reflux is the underlying cause for their symptoms.

Alternative medicine

The value of acupuncture has been evaluated in GERD patients who failed on once-daily PPI. When compared with doubling the PPI dose, adding acupuncture was significantly better in controlling regurgitation, and daytime and nighttime heartburn. This is the first study to suggest that alternative approaches for treating visceral pain may have a role in patients with refractory GERD [48].

Psychological treatment

Patients with poor correlation of symptoms with acid reflux events display a high level of anxiety compared with patients who demonstrate a close correlation between symptoms and acid-reflux events [49]. Anxiety and depression have been shown to increase GERD-related symptoms in population-based studies. A recent study provided the first evidence that response to PPI treatment may depend on the level of psychological distress [50]. Thus, it has been proposed that patients who did not respond to PPI therapy are more likely to have psychosocial comorbidity than those who were successfully treated with a PPI. In these patients, treatment directed toward underlying psychosocial abnormality may improve patients' response to PPI therapy.

Case continuation

The patient presented had failed a full course of once-daily PPI. In addition to lifestyle modifications, and after excluding poor compliance and improper dosage timing, she could be offered a switch to another PPI or a double dose of the current PPI. The latter therapeutic strategy is commonly pursued by practicing physicians and has become the standard of care. It has yet to be determined how long the patient should remain on the new PPI regimen before treatment success or failure can be declared. Many physicians will elect to repeat a 2-month course of treatment, but this time with twice-daily PPI (given half an hour before breakfast and half an hour before dinner) and re-evaluation of the patient's symptomatic response.

Invasive testing should be considered only if the patient failed twice-daily PPI. If alarm symptoms emerge, an upper endoscopy should be immediately entertained. If the patient becomes asymptomatic on twice-daily PPI, maintenance treatment should be offered. For maintenance, it is likely that the patient will require the same PPI dose that induced symptom remission, although titration to once-daily PPI might be considered.

If the patient continues to report incomplete symptom improvement, two management approaches are available (Figure 2.2). If the treating physician has access to MII-pH testing, the test should be performed on treatment. If the esophageal impedance test is positive for symptoms related to weakly acidic reflux, treatment with baclofen should be considered. There are no clear rules on how to dose baclofen in this clinical situation, although the extensive side-effect profile of the drug might suggest a low (dose) and slow (increase in dose) approach. Antireflux surgery should be offered only to a carefully selected patient with clear documentation of symptoms that are associated with weakly acidic reflux by using SI and/or SAP. If the esophageal impedance is negative, then pain modulators might be considered. They include tricyclic antidepressants, trazodone, and SSRIs. If the esophageal impedance is positive for acid reflux-related symptoms (the least common scenario), the patient's dosing time of PPI and compliance should be reviewed again. In some cases, adding an H_2-receptor antagonist at bedtime could be helpful.

In many cases, esophageal impedance is not available and empiric therapy is used. In this situation, the patient's predominant symptom might guide treatment. If the patient presents with primarily regurgitation and/or a bitter or sour taste in the mouth, baclofen should be initially prescribed. If the predominant symptom is heartburn, adding an H_2-receptor antagonist at bedtime should be considered first, and, if the patient still exhibits lack of response, pain modulators might be considered.

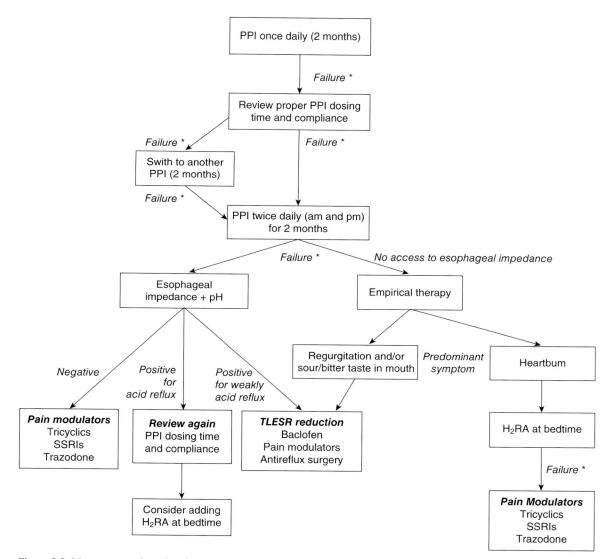

Figure 2.2 Management algorithm for patient with gastroesophageal reflux disease (GERD) who failed treatment with once-daily proton pump inhibitor (PPI). *Partial or incomplete relief of symptoms. H₂RA, H₂-receptor antagonist; SSRIs, selective serotonin reuptake inhibitors; TLESR, transient lower esophageal sphincter relaxation. (Redrawn with permission after Fass R. Proton pump inhibitor failure – what are the therapeutic options? *Am J Gastroenterol* 2009;**104**(suppl 2):S33–8.)

Case 2: patient with atypical chest pain

Case presentation

A 45-year-old woman was referred to the outpatient gastrointestinal clinic by her primary care physician for the evaluation of a 4-year history of unexplained, intermittent, substernal chest pain. The patient describes the pain as squeezing, pressure like, or heavy. It does not radiate to the back, neck, arms, or jaws. The pain is continuous and unrelated to exertion, emotion, or exposure to cold, and can occur several times a week. The pain can last for hours and is not relieved by rest or nitroglycerin.

The patient was admitted twice during the last year to the cardiac care unit but ruled out for myocardial infarction. Before referral to the gastrointestinal clinic, the patient underwent a cardiac workup that included a stress test and a cardiac catheterization; all were within normal limits.

The patient denies dysphagia, odynophagia, anorexia, nausea, vomiting, weight loss, or a history of hematemesis or anemia.

Past medical history: recently diagnosed hypertension, currently well controlled

Past surgical history: none

Current medications: lisinopril for hypertension

Social history: employed; considers her work to be very stressful. She is married and has two children at home. Both of her pregnancies were unremarkable

Family history: unremarkable

Habits: she denies smoking or drinking alcohol. However, she admits to occasional late-night business meals

Physical examination: BP 137/85 mmHg; heart rate 78/min; weight 65 kg; height: 170 cm; BMI: 22.5

General appearance: well appearing woman, sitting comfortably. Oral cavity without mucosal abnormalities

Neck: no masses, lymphadenopathy or goiter

Heart: regular rhythm, normal heart sounds without murmurs

Lungs: clear to auscultation

Abdomen: soft and not distended. No masses or tenderness. Normal bowel sounds

Extremities: no edema or cyanosis.

Her primary care physician found no specific cause for her recurrent chest pain and thus initially treated the patient with NSAIDs without symptom relief. Subsequently the patient was treated with 300 mg ranitidine twice a day for 2 months. When this failed, it was followed by 20 mg omeprazole once a day for an additional 2 months without symptom relief.

An upper endoscopy by another gastroenterologist showed a non-dilated, normal-appearing esophagus, as well as normal gastric and duodenal mucosa.

Questions

• What are the diagnostic considerations in this patient?

• What is the pathophysiolopgy of this condition?
• What diagnostic tests are useful in this condition?
• What therapeutic options can be offered to this patient?

The problem

Non-cardiac chest pain (NCCP) is defined as recurring angina-like retrosternal chest pain of non-cardiac origin. NCCP is very common in the general population, with a mean annual prevalence of approximately 25%.

An important step toward understanding the underlying mechanisms of NCCP was the recognition that GERD is its most common contributing factor. although chest pain has been considered an atypical manifestation of GERD, it is an integral part of the limited repertoire of esophageal symptoms. In patients with non-GERD-related NCCP, esophageal motility disorders and functional chest pain of presumed esophageal origin are the main underlying mechanisms for symptoms.

The Rome III Committee did not specifically address NCCP. The term "functional chest pain of presumed esophageal origin" is used to describe recurrent episodes of substernal chest pain of visceral quality with no apparent explanation (Box 2.1). As with all other functional esophageal disorders, GERD and esophageal dysmotility should be ruled out first before the diagnosis is established [51]. However, up to 20% of patients with functional chest pain exhibit other functional disorders, primarily irritable bowel syndrome (27%) and abdominal bloating (22%) [52].

Box 2.1 The Rome III diagnostic criteria for functional chest pain of presumed esophageal origin [1]

Midline chest pain or discomfort that is not of burning quality

Absence of evidence that gastroesophageal reflux is the cause of the symptom

Absence of histopathology-based esophageal motility disorders

All criteria fulfilled for the last 3 months with symptoms onset at least 6 months before diagnosis.

Differential diagnosis

Cardiac or non-cardiac chest pain?

Chest pain may be the manifestation of GI or non-GI-related disorders (Box 2.2). A patient's history and characteristics do not reliably distinguish between cardiac and esophageal causes of chest pain [53]. It should be noted that 30% of the patients thought to have chest pain caused by coronary artery disease have normal coronary angiography. In addition, coronary artery disease was found in up to 25% of the patients defined as having an atypical chest pain.

Therefore, all patients who present with chest pain, regardless of its character, should initially undergo a proper cardiac evaluation before being referred to a gastroenterologist. The cardiologist's first priority is to exclude any acute life-threatening cardiovascular condition [54], including acute coronary syndrome, aortic dissection, pulmonary thromboembolism, and pericardial tamponade. If these acute conditions have been excluded, evaluation for chronic ischemic heart disease or pericardial disease must be pursued. Various tests can help determine the presence and severity of ischemia, left ventricular function, appearance of the coronary arteries, and functional capacity. They include exercise ECG, echocardiography, or nuclear SPECT (single photon emission computed tomography) and – if patients are unable to exercise – pharmacological echocardiography, nuclear SPECT, or cardiac MRI (magnetic resonance imaging). The decision of what tests to pursue should be left to the discretion of the treating cardiologist.

Pathophysiology of NCCP

The pathophysiology of NCCP remains to be fully elucidated. Identified underlying mechanisms are diverse and often overlapping. Of the GI causes, GERD is by far the most common cause of NCCP. Other GI-related etiological factors that have been proposed include esophageal motility disorders, abnormal mechanophysical properties of the esophagus, sustained esophageal longitudinal muscle contractions, esophageal hypersensitivity, and psychological comorbidities.

Gastroesophageal reflux disease

GERD has been reported to be the most common esophageal cause for NCCP. Reports of typical GERD

Box 2.2 Common non-cardiac etiologies for chest pain

Musculoskeletal
  Costochondritis
  Fibromyalgia
  Precordial catch syndrome
  Slipping rib syndrome
  Xyphoditis
  Thoracic outlet syndrome
  Cervical or thoracic spinal disease

Gastrointestinal
  Gastroesophageal reflux disease
  Esophageal dysmotility
  Peptic ulcer disease
  Biliary disease
  Pancreatitis
  Intra-abdominal masses (benign and malignant].

Pulmonary or intrathoracic
  Pneumonia
  Pleurisy
  Pulmonary embolism
  Lung cancer
  Sarcoidosis
  Pneumothorax or pneumomediastinum
  Pleural effusions
  Mediastinitis
  Aortic aneurysm
  Pericarditis or myocarditis
  Pulmonary hypertension
  Intrathoracic masses (benign and malignant].

Psychiatric causes
  Panic disorder
  Anxiety
  Depression
  Somatization
  Hypochondriasis
  Munchausen's syndrome

Miscellaneous
  Herpes zoster
  Drug-induced pain
  Sickle cell crisis

symptoms (heartburn and acid regurgitation) might be present in up to 70% of the patients and are highly predictive of GERD-related NCCP. Erosive esophagitis has been documented in 10–70% and abnormal esophageal acid exposure in 40–60% of the GERD-related NCCP patients. Several studies have found that patients with GERD-related NCCP often report chest pain that is provoked by meals or recumbency, and might be relieved by antacids. The presence of abnormal esophageal acid exposure or erosive esophagitis in patients with NCCP might suggest association only. However, review of therapeutic studies in NCCP revealed that up to 80% of the patients with either EE or abnormal pH testing responded to potent antireflux treatment. Consequently, the presence of esophageal mucosal injury and/or abnormal esophageal acid exposure is highly predictive that GERD is the likely underlying cause of a patient's symptoms.

Esophageal dysmotility
Although often entertained as an etiology of NCCP in the absence of GERD, the role of esophageal dysmotility in NCCP is likely very limited. Over 70% of patients with non-GERD-related NCCP have normal esophageal motility [55,56]. Esophageal dysmotility when documented by esophageal manometry is rarely associated with chest pain [57]. Furthermore, in NCCP patients who underwent simultaneous esophageal manometry and pH testing, chest pain was more commonly associated with acid reflux events than motility abnormalities [58,59]. Studies have shown that chest pain will often improve without any normalization of the esophageal motor abnormalities. Unlike GERD, in which PPIs are generally highly effective in alleviating symptoms, we are still devoid of pharmacological agents that can effectively treat esophageal dysmotility. The latter further complicates our ability to determine any relationship between chest pain and manometric findings. That being said, esophageal motility disorders can still be demonstrated in 30% of the patients with non-GERD-related NCCP.

Hypotensive lower esophageal sphincter (LES) was the most common (61%) esophageal motor disorder found in patients with NCCP in a study using the Clinical Outcomes Research Initiative (CORI) database [56]. Spastic esophageal motility disorders were shown to be the second most common cause, with nutcracker esophagus affecting 10%, hypertensive LES 10%, and diffuse esophageal spasm 2% of the NCCP cases with esophageal dysmotility. However, in another study of non-GERD-related NCCP, nutcracker esophagus was the most common motor disorder documented during esophageal manometry, followed by non-specific esophageal motility disorders, diffuse esophageal spasm, hypertensive LES, and achalasia [55].

As a result of the weak correlation between documented esophageal dysmotility during manometry and chest pain, some have postulated that motility disorders serve more as a marker for a currently poorly understood esophageal abnormality that contributes to the patient's NCCP.

Esophageal hypersensitivity
Visceral hypersensitivity is a phenomenon in which the conscious perception of a visceral stimulus is enhanced independent of the intensity of the stimulus [60,61]. Peripheral and central mechanisms have been proposed to be responsible for esophageal hypersensitivity in patients with NCCP.

Peripheral sensitization of esophageal sensory afferents may lead to subsequently heightened responses to physiological or pathological stimuli of the esophageal mucosa. In addition, central sensitization at the level of the brain or dorsal horn of the spinal cord may modulate afferent neural function and thus enhance perception of intraluminal stimuli [62]. What causes peripheral or central sensitization remains to be elucidated. Studies have shown that acute tissue irritation results in subsequent peripheral and central sensitization, which is manifested as increased background activity of sensory neurons, the lowering of nociceptive thresholds, changes in stimulus response curves, and enlargements of receptive fields [63]. Peripheral sensitization involves the reduction of the esophageal pain threshold and an increase in the transduction processes of primary afferent neurons. Esophageal tissue injury, inflammation, spasm, or repetitive mechanical stimuli can all sensitize peripheral afferent nerves.

The presence of esophageal hypersensitivity can be subsequently demonstrated long after the original stimulus is no longer present and the esophageal mucosa has healed. Several studies have demonstrated that patients with non-GERD-related NCCP have lower perception thresholds for pain. Richter et al.

used balloon distension in the distal esophagus, and found that 50% of the patients with NCCP developed pain at volumes of 8 mL or less in comparison with 9 mL or more in healthy individuals who developed pain [64]. The authors found no difference in the pressure–volume curve of the two groups, as well as no difference in esophageal motility. When the balloon was inflated to 10 mL, patients with a history of NCCP were more likely to experience pain (18 of 30) than the control individuals (6 of 30). Barish et al. evaluated 50 patients with NCCP and 30 healthy volunteers using a graded balloon distension protocol [65]. Of the patients with NCCP, 56% experienced their "typical" chest pain during balloon distension compared with 20% of control individuals. Of those with NCCP who experienced pain, 86% reported it at volumes less than 8 mL while all normal volunteers experienced pain with 9 mL or greater.

Investigators have used cerebral-evoked potentials as an objective measurement to assess central sensitization in NCCP patients [61,66,67]. In response to esophageal balloon distension, evoked potential quality scores and amplitude of the major peaks increased significantly with increased sensation, in both NCCP patients and healthy control individuals. However, in the NCCP patients, quality score and amplitude of the evoked potentials were lower and latencies were longer than in the control individuals. The volumes of air required to produce the various sensations were lower in the patients. Because of the smaller cortical-evoked potentials, it was hypothesized that the increased perception of esophageal stimuli might in fact be the result of enhanced cerebral processing of visceral sensory input rather than hyperalgesic responses of visceral afferent pathways.

Positron emission tomography (PET) and functional MRI (fMRI) have been increasingly used to evaluate brain–gut relationships in patients with reflux symptoms. However, there are no studies that particularly explored the role of functional brain imaging in NCCP.

Psychological comorbidities
Between 17% and 43% of patients with NCCP may have some type of psychological abnormality [68]. Psychological comorbidity can modulate esophageal perception and cause individuals to perceive low-intensity esophageal stimuli as being painful [69–72]. Anxiety, depression, neuroticism, and hypochondriac

behavior have all been described in NCCP patients [73–76]. However, these findings have been inconsistent when NCCP patients were compared with patients with coronary artery disease, with some authors reporting increased anxiety and depression in NCCP patients whereas others reported no significant difference between the two disorders. In a recent study of 167 patients with NCCP and 32 with chest pain and coronary artery disease, there was no significant difference in the incidence of depression, anxiety, or neuroticism between the two groups [77]. The authors stated that the discrepancy in their results with previous findings might be secondary to different inclusion criteria or an overall low prevalence of major depression. The study did find that panic disorder was more common in NCCP patients (41%) compared with those with coronary artery disease.

NCCP patients with psychological disorders show diminished quality of life, more frequent chest pain, and less treatment satisfaction than NCCP patients without psychological comorbidity [78].

Natural history

The long-term prognosis of NCCP patients is excellent and very few eventually succumb to coronary artery disease or other cardiovascular-related disorders. However, most NCCP patients continue to report episodes of chest pain. In one study, 75% of the surviving NCCP patients continued to report chest pain 11 years later, and 34% reported weekly chest pain. NCCP patients demonstrate poor quality of life primarily due to continuation of symptoms many years after diagnosis. In a study from Norway, NCCP patients reported a significantly greater impairment of health-related quality of life compared with the general population [79]. NCCP patients demonstrate long-term impaired functional status and frequently utilize healthcare resources because of their chest pain [80]. Consequently, NCCP is a costly disorder, resulting in a significant economic burden on the health care system.

Diagnostic strategies

The currently available diagnostic tests in NCCP are primarily designed to evaluate patients for GERD, esophageal dysmotility, and esophageal hypersensitivity as the potential underlying mechanisms for symptoms. The role of the different diagnostic tests in NCCP has evolved over the years, primarily due to the introduction of the PPI test and the recognition that provocative tests have limited sensitivity.

PPI test

The PPI test (or short therapeutic trial) is defined as a short course (1–4 weeks) of high-dose PPI for diagnosing GERD-related NCCP. The test is considered positive if the symptom assessment score for chest pain improves by more than 50% relative to the baseline. The test is highly sensitive, specific, and accurate for diagnosing GERD-related NCCP. The PPI test could be used by primary care physicians due to its simplicity and availability.

The doses used in the PPI test in patients with symptoms suggestive of NCCP have ranged from 60 mg to 80 mg daily for omeprazole, 30 mg to 90 mg daily for lansoprazole, and 40 mg daily for rabeprazole, over a period of 1–28 days [81]. In different studies, the sensitivity of the PPI test for GERD-related NCCP ranged from 69% to 95% and the specificity from 67% to 86% [82,83].

There is evidence that, when using the PPI test, there is a significant correlation between the severity of esophageal acid exposure in the distal esophagus as determined by ambulatory 24-hour esophageal pH monitoring and the change in SI score after treatment. In other words, the higher the esophageal acid exposure, the greater the response to the PPI test in patients with GERD-related NCCP [84].

Economic analysis also showed that the use of the PPI test in GERD-related NCCP is a cost-saving approach primarily due to significant reduction in the utilization of various invasive diagnostic tests that are of unproven utility in the diagnosis and subsequent management of patients with NCCP [85].

Upper endoscopy

Upper endoscopy is the gold standard for diagnosing anatomic and mucosal abnormalities of the upper GI tract. In GERD-related NCCP, upper endoscopy can detect erosive esophagitis, stricture, ulceration, and Barrett's esophagus.

In NCCP patients with alarm features (weight loss, dysphagia, anorexia, upper GI bleeding, and anemia) upper endoscopy should be considered as the initial diagnostic tool. Otherwise, the value of upper endoscopy in NCCP has been an area of controversy. In the largest study thus far (assessing 3688 consecutive NCCP patients), 44% had a normal endoscopy. The findings in those with abnormal endoscopy included hiatal hernia (28.6%), EE (19.4%), Barrett's esophagus (4.4%), esophageal stricture or stenosis (3.6%), and peptic ulcer (2%) [86]. In this study, most of the mucosal findings in NCCP patients were GERD related. Overall, it appears that the value of upper endoscopy in NCCP is limited, because findings are primarily related to GERD. Potentially, the test may be indicated as a screening tool for Barrett's esophagus in GERD-related NCCP patients.

Esophageal pH monitoring

Ambulatory 24-hour esophageal pH monitoring with symptom correlation is still commonly used to evaluate patients with NCCP [87]. However, the presence of abnormal distal esophageal acid exposure during pH monitoring does not always mean that the patient's chest pain is GERD related.

The pH monitoring is invasive, inconvenient to patients, costly, and not readily available for many physicians. In addition, the yield of the test in NCCP has not been rigorously studied. This is compounded by the rarity of chest pain symptoms during the test in many patients, making it difficult to determine the relationship between patients' symptoms and acid reflux events [88].

Off therapy pH monitoring appears to have value in patients with NCCP in whom objective evidence of acid reflux is required. For example, pH testing is indicated in GERD-related NCCP patients with unremarkable upper endoscopy who are candidates for antireflux surgery. The value of pH testing, off or on therapy, in patients with an equivocal or negative PPI test remains unknown. However, it appears that the test has a therapeutic predictive value in addition to its diagnostic merit [84]. Patients with greater esophageal acid exposure appear to have a better response rate to antireflux treatment.

The wireless pH capsule is attached to the esophageal wall and transmits pH data to a recording device. This system collects pH data for 48 hours and potentially for up to 96 hours. It is better tolerated than catheter-based pH systems, is highly reliable, and provides reproducible results [89]. The wireless pH capsule increases the detection of patients with abnormal pH test and/or positive SAP. In one study extending the pH monitoring time to 48 hours, the number of NCCP patients with diagnosis of GERD increased by 19.4% [90].

Esophageal manometry

In NCCP, esophageal manometry is commonly performed if GERD has been excluded as the underlying cause [52]. Esophageal manometry can identify an esophageal motility disorder in approximately a third of NCCP patients. Hypotensive LES (61%) is the most common motility abnormality diagnosed, followed by hypertensive LES, non-specific esophageal motor disorder, and nutcracker esophagus (10% each). Achalasia and diffuse esophageal spasm are very uncommon in NCCP [56]. The presence of a motility abnormality during esophageal manometry is rarely associated with reports of chest pain, raising a question about the exact relationship between the aforementioned motility findings and chest pain. As most spastic motility disorders respond the best to visceral analgesics, the test is reserved primarily to diagnose NCCP caused by achalasia.

Other tests

Some patients with NCCP require evaluation by an expert psychologist or psychiatrist because of the high prevalence rate of psychological abnormalities. Deciding who should be referred is determined individually, but likely candidates are those who appear to be refractory to therapeutic interventions or those who display clear features of a psychological disorder.

Provocative testing – such as the edrophonium test, acid perfusion test, balloon distension test, ergonovine test, and bethanechol test – have all fallen out of favor because of their low sensitivity and potential side effects.

Treatment

Treatment for NCCP should be targeted toward the specific underlying mechanism responsible for a patient's symptoms. As GERD is by far the most common condition observed in patients with NCCP, treatment for GERD is indicated in all patients presenting with NCCP unless a specific alternative diagnosis is present [91]. Table 2.1 provides a general

Table 2.1 General treatment plan for non-cardiac chest pain (NCCP)

GERD-related NCCP	PPIs, twice-daily for at least 2 months
Non-GERD-related NCCP	Muscle relaxants (nitrates, calcium channel blockers)
	Botulinum toxin injection
	Pain modulators (TCAs, SSRIs or trazodone), non-mood altering low dose, given at bedtime
	Surgery for achalasia
	Cognitive–behavioral therapy/ hypnotherapy

GERD, gastroesophageal reflux disease; PPI, proton pump inhibitor; SSRI, selective serotonin reuptake inhibitors; TCA, tricyclic antidepressant.

treatment plan and Figure 2.3 provides a proposed management algorithm for NCCP.

GERD-related NCCP

Acid-suppressive therapy results in significant symptom improvement in most patients with GERD-related NCCP. Such patients should be treated with at least double the standard dose of PPI until symptoms remit, followed by dose tapering to determine the lowest PPI dose that can control symptoms. Thus far, most studies assessing the efficacy of PPIs in NCCP used omeprazole. However, it is likely that all PPIs would demonstrate similar efficacy. The duration of treatment for GERD-related chest pain has not been critically evaluated. Most available studies followed patients for 6–8 weeks only [92–95]. As with other extraesophageal manifestations of GERD, NCCP patients may require more than 2 months of therapy for optimal symptom control.

The value of antireflux surgery in GERD-related NCCP is unclear. Several studies have demonstrated significant improvement in symptoms after laparoscopic fundoplication in patients with GERD-related NCCP [96–99]. Unfortunately, these studies evaluated the effect of surgery on all GERD-related atypical/extraesophageal symptoms and did not specifically target NCCP. None of the surgical studies

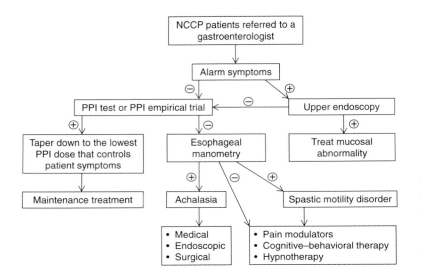

Figure 2.3 Proposed management algorithm for non-cardiac chest pain (NCCP). PPI, proton pump inhibitor. (Redrawn with permission after Fass R, Navarro-Rodriguez T. Noncardiac chest pain. *J Clin Gastroenterol* 2008;42:636–46.)

was a randomized controlled trial. All studies originated from tertiary referral centers specializing in the management of esophageal disorders.

Non-GERD-related NCCP

The treatment of non-GERD-related NCCP is primarily based on esophageal pain modulation (see Table 2.1). An important development in this field was the recognition that NCCP patients with spastic esophageal motor disorders (except achalasia) are more likely to respond to pain modulators than to muscle relaxants. Unfortunately, no large, well-designed studies to assess pain modulators in patients with non-GERD-related NCCP have been performed thus far.

Pain modulators

Esophageal hypersensitivity is thought to be the primary underlying mechanism of non-GERD-related NCCP, regardless of the presence or absence of an esophageal motor disorder (except achalasia). Consequently, drugs that can alter esophageal pain perception have become the mainstay of treatment in these patients.

Tricyclic antidepressants

Tricyclic antidepressants (TCAs) have both central neuromodulatory and peripheral visceral analgesic effects. Several clinical trials have found favorable effects of low-dose TCA treatment on esophageal pain perception in both healthy individuals [100] and patients with NCCP [101]. The long-term effects of TCAs in NCCP were assessed in a retrospective analysis of 21 patients with an incomplete response to antireflux treatment [102]. Three-quarters of the patients with NCCP continued to experience symptomatic relief during long-term use of the medications for up to 3 years. The use of a low-dose TCA in these trials suggests that the benefit of this class of drugs is mediated through their visceral rather than their antidepressant properties.

It is recommended that TCA doses are slowly titrated to a maximum of 50–75 mg daily. The incremental increase in dosing should be based on symptom improvement and development of side effects. TCAs are commonly administered at nighttime due to their anticholinergic side effects. Because of the varied effects of TCAs on their respective receptors, failure of one agent to improve symptoms is not indicative of future failure of other TCAs.

Trazodone, a tetracyclic antidepressant and anxiolytic, in doses of 100–150 mg/day can also produce improvement in NCCP [103]. However, esophageal motility abnormalities remain unchanged.

Selective serotonin reuptake inhibitors

Sertraline induced a significant reduction in chest pain scores compared with placebo in 30 patients with

NCCP, when started at 50 mg and adjusted to a maximum of 200 mg/day for 8 weeks. Side effects occurred in 27% of the patients and included delayed ejaculation, decreased libido, and restlessness [104]. Paroxetine administered for 8 weeks provided greater improvement in physician-rated chest pain but not in patients' self-rated chest pain scores, compared with placebo [105]. These studies are relatively small but suggest a visceral analgesic effect of SSRIs in NCCP patients that is somewhat limited by their side-effect profiles.

Muscle relaxants

Studies that evaluated the value of nitrates (short and long acting) in NCCP are limited due to small numbers of patients, and are inconsistent with regard to drug efficacy [106–110]. However, side effects such as headache and hypotension limit their clinical use. It is also possible that patients may become refractory to therapy after long-term use. There have been no placebo-controlled trials of nitrate treatment for non-GERD-related NCCP.

Calcium channel blocking agents (such as diltiazem, nifedipine, and verapamil) appear to be of limited value and their use might be complicated by side effects, such as hypotension, constipation, and pedal edema.

Psychological treatment

Reassurance about the benign nature of NCCP has been emphasized as an important early therapeutic intervention. However, patients' symptoms are seldom relieved by reassurance only, resulting in the need for additional treatment. In patients who have panic disorder, treatment with alprazolam and clonazepam has been demonstrated to reduce panic attack frequency, chest pain episodes, and anxiety scores. Benzodiazepines should be used cautiously in NCCP patients, primarily because of their addictive effect.

Cognitive–behavioral therapy (CBT) has been reported to be effective in the treatment of NCCP. NCCP patients receiving CBT reported significant improvement in frequency and intensity of chest pain when compared with "usual care." The improvement was long lasting (4–12 months after therapy) [111–112]. CBT has also been successfully used for the treatment of NCCP patients without an existing panic disorder [113].

Hypnotherapy has been associated with an 80% improvement in symptoms and a significant reduction in pain intensity in NCCP. Patients received 12 sessions of hypnotherapy. In comparison, only 23% symptom improvement was demonstrated in the control group. Hypnotherapy also resulted in a significantly greater improvement in overall wellbeing in addition to a reduction in medication usage [114].

In a Cochrane analysis of all the psychological interventions in NCCP, the authors found a significant reduction in chest pain in the first 3 months after the intervention which was maintained for 3–9 months afterwards [115].

Case continued

The patient presented should initially be treated with a PPI given twice daily until symptoms remit, followed by dose tapering to determine the lowest dose that can control the patient's symptoms. Duration of treatment should be at least 2 months, although longer duration of treatment (3–6 months) might be required in a subset of patients.

If the patient does not respond to twice-daily PPI after at least 2 months of treatment, performing pH testing on therapy would be a low-yield procedure. Esophageal manometry should be considered only if achalasia is suspected. Otherwise, a trial of a pain modulator is recommended. A low dose (10–25 mg) of a TCA can be administered at bedtime and increased by 10–25 mg increments per week to a maximal, non-mood-altering dose of 50–75 mg/day.

Finally, evaluating psychological comorbidity is important, especially in patients who appear to be refractory to current therapeutic management. Referral to a psychologist or psychiatrist who is an expert in the field of functional bowel disorders could be of benefit.

Take-home points

• Patients presenting for the first time with chest pain should be initially evaluated by a cardiologist in order to rule out a cardiac source.
• GERD is the most common esophageal cause of NCCP.
• Diagnostic methods should be used in a logical and systematic step-by-step approach with each patient

assessed, based on presenting symptoms and medical history.

• The PPI test is an excellent first diagnostic step for NCCP.

• Acid-suppressive therapy induces a significant clinical improvement in most patients with GERD-related NCCP.

• Drugs that can alter esophageal pain perception have become the mainstay of therapy in non-GERD-related NCCP.

• Psychological comorbidities should be assessed and treated in those NCCP patients with signs of psychological disorders or who are refractory to treatment.

References

1 Inadomi JM, McIntyre L, Bernard L, Fendrick AM. Step-down from multiple- to single-dose proton pump inhibitors (PPIs): a prospective study of patients with heartburn or acid regurgitation completely relieved with PPIs. *Am J Gastroenterol* 2003;**98**:1940–4.

2 Gallup Organization. *2000 Gallup Study of Consumers' Use of Stomach Relief Products*. Princeton: Gallup Organization, 2000.

3 Dean BB, Gano Jr. AD, Knight K, Ofman JJ, Fass R. Effectiveness of proton pump inhibitors in nonerosive reflux disease. *Clin Gastroenterol Hepatol* 2004;**2**: 656–64.

4 Chey WD, Mody RR, Wu EQ, et al. Treatment patterns and symptom control in patients with GERD: US community-based survey. *Curr Med Res Opin* 2009;**25**:1869–78.

5 Fass R. Proton pump inhibitor failure – what are the therapeutic options? *Am J Gastroenterol* 2009;**104** (suppl 2):S33–8.

6 Fass R, Sampliner RE. Barrett's oesophagus: optimal strategies for prevention and treatment. *Drugs* 2003;**63**:555–64.

7 Fass R, Sifrim D. Management of heartburn not responding to proton pump inhibitors. *Gut* 2009;**58**:295–309.

8 Hatlebakk JG, Katz PO, Camacho-Lobato L, Castell DO. Proton pump inhibitors: better acid suppression when taken before a meal than without a meal. *Aliment Pharmacol Ther* 2000;**14**:1267–72.

9 Gunaratnam NT, Jessup TP, Inadomi J, Lascewski DP. Sub-optimal proton pump inhibitor dosing is prevalent in patients with poorly controlled gastro-oesophageal reflux disease. *Aliment Pharmacol Ther* 2006;**23**:1473–7.

10 Vela MF, Camacho-Lobato L, Srinivasan R, Tutuian R, Katz PO, Castell DO. Simultaneous intraesophageal impedance and pH measurement of acid and nonacid gastroesophageal reflux: effect of omeprazole. *Gastroenterology* 2001;**120**:1599–606.

11 Katz P, Gideon RM, Tutuian R. Reflux symptoms on twice daily (BID) proton pump inhibitor (PPI) associated with non acid reflux; a manifestation of hypersensitive esophagus? (abstract). *Am J Gastroenterol* 2005;**128**(4 suppl 2):925, A-130.

12 Mainie I, Tutuian R, Shay S, et al. Acid and non-acid reflux in patients with persistent symptoms despite acid suppressive therapy: a multicentre study using combined ambulatory impedance-pH monitoring. *Gut* 2006;**55**:1398–402.

13 Zerbib F, Roman S, Ropert A, et al. Esophageal pH-impedance monitoring and symptom analysis in GERD: a study in patients off and on therapy. *Am J Gastroenterol* 2006;**101**:1956–63.

14 Zerbib F, Duriez A, Roman S, Capdepont M, Mion F. Determinants of gastro-oesophageal reflux perception in patients with persistent symptoms despite proton pump inhibitors. *Gut* 2008;**57**:156–60.

15 Tutuian R, Vela MF, Hill EG, Mainie I, Agrawal A, Castell DO. Characteristics of symptomatic reflux episodes on Acid suppressive therapy. *Am J Gastroenterol* 2008;**103**:1090–6.

16 Karamanolis G, Stevens W, Vos R, Tack J, Clave P, Sifrim D. Oesophageal tone and sensation in the transition zone between proximal striated and distal smooth muscle oesophagus. *Neurogastroenterol Motil* 2008;**20**:291–7.

17 Tack J, Koek G, Demedts I, Sifrim D, Janssens J. Gastroesophageal reflux disease poorly responsive to single-dose proton pump inhibitors in patients without Barrett's esophagus: acid reflux, bile reflux, or both? *Am J Gastroenterol* 2004;**99**:981–8.

18 Gasiorowska A, Navarro-Rodriguez T, Wendel C, et al. Comparison of the degree of duodenogastroesophageal reflux and acid reflux between patients who failed to respond and those who were successfully treated with a proton pump inhibitor once daily. *Am J Gastroenterol* 2009;**104**:2005–13.

19 Emerenziani S, Sifrim D, Habib FI, et al. Presence of gas in the refluxate enhances reflux perception in non-erosive patients with physiological acid exposure of the oesophagus. *Gut* 2008;**57**:443–7.

20 Hobson AR, Furlong PL, Aziz Q. Oesophageal afferent pathway sensitivity in non-erosive reflux disease. *Neurogastroenterol Motil* 2008;**20**:877–83.

21 Vela M, Camacho-Lobato L, Srinivasan R, Tutuian R, Katz P, Castell D. Simultaneous intraesophageal impedance and pH measurement of acid and

nonacid gastroesophageal reflux: effect of omeprazole. *Gastroenterology* 2001;**120**:1599–606.

22 Lichtenstein DR, Cash BD, Davila R, et al. Role of endoscopy in the management of GERD. *Gastrointestinal endoscopy* 2007;**66**:219–24.

23 Richter JE. How to manage refractory GERD. *Nat Clin Pract Gastroenterol Hepatol* 2007;**4**:658–64.

24 Poh CH, Gasiorowska A, Navarro-Rodriguez T, et al. Upper GI tract findings in patients with heartburn in whom proton pump inhibitor treatment failed versus those not receiving antireflux treatment. *Gastrointest Endosc* 2009.

25 Fass R, Hell R, Sampliner RE, et al. Effect of ambulatory 24-hour esophageal pH monitoring on reflux-provoking activities. *Dig Dis Sci* 1999;**44**:2263–9.

26 Bautista JM, Wong WM, Pulliam G, Esquivel RF, Fass R. The value of ambulatory 24 hr esophageal pH monitoring in clinical practice in patients who were referred with persistent gastroesophageal reflux disease (GERD)-related symptoms while on standard dose anti-reflux medications. *Dig Dis Sci* 2005;**50**:1909–15.

27 Charbel S, Khandwala F, Vaezi MF. The role of esophageal pH monitoring in symptomatic patients on PPI therapy. *Am J Gastroenterol* 2005;**100**:283–9.

28 Koek GH, Tack J, Sifrim D, Lerut T, Janssens J. The role of acid and duodenal gastroesophageal reflux in symptomatic GERD. *Am J Gastroenterol* 2001;**96**:2033–40.

29 Sharma N, Agrawal A, Freeman J, Vela MF, Castell D. An analysis of persistent symptoms in acid-suppressed patients undergoing impedance-pH monitoring. *Clin Gastroenterol Hepatol* 2008;**6**:521–4.

30 Hirano I, Zhang X, Pandolfino JE, Kahrilas P. Bravo pH capsule monitoring with and without proton pump inhibitor therapy. *Clin Gastroenterol Hepatol* 2005;**3**:1083–8.

31 Kaltenbach T, Crockett S, Gerson L. Are lifestyle measures effective in patients with gastroesophageal reflux disease? An evidence-based approach. *Arch Intern Med* 2006;**166**:965–71.

32 Peghini PL, Katz PO, Castell DO. Ranitidine controls nocturnal gastric acid breakthrough on omeprazole: a controlled study in normal subjects. *Gastroenterology* 1998;**115**:1335–9.

33 Fackler WK, Ours TM, Vaezi MF, Richter JE. Long-term effect of H2RA therapy on nocturnal gastric acid breakthrough. *Gastroenterology* 2002;**122**:625–32.

34 Mainie I, Tutuian R, Castell DO. Addition of a H_2 receptor antagonist to PPI improves acid control and decreases nocturnal acid breakthrough. *J Clin Gastroenterol* 2008;**42**:676–9.

35 Rackoff A, Agrawal A, Hila I, Mainie I, Tutuian R, Castell DO. Histamine-2 receptor antagonists at night

36 Kahrilas PJ, Shaheen NJ, Vaezi MF, et al. American Gastroenterological Association Medical Position Statement on the management of gastroesophageal reflux disease. *Gastroenterology* 2008;**135**:1383–91, 1391 e1–5.

37 Khan M, Santana J, Donnellan C, Preston C, Moayyedi P. Medical treatments in the short term management of reflux oesophagitis. *Cochrane Database System Rev* 2007;(**2**):CD003244.

38 Fass R, Sontag SJ, Traxler B, Sostek M. Treatment of patients with persistent heartburn symptoms: a double-blind, randomized trial. *Clin Gastroenterol Hepatol* 2006;**4**:40–56.

39 Hatlebakk J, Katz P, Kuo B, Castell DO. Nocturnal gastric acidity and acid breakthrough on different regimens of omeprazole 40 mg daily. *Aliment Pharmacol Ther* 1998;**12**:1235–40.

40 Sharma P, Shaheen NJ, Perez MC, et al. Clinical trials: healing of erosive oesophagitis with dexlansoprazole MR, a proton pump inhibitor with a novel dual delayed-release formulation – results from two randomized controlled studies. *Aliment Pharmacol Ther* 2009;**29**:731–41.

41 Fass R, Chey WD, Zakko SF, et al. Clinical trial: the effects of the proton pump inhibitor dexlansoprazole MR on daytime and nighttime heartburn in patients with non-erosive reflux disease. *Aliment Pharmacol Ther* 2009;**29**:1261–72.

42 Zhang Q, Lehmann A, Rigda R, Dent J, Holloway RH. Control of transient lower oesophageal sphincter relaxations and reflux by the GABA(B) agonist baclofen in patients with gastro-oesophageal reflux disease. *Gut* 2002;**50**:19–24.

43 Koek GH, Sifrim D, Lerut T, Janssens J, Tack J. Effect of the GABA(B) agonist baclofen in patients with symptoms and duodeno-gastro-oesophageal reflux refractory to proton pump inhibitors. *Gut* 2003;**52**:1397–402.

44 Vela MF, Tutuian R, Katz PO, Castell DO. Baclofen decreases acid and non-acid post-prandial gastro-oesophageal reflux measured by combined multichannel intraluminal impedance and pH. *Aliment Pharmacol Ther* 2003;**17**:243–51.

45 Fass R, Shapiro M, Dekel R, Sewell J. Systematic review: proton-pump inhibitor failure in gastro-oesophageal reflux disease – where next? *Aliment Pharmacol Ther* 2005;**22**:79–94.

46 Clouse RE, Lustman PJ, Eckert TC, et al. Low-dose trazodone for symptomatic patients with esophageal contraction abnormalities. A double-blind,

placebo-controlled trial. *Gastroenterology* 1987;**92**: 1027–36.

47 Handa M, Mine K, Yamamoto H, Smith. Antidepressant treatment of patients with diffuse esophageal spasm: a psychosomatic approach. *J Clin Gastroenterol* 1999;**28**:228–32.

48 Dickman R, Schiff E, Holland A, et al. Clinical trial: acupuncture vs. doubling the proton pump inhibitor dose in refractory heartburn. *Aliment Pharmacol Ther* 2007;**26**:1333–44.

49 Rubenstein JH, Nojkov B, Korsnes S, Adlis SA, Shaw MJ, Weinman B, et al. Oesophageal hypersensitivity is associated with features of psychiatric disorders and the irritable bowel syndrome. *Aliment Pharmacol Ther* 2007;**26**:443–53.

50 Nojkov B, Rubenstein JH, Adlis SA, et al. The influence of co-morbid IBS and psychological distress on outcomes and quality of life following PPI therapy in patients with gastro-oesophageal reflux disease. *Aliment Pharmacol Ther* 2008;**27**:473–82.

51 Galmiche JP, Clouse RE, Balint A, et al. Functional esophageal disorders. *Gastroenterology* 2006;**130**: 1459–65.

52 Mudipalli RS, Remes-Troche JM, Andersen L, Rao SSC. Functional chest pain – esophageal or overlapping functional disorder. *J Clin Gastroenterol* 2007;**41**: 264–9.

53 Jerlock M, Welin C, Rosengren A, Gaston-Johannson F. Pain characteristics in patients with unexplained chest pain and patients with ischemic heart disease. *Eur J Cardiovasc Nurs* 2007;**6**:130–6.

54 Fenster PE. Evaluation of chest pain: a cardiology perspective for gastroenterologists. *Gastroenterol Clin North Am* 2004;**33**:35–40.

55 Katz PO, Dalton CB, Richter JE, Wu WC, Castell DO. Esophageal testing of patients with noncardiac chest pain or dysphagia. Results of three years' experience with 1161 patients. *Ann Intern Med* 1987;**106** :593–7.

56 Dekel R, Pearson T, Wendel C, DeGarmo P, Fennerty MB, Fass R. Assessment of oesophageal motor function in patients with dyspepsia or chest pain – the Clinical Outcomes Research Initiative experience. *Aliment Pharmacol Ther* 2003;**18**:1083–9.

57 Fass R, Winters GF. Evaluation of the patient with noncardiac chest pain: is gastroesophageal reflux disease or an esophageal motility disorder the cause? *Medscape Gastroenterol* 2001;**3**:1–10.

58 Lam HG, Dekker W, Kan G, Breedijk M, Smout AJ. Acute noncardiac chest pain in a coronary care unit. Evaluation by 24-hour pressure and pH recording of the esophagus. *Gastroenterology* 1992;**102**:453–60.

59 Peters L, Maas L, Petty D, et al. Spontaneous noncardiac chest pain. Evaluation by 24-hour ambulatory esopha-geal motility and pH monitoring. *Gastroenterology* 1988;**94**:878–86.

60 Lembo AJ. Visceral hypersensitivity in noncardiac chest pain. *Gastroenterol Clin North Am* 2004;**33**:55–60.

61 Hollerbach S, Bulat R, May A, et al. Abnormal cerebral processing of oesophageal stimuli in patients with non-cardiac chest pain (NCCP). *Neurogastroenterol Motil* 2000;**12**:555–65.

62 Fass R, Naliboff B, Higa L, et al. Differential effect of long-term esophageal acid exposure on mechanosensi-tivity and chemosensitivity in humans. *Gastroenterology* 1998;**115**:1363–73.

63 Handwerker HO, Reeh PW. Nociceptors: chemosensi-tivity and sensitization by chemical agents. In: Willis WD Jr (ed.), *Hyperalgesia and Allodynia*. New York: Raven Press, 1992: 107.

64 Richter JE, Barish CF, Castell DO. Abnormal sensory perception in patients with esophageal chest pain. *Gastroenterology* 1986;**91**:845–52.

65 Barish CF, Castell DO, Richter JE. Graded esophageal balloon distention. A new provocative test for noncar-diac chest pain. *Dig Dis Sci* 1986;**31**:1292–8.

66 DeVault KR, Castell DO. Esophageal balloon disten-tion and cerebral evoked potential recording in the evaluation of unexplained chest pain. *Am J Med* 1992; **92**:20S–26S.

67 Kamath MV, May A, Hollerbach S, et al. Effects of esophageal stimulation in patients with functional dis-orders of the gastrointestinal tract. *Crit Rev Biomed Eng* 2000;**28**:87–93.

68 Aziz Q. Acid sensors in the gut: the taste of things to come. *Eur J Gastroenterol Hepatol* 2001;**13**:885–8.

69 Bass C, Wade C. Chest pain with normal coronary arteries: a comparative study of psychiatric and social morbidity. *Psychol Med* 1984;**14**:51–61.

70 Channer KS, Papouchado M, James MA, Rees JR. Anxiety and depression in patients with chest pain referred for exercise testing. *Lancet* 1985;**ii**:820–3.

71 Costa PT Jr. Influence of the normal personality dimen-sion of neuroticism on chest pain symptoms and coro-nary artery disease. *Am J Cardiol* 1987;**60**(18): 20J–26J.

72 McCroskery JH, Schell RE, Sprafkin RP, Lantinga LJ, Warner RA, Hill N. Differentiating anginal patients with coronary artery disease from those with normal coronary arteries using psychological measures. *Am J Cardiol* 1991;**67**:645–6.

73 Flugelman MY, Weisstub E, Galun E, et al. Clinical, psychological and thallium stress studies in patients with chest pain and normal coronary arteries. *Int J Cardiol* 1991;**33**:401–8.

74 Mayou R, Bryant B, Forfar C, Clark D. Non-cardiac chest pain and benign palpitations in the cardiac clinic. *Br Heart J* 1994;**72**:548–53.

75 Chignon JM, Lepine JP, Ades J. Panic disorder in cardiac outpatients. *Am J Psychiatry* 1993;**150**: 780–5.

76 Tennant C, Mihailidou A, Scott A, et al. Psychological symptom profiles in patients with chest pain. *J Psychosom Res* 1994;**38**:365–71.

77 Dammen T, Ekeberg O, Arnesen H, Friis S. Personality profiles in patients referred for chest pain. Investigation with emphasis on panic disorder patients. *Psychosomatics* 2000;**41**:269–76.

78 Demiryoguran NS, Karcioglu O, Topacoglu H, et al. Anxiety disorder in patients with non-specific chest pain in the emergency setting. *Emerg Med J* 2006; **23**:99–102.

79 Dammen T, Ekeberg O, Arnesen H, Friis S. Health-related quality of life in non-cardiac chest pain patients with and without panic disorder. *Int J Psychiatry Med* 2008;**38**:271–86.

80 Eslick GD. Noncardiac chest pain: epidemiology, natural history, health care seeking, and quality of life. *Gastroenterol Clin North Am* 2004;**33**:1–23.

81 Gasiorowska A, Fass R. The proton pump inhibitor (PPI) test in GERD: does it still have a role? *J Clin Gastroenterol* 2008;**42**:867–74.

82 Cremonini F, Wise J, Moayyedi P, Talley NJ. Diagnostic and therapeutic use of proton pump inhibitors in non-cardiac chest pain: a meta-analysis. *Am J Gastroenterol* 2005;**100**:1226–32.

83 Wang W, Huang J, Zheng G, et al. Is proton pump inhibitor testing an effective approach to diagnose gastroesophageal reflux disease in patients with non-cardiac chest pain? *Arch Intern Med* 2005;**165**: 1222–8.

84 Fass R, Fennerty MB, Johnson C, Camargo L, Sampliner RE. Correlation of ambulatory 24-hour esophageal pH monitoring results with symptom improvement in patients with noncardiac chest pain due to gastroesophageal reflux disease. *J Clin Gastroenterol* 1999;**28**:36–9.

85 Fass R, Fennerty MB, Ofman JJ, et al. The clinical and economic value of a short course of omeprazole in patients with noncardiac chest pain. *Gastroenterology* 1998;**115**:42–9.

86 Dickman R, Mattek N, Holub J, Peters D, Fass R. Prevalence of upper gastrointestinal tract findings in patients with noncardiac chest pain versus those with gastroesophageal reflux disease (GERD)-related symptoms: results from a national endoscopic database. *Am J Gastroenterol* 2007;**102**:1173–9.

7 Richter JE, Hewson EG, Sinclair JW, Dalton CB. Acid perfusion test and 24-hour esophageal pH monitoring with symptom index. Comparison of sts for esophageal acid sensitivity. *Dig Dis Sci* 1;**36**:56571.

88 Paterson WG. Canadian Association of Gastroenterology Practice Guidelines: management of noncardiac chest pain. *Can J Gastroenterol* 1998;**12**:401–7.

89 Pandolfino JE, Richter JE, Ourts T, Guardino JM, Chapman J, Karhrilas PJ. Ambulatory esophageal pH monitoring using a wireless system. *Am J Gastroenterol* 2003;**98**:740–9.

90 Prakash C, Clouse RE. Wireless pH monitoring in patients with non-cardiac chest pain. *Am J Gastroenterol* 2006;**101**:446–52.

91 Fass R, Navarro-Rodriguez T. Noncardiac chest pain. *J Clin Gastroenterol* 2008;**42**:636–46.

92 Achem SR, Kolts BE, Wears R, Burton L, Richter JE. Chest pain associated with nutcracker esophagus: a preliminary study of the role of gastroesophageal reflux. *Am J Gastroenterol* 1993;**88**:187–92.

93 Stahl WG, Beton RR, Johnson CS, Brown CL, Waring JP. Diagnosis and treatment of patients with gastro-esophageal reflux and noncardiac chest pain. *South Med J* 1994;**87**:739–42.

94 Achem SR, Kolts BE, MacMath T, et al. Effects of omeprazole versus placebo in treatment of noncardiac chest pain and gastroesophageal reflux. *Dig Dis Sci* 1997;**42**:2138–45.

95 Chambers J, Cooke R, Anggiansah A, Owen W. Effect of omeprazole in patients with chest pain and normal coronary anatomy: initial experience. *Int J Cardiol* 1998;**65**:51–5.

96 Patti M, Molena D, Fisichella P, Smith. Gastroesophageal reflux disease (GERD) and chest pain. Results of laparoscopic antireflux surgery. *Surg Endosc* 2002;**16**: 563–6.

97 Farrell T, Richardson W, Trus T, Smith. Response of atypical symptoms of gastro-oesophageal reflux to antireflux surgery. *Br J Surg* 2001;**88**:1649–52.

98 Rakita S, Villadolid D, Thomas A, et al. Laparoscopic Nissen fundoplication offers high patient satisfaction with relief of extraesophageal symptoms of gastroesophageal reflux disease. *Am Surg* 2006;**72**: 207–12.

99 So J, Zeitels S, Rattner D. Outcomes of atypical symptoms attributed to gastroesophageal reflux treated by laparoscopic fundoplication. *Surgery* 1998;**124**: 28–32.

100 Peghini PL, Katz PO, Castell DO. Imipramine decreases oesophageal pain perception in human male volunteers. *Gut* 1998;**42**:807–13.

101 Cannon 3rd RO, Quyyumi AA, Mincemoyer R, et al. Imipramine in patients with chest pain despite normal coronary angiograms. *N Engl J Med* 1994;**330**: 1411–17.

102 Prakash C, Clouse RE. Long-term outcome from tricyclic antidepressant treatment of functional chest pain. *Dig Dis Sci* 1999;**44**:2373–9.

103 Clouse RE, Lustman PJ, Eckert TC, et al. Low-dose trazodone for symptomatic patients with esophageal contraction abnormalities. A double-blind, placebo-controlled trial. *Gastroenterology* 1987;**92**:1027–36.

104 Varia I, Logue E, O'Connor C, Smith. Randomized trial of sertraline in patients with unexplained chest pain of noncardiac origin. *Am Heart J* 2000;**140**:367–72.

105 Doraiswamy PM, Varia I, Hellegers C, et al. A randomized controlled trial of paroxetine for noncardiac chest pain. *Psychopharmacol Bull* 2006;**39**:15–24.

106 Orlando R, Bozymski E. Clinical and manometric effects of nitroglycerin in diffuse esophageal spasm. *N Engl J Med* 1989;**289**:23–5.

107 Millaire A, Ducloux G, Marquand A, Vaksmann G. [Nitroglycerin and angina with angiographically normal coronary vessels. Clinical effects and effects on esophageal motility]. *Arch Mal Coeur Vaiss* 1989;**82**:63–8.

108 Swamy N. Esophageal spasm: clinical and manometric response to nitroglycerine and long acting nitrites. *Gastroenterology* 1977;**72**:23–7.

109 Kikendall J, Mellow M. Effect of sublingual nitroglycerin and long-acting nitrate preparations on esophageal motility. *Gastroenterology* 1980;**79**:7036.

110 Mellow M. Effect of isosorbide and hydralazine in painful primary esophageal motility disorders. *Gastroenterology* 1982;**83**:364–70.

111 van Peski-Oosterbaan AS, Spinhoven P, van Rood Y, van der Does JW, Bruschke AV, Rooijmans HG. Cognitive-behavioral therapy for noncardiac chest pain: a randomized trial. *Am J Med* 1999;**106**:424–9.

112 Klimes I, Mayou RA, Pearce MJ, Coles L, Fagg JR. Psychological treatment for atypical non-cardiac chest pain: a controlled evaluation. *Psychol Med* 1990;**20**:605–11.

113 van Peski-Oosterbaan A, Spinhoven P, van Rood Y, Smith. Cognitive-behavioral therapy for noncardiac chest pain: a randomized trial. *Am J Med* 1999;**106**: 424–9.

114 Jones H, Cooper P, Miller V, Smith. Treatment of non cardiac chest pain: a controlled trial of hypnotherapy. *Gut* 2006;**55**:1403–8.

115 Kisely S, Campbell LA, Skerritt P. Psychological interventions for symptomatic management of non-specific chest pain in patients with normal coronary anatomy. *Cochrane Database Syst Rev* 2005;(1):CD004101.

3

The Clinical Approach to Dyspepsia

Mary Farid[1] and Brennan Spiegel[2]

[1]UCLA Affiliated Training Program in Digestive Diseases, Los Angeles, California, USA
[2]VA Greater Los Angeles Healthcare System, David Geffen School of Medicine at UCLA and UCLA/VA Center for Outcomes Research and Education, Los Angeles, California, USA

Case 1: intermittent epigastric pain

Case presentation

A 47-year-old woman presents to your office complaining of intermittent epigastric pain occurring at least once weekly for the last 12 months. The pain lasts approximately 30 min and is not relieved or exacerbated by food. She has no heartburn, nausea, bloating, dysphagia, or vomiting. Her weight has been stable. She has no history of peptic ulcer disease. She has no history of fever, chills, night sweats, melena, or hematochezia.

Her past medical history is significant for chronic low back pain, for which she has been taking 800 mg ibuprofen three times daily. She does not take any other medicines.

She does not smoke and reports only social alcohol use. She has no family history of gastrointestinal (GI) malignancy.

Physical examination: she is 5′ 2″ (157 cm) and 130 lb (59 kg). Her vital signs are normal. She has no abdominal tenderness to palpation, has normal bowel sounds, and no masses are palpated. Her fecal occult blood test is negative. The remainder of her examination is normal.

Questions

• Based upon the information provided to this point, what is the patient's most likely diagnosis?

• What, if any, tests would you order at this time?
• How would you treat this patient?

Differential diagnosis

The differential diagnosis of chronic abdominal pain is broad but the authors focus on this patient's presentation in an attempt to determine the most likely diagnosis. Her main complaint is chronic intermittent epigastric pain, which is not associated with heartburn or other reflux symptoms, making gastroesophageal reflux disease (GERD) less likely. She does not describe postprandial pain, nausea, or vomiting, nor does she localize the pain to the right upper quadrant or right shoulder, which would also make biliary colic less likely. She does not report weight loss, melena, or change in stool frequency or form, and she has no family history or other risk factors for malignancy. Furthermore, she is younger than 55 years which, according to guidelines, makes malignancy a less likely etiology of her symptoms. Functional dyspepsia is certainly a possibility. However, she is taking a high dose of a non-steroidal anti-inflammatory drug (NSAID), which puts her at risk for developing peptic ulcer disease. Thus, although functional dyspepsia is the most common cause of dyspepsia, we should put NSAID-induced dyspepsia, with possible underlying peptic ulcer, high on the list.

Problem-based Approach to Gastroenterology and Hepatology, First Edition. Edited by John N. Plevris, Colin W. Howden.
© 2012 Blackwell Publishing Ltd. Published 2012 by Blackwell Publishing Ltd.

Patient management

As this patient has a strong risk factor for developing peptic ulcer disease, she should have an upper endoscopy to confirm the diagnosis. An alternative strategy would be to empirically treat with a proton pump inhibitor (PPI) for 6–8 weeks to ensure healing of any possible underlying ulcer. However, an upper endoscopy would allow not only confirmation of the diagnosis, but also an opportunity to biopsy the ulcer to rule out malignancy, as well as to biopsy for *Helicobacter pylori*. NSAIDs can cause dyspeptic symptoms in the absence of an ulcer, so a key intervention in the management of this patient would be to address the need for ongoing NSAID use. If a non-NSAID pain reliever can be substituted for her chronic back pain, this should be done. If an NSAID is required, the patient should be placed on PPI co-therapy, not only to treat her symptoms but also to help prevent the development of peptic ulcer.

Case 2: intermittent abdominal discomfort

Case presentation

A 44-year-old man presents to your office complaining of intermittent abdominal discomfort for the last 12 months. He describes the discomfort as "fullness" after meals, which he localizes to the epigastrium. He does not have a history of heartburn, epigastric pain, dysphagia, or vomiting. His weight has been stable. He is not taking any NSAIDs or aspirin and has no history of peptic ulcer disease. He has no history of fever, chills, night sweats, melena, or hematochezia.

He has no significant past medical history. He has no allergies and takes no medicines. He does not smoke. He reports only social alcohol use. He has no family history of GI malignancy.

Physical examination: he is 5′ 8″ (173 cm) and 190 lb (77 kg). His vital signs are normal. His abdominal examination is normal. His fecal occult blood test is negative. The remainder of his examination is normal.

Questions

Based on the information provided to this point, what is the most likely diagnosis in this patient?

- What, if any, tests would you order at this time?
- What is the role of testing for *H. pylori* in this patient?
- How would you check for *H. pylori*?
- What is the role of upper endoscopy in this patient?
- How would you treat this patient?

Differential diagnosis

This patient presents with epigastric discomfort and a sensation of "fullness" after meals. The most common cause of dyspepsia in this setting is underlying functional dyspepsia. Other possibilities include peptic ulcer disease, non-reflux-predominant GERD, or foregut malignancy. Given that he is under 55 years and has no alarm features, malignancy is less likely. He is not taking an NSAID or any other medicine that could be causing his symptoms. He has no obvious risk factors for peptic ulcer, although it is still a possibility, particularly if the *H. pylori* prevalence in his community is high. However, given his overall presentation, the most likely diagnosis in this patient is functional or non-ulcer dyspepsia. The presence of "fullness" but no epigastric pain implies the variant of postprandial distress syndrome (PDS) rather than epigastric pain syndrome (EPS); these are discussed further below.

Patient management

Functional dyspepsia requires a negative upper endoscopy before the diagnosis can be confirmed. However, as this patient is aged under 55 and has no alarm features, empiric implementation of one of two treatment strategies may be employed first before proceeding to endoscopy. The first strategy would be to test for *H. pylori* and treat if positive. This would be the most cost-effective strategy if this patient were from a population where the *H. pylori* prevalence was >10%. The optimal method of testing for *H. pylori* would be either a stool antigen test or a urea breath test. The second strategy would apply if the patient came from a population where the *H. pylori* prevalence is <10%; in that case, an empiric trial of a PPI for 6–8 weeks is suggested. If his symptoms improve or resolve, the PPI can be continued or a trial off the PPI can be considered to see if the symptoms recur. If the patient continues to have symptoms despite a trial of PPI therapy, the next step would be consideration of the test-and-treat strategy for *H. pylori* or proceeding with upper endoscopy. Trials of other medicine such as H_2-receptor blockers, prokinetics, tricyclic antidepressants, and selective serotonin receptor blockers can also be considered.

Commentary

One-third of adults experience pain or discomfort in the upper abdomen during a given year [1,2]. Of these, a quarter seek treatment, making dyspepsia the presenting complaint in 4% of primary care visits and 20% of outpatient gastroenterology consultations [1,2]. The large burden of illness of dyspepsia, including its high population prevalence and impact on quality of life, leads to over US$14 billion annually in direct costs of care [3]. In light of this high health economic burden, it is important that providers follow "best practice" evidence-based management guidelines in order to improve patient outcomes while minimizing resource utilization.

Dyspepsia is defined as chronic or recurrent pain or discomfort centered in the upper abdomen [2]. Discomfort is defined as a subjective negative feeling that is non-painful, and can incorporate a variety of symptoms including early satiety, bloating, upper abdominal fullness, or nausea. Patients with predominant or frequent symptoms of heartburn or acid regurgitation should be considered to have GERD until proven otherwise. This is an important clinical distinction, because reflux-predominant symptoms imply underlying GERD, whereas non-reflux-predominant symptoms remain within the dyspepsia spectrum. This is confusing to some providers, although it need not be. The confusion stems from the fact that GERD can indeed underlie non-reflux-predominant dyspepsia, i.e. GERD need not present with reflux-predominant symptoms alone – it sometimes presents with epigastric pain or discomfort in the absence of reflux. Yet in the presence of reflux predominance, GERD would be the leading diagnosis and the clinical picture would be inconsistent with dyspepsia – a *non*-reflux-predominant syndrome.

Dyspepsia is divided into "complicated" and "uncomplicated" forms. Uncomplicated dyspepsia refers to symptoms in the absence of alarming features, including unintended weight loss, dysphagia, gastrointestinal bleeding, anemia, occult GI bleeding,

physical evidence of malignancy (e.g. abdominal mass, lymphadenopathy), and other concerning signs or symptoms. Complicated dyspepsia refers to the presence of any of these alarming features. The most common etiology for uncomplicated dyspepsia is "functional dyspepsia," defined further below. Functional dyspepsia accounts for roughly 60% of dyspepsia. Up to 25% of cases are due to underlying peptic ulcer disease and 10% are from non-reflux-predominant GERD. Less than 1% of uncomplicated dyspepsia in the USA is from gastric malignancy. It can be difficult to distinguish these disorders on the basis of symptoms alone. Ulcer pain may be burning or gnawing in quality, but often the patient may simply have vague discomfort or cramping. Patients on concurrent aspirin or other NSAIDs have a higher pre-test likelihood for peptic ulcer. Epigastric burning might be a sign of GERD, but also occurs with functional dyspepsia and peptic ulcer. Only the presence of "heartburn" or "regurgitation" is sufficiently specific for GERD. Other symptoms within the dyspepsia spectrum have poor sensitivity and specificity and cannot be relied upon to accurately discriminate between conditions.

Functional dyspepsia deserves special comment because of its high population prevalence and high pre-test likelihood in uncomplicated dyspepsia. The Rome III committee applies the following definition of functional dyspepsia [3]:

"The following criteria should be fulfilled for the last three months with symptom onset at least six months before diagnosis:

Bothersome postprandial fullness

Early satiation

Epigastric pain

Epigastric burning

No evidence of structural disease (including at upper endoscopy) that is likely to explain the patient's symptoms."

The guidelines further divide functional dyspepsia into two syndromes: (1) EPS and (2) PDS. EPS is marked by pain and burning, but not fullness or early satiety. In contrast, PDS is marked by fullness and satiety, but not pain or burning. The concept is that EPS may arise from visceral hypersensitivity, whereas PDS may arise from abnormalities in gastric motility and accommodation. This suggests that treatment varies for EPS and PDS, as described below. In short, functional dyspepsia is marked by dyspepsia in the absence of structural disease on endoscopy, and has "pain-predominant" (EPS) and "dysmotility-predominant" (PDS) forms.

A common dilemma in uninvestigated dyspepsia is whether or not to perform upper endoscopy early in the diagnostic evaluation. Because of the uncommon but important possibility that gastric cancer may be the underlying cause for dyspepsia, it is recommended that those patients who are at increased risk for developing gastric cancer undergo upper endoscopy [2]. This includes patients over the age 55 or those who have "alarm features" including bleeding, anemia, unexplained weight loss of >10% of body weight, progressive dysphagia, odynophagia, persistent vomiting, a family history of gastrointestinal cancer, previous esophagogastric malignancy, previous documented peptic ulcer, lymphadenopathy, or an abdominal mass. Patients fulfilling any of these criteria should undergo prompt upper endoscopy to rule out cancer and peptic ulcer disease.

In patients younger than 55 with no alarm features, two main treatment strategies may be considered. The first is to test for *H. pylori* and treat if positive; if eradication is successful but symptoms persist, then a trial of acid suppression should be offered. The rationale behind this "test-and-treat" approach is that *H. pylori* eradication is highly effective in peptic ulcer disease, and has some (albeit modest) efficacy in functional dyspepsia. This strategy is most cost-effective in high prevalence populations (e.g. recent immigrants from developing countries), where the prevalence of *H. pylori* typically exceeds 10% [4]. The most accurate non-invasive methods of testing for *H. pylori* are the urea breath test and the stool antigen test. If the patient tests positive, the current treatment of choice is a combination of a PPI (standard dose twice daily) with amoxicillin (1 g twice daily) and clarithromycin (500 mg twice daily) administered for 7–14 days. Metronidazole (500 mg twice daily) may be substituted for amoxicillin in this regimen if the patient is allergic to penicillin. The main disadvantage of the test-and-treat strategy is that cure of *H. pylori* infection will lead to symptom improvement only in a minority of patients [5–9]. However, there is evidence that "test and treat" is at least equivalent to prompt endoscopy in terms of outcomes. Several trials comparing the two have shown no differences in symptomatic outcomes or quality of life between the two groups at 1 year. Because of the cost of upper endoscopy, it is reasonable to pursue the test-and-treat strategy first in patients who are younger than 55 and without alarm features.

The second main treatment strategy for patients younger than 55 without alarm features is to prescribe a course of antisecretory therapy empirically for 4–8 weeks. If the patient fails to respond or relapses rapidly after stopping the antisecretory therapy, the test-and-treat approach should be applied before consideration of referral for upper endoscopy. This strategy has been found to be most cost-effective in low prevalence populations (e.g. high socioeconomic areas, where the background prevalence of ulcer or *H. pylori* is low). If an initial trial of acid suppression fails and the patient is *H. pylori* negative, it is reasonable to step up therapy by increasing the dose. Although previous guidelines have recommended an empiric trial of H_2-receptor blockers for 6–8 weeks, recent studies have demonstrated that PPI therapy has better symptomatic outcomes compared with H_2-receptor blockers in patients with dyspepsia [10].

In those patients who have failed both the test-and-treat approach and an empiric trial of antisecretory therapy, the next step may be referral for upper endoscopy (if not already performed). However, endoscopy is not mandatory in these patients who do not have alarm features, and its diagnostic yield is low. Therefore, the decision whether or not to use endoscopy must be based on clinical judgment.

Once a diagnosis of functional dyspepsia is confirmed by a negative endoscopy, an empiric trial of therapy is commonly prescribed. Some patients may not require medication after they have had reassurance with a negative endoscopy. Simple lifestyle modifications should also be tried, including avoiding high-fat meals, eating frequent and smaller meals throughout the day, and avoiding specific foods that precipitate symptoms. Medication therapy may also be initiated with either an H_2-receptor blocker or a PPI. PPI therapy, in particular, may be effective for pain-predominant functional dyspepsia, but not "dysmotility-predominant" functional dyspepsia. Thus, patients fulfilling the criteria for EPS should be tried on a 4- to 8-week course of PPI therapy before moving to other modalities. However, those with PDS are less likely to respond.

The management of endoscopy-proven functional dyspepsia is challenging when initial antisecretory therapy and *H. pylori* eradication fails. Patients who fail to respond to simple measures should have their diagnosis reconsidered. Other diagnoses to consider include abdominal wall pain, biliary pain, delayed gastric emptying, irritable bowel syndrome, and other more rare causes of chronic upper abdominal pain. Further testing (e.g. ultrasonography, computed tomography, gastric emptying study) can be considered, but usually is of low yield.

Patients with EPS might be tried on a low dose of a tricyclic antidepressant if they fail test-and-treat and PPI therapy. This is based on the theory that tricyclic antidepressants modify visceral hypersensitivity. Those with PDS, particularly if there is fullness or nausea, might be treated with a prokinetic (e.g. metoclopramide, erythromycin, or domperidone), or with an agent known to promote gastric accommodation (e.g. paroxetine or buspirone). The latter agents are most relevant for patients with early satiety – a symptom that may denote impaired gastric accommodation. If these therapies fail in PDS, low-dose tricyclic antidepressants should be considered. If this fails, cognitive–behavioral therapies such as psychotherapy or hypnotherapy have proven effective in recalcitrant functional dyspepsia.

References

1 Talley NJ, Zinsmeister AR, Schleck CD, et al. Dyspepsia and dyspepsia subgroups: A population-based study. *Gastroenterology* 1992;**102**(4 Pt 1):1259–68.
2 Talley NJ, Vakil N. Guidelines for the management of dyspepsia. Practice guidelines. *Am J Gastroenterol* 2005;**100**:2324–37.
3 Tack J, Talley NJ, Camilleri M, et al. Functional gastroduodenal disorders. *Gastroenterology* 2006;**130**:1466.
4 Spiegel BM, Vakil NB, Ofman JJ. Dyspepsia management in primary care: A decision analysis of competing strategies. *Gastroenterology* 2002;**122**:1270–85.
5 Moayyedi P, Feltbower R, Brown J, et al. Effect of population screening and treatment for *Helicobacter pylori* on dyspepsia and quality of life in the community: A randomized controlled trial. Leeds HELP Study Group. *Lancet* 2000;**355**:1665–9.
6 Chiba N, Van Zanten SJ, Sinclair P, et al. Treating *Helicobacter pylori* infection in primary care patients with uninvestigated dyspepsia: The Canadian adult dyspepsia empiric treatment – *Helicobacter pylori* positive (CADETHp) randomised controlled trial. *BMJ* 2002;**324**:1012–16.
7 Allison JE, Hurley LB, Hiatt RA, et al. A randomized controlled trial of test-and-treat strategy for *Helicobacter pylori*: Clinical outcomes and health care costs in a managed care population receiving long-term acid suppression therapy for physician-diagnosed peptic ulcer disease. *Arch Intern Med* 2003;**163**:1165–71.
8 Ladabaum U, Fendrick AM, Glidden D, et al. *Helicobacter pylori* test-and-treat intervention compared to usual care in primary care patients with suspected peptic ulcer disease in the United States. *Am J Gastroenterol* 2002;**97**:3007–14.
9 Lassen AT, Pedersen FM, Bytzer P, et al. *Helicobacter pylori* test-and-eradicate versus prompt endoscopy for management of dyspeptic patients: A randomised trial. *Lancet* 2000;**356**:455–60.
10 Delaney BC, Moayyedi P, Forman D. Initial management strategies for dyspepsia. *Cochrane Database of Syst Rev* 2003;(**2**):CD001961.

4 Acute, Recurrent, and Chronic Abdominal Pain

Brian E. Lacy and Chad C. Spangler

Division of Gastroenterology & Hepatology Dartmouth-Hitchcock Medical Center, Lebanon NH, USA.

Evaluation of the patient with abdominal pain, whether acute, recurrent, or chronic in nature, can at times overwhelm the physician, due to the multiple symptoms that are often quite non-specific. However, a careful history and physical examination, combined with the judicious use of diagnostic tests, usually lead to the correct diagnosis. In this chapter, three different patients with abdominal pain are presented in order to illustrate a stepwise approach to the management of patients with abdominal pain.

Case 1: severe abdominal pain

Case presentation

Lorraine is an 82-year-old retired educator who presents to the emergency department for the evaluation of severe abdominal pain. She was in her usual state of health until earlier in the day when she developed severe pain throughout her abdomen, which has persisted for the last 12 hours. She awoke feeling well. Her symptoms began approximately 30 min after the morning meal. She describes left-sided abdominal pain that is constant, sharp, severe, and without radiation. Lorraine initially tried to ignore the pain; however, it increased in intensity during the 3–4 hours after onset. Lorraine then became nauseous and vomited a small volume of bilious, non-bloody fluid.

Seven hours after the onset of her pain, she developed diarrhea. The stool was initially liquid and

brown in color; however, it quickly changed to bright red blood. At this point, Lorraine's family transported her to the local emergency department.

A review of systems reveals that the abdominal pain is associated with chills and diaphoresis. She is weak and gets lightheaded when standing. Her medical problems include chronic atrial fibrillation, hypertension, hyperlipidemia, and a previous transient ischemic attack (in the distribution of the right middle cerebral artery or MCA). Her medications include low-dose daily aspirin, a thiazide diuretic, and a lipid-lowering agent. She is not allergic to any medications. She has never experienced symptoms like this before. She was a college professor of English for many years, but is now retired, widowed, and lives alone. She smoked one pack of cigarettes per day for many years but quit 7 years ago. She enjoys a single glass of sherry each evening before dinner; she has never used illicit substances. Her only surgery was a cholecystectomy more than 20 years ago.

Physical examination reveals her to be in acute distress. Her vital signs are notable for fever to 101°F (38.3°C), tachycardia to 120 beats/min, a blood pressure of 90/45 mmHg, and a respiratory rate of 28/min. Head, ears, eyes, and nose and throat examination are normal. Her cardiac examination is significant for a soft systolic cardiac murmur and tachycardia; her lungs are clear on auscultation. Lorraine's abdomen is distended, firm, and quite tender to light pressure; bowel sounds are decreased

---

Problem-based Approach to Gastroenterology and Hepatology, First Edition. Edited by John N. Plevris, Colin W. Howden.
© 2012 Blackwell Publishing Ltd. Published 2012 by Blackwell Publishing Ltd.

on auscultation. She actively guards palpation, and shows signs of rebound tenderness with pain referred to the right upper quadrant. A non-painful rectal examination reveals maroon blood mixed with brown stool.

Questions

The clinical questions that need to be answered when evaluating this patient's case include:
• Does Lorraine require emergency medical attention?
• What diagnostic evaluation is required?
• What is the optimal treatment for her illness?

Differential diagnosis

In evaluating the patient with the acute onset of abdominal pain, formulating a narrow differential diagnosis can be challenging, given all the structures not only within the abdominal cavity, but also within the pelvis, thorax, and abdominal wall, that can elicit symptoms of pain. It is important to first localize the abdominal pain and then use the patient's clinical history, disease prevalence, as well as physical examination and diagnostic test findings, in order to narrow the list of disease processes.

In this case, Lorraine describes pain that is isolated to the left side of the abdomen. Pain in this location that is acute in onset, and sharp and severe in nature, could potentially involve structures in the abdomen such as the small bowel, transverse or descending colon, spleen, pancreas, or aorta. Alternatively, thoracic structures, including the left hemidiaphragm, lung, or heart, retroperitoneal structures such as the kidney, and pelvic organs such as the ovary or fallopian tube, should be included when formulating the differential diagnosis. Finally, extracavitary structures such as muscle, bone, and integument must also be considered.

Lorraine's other symptoms of bloody diarrhea, nausea, vomiting, and fever dramatically narrow the differential diagnosis. These factors increase the likelihood of an intra-abdominal process, with a gastrointestinal (GI) source being most likely, although vascular and genitourinary lesions also need to be considered. Typical illnesses associated with the GI tract that are consistent with her symptoms and age include a perforated viscus, an inflammatory process

such as diverticulitis or colitis (either ischemic or infectious), intussusception, volvulus, abscess, ileus, or an acute ischemic process. Vascular causes to consider include vasculitis, arterial dissection, embolic or thrombotic vascular obstruction, or splenic rupture/infarction. A more comprehensive differential diagnosis for the abrupt onset of abdominal pain is provided in Table 4.1.

In Lorraine's case, the attending physician in the emergency department ordered a full panel of lab tests including a complete blood count (CBC), complete metabolic profile, blood cultures, lipase, and an L-lactate. A computed tomography (CT) scan of the abdomen, ECG, and chest radiograph were ordered and consultation was requested from the general surgery and gastroenterology services.

Diagnostic findings and final diagnosis

Evaluating the patient with acute abdominal pain can be quite difficult for the initial examiner, given the prevalence of benign pain syndromes [1]. Thus, it is critical for the responsible caregiver to distinguish an emergency situation from one that may be observed over time with minimal intervention. The clinical history and initial physical examination are notable for several significant warning signs (abrupt onset of pain, progression of symptoms, associated GI bleeding, presence of peritoneal signs with hemodynamic instability) that should prompt triage of this patient as her underlying illness could be life threatening. The emergency room physician appropriately recognized the acuity of the situation, and ordered a panel of lab tests (Box 4.1) as well as radiological studies to help identify Lorraine's problem. Urgent radiological studies are often necessary in the setting of acute abdominal pain because symptoms do not always correlate well with the final diagnosis [2].

The CBC revealed slightly depressed hemoglobin, a leukocytosis, and a normal platelet count. Her serum lipase was normal which argues against acute pancreatitis. The serum L-lactate is elevated as is the blood urea nitrogen (BUN) and creatinine (see Box 4.1 for specific lab values). The leukocytosis indicates an acute inflammatory or infectious process. The elevated L-lactate is concerning for either an intestinal perforation or an acute ischemic insult. This test has a high sensitivity in the setting of ischemic/infracted bowel, but is quite non-specific [3].

Intestinal causes	Extraintestinal causes
Abrupt onset (instantaneous)	
Ruptured esophagus	Pulmonary infarct
Perforated ulcer	Ruptured or dissecting aneurysm
Ruptured abscess or hematoma	Ruptured ectopic pregnancy
Intestinal infarct (may also be gradual)	Pneumothorax
Ruptured spleen	Myocardial infarct
Rapid onset (minutes)	
Perforated viscus	Ureteral colic
Strangulated viscus	Renal colic
Volvulus	Ectopic pregnancy
Pancreatitis	Splenic infarct
Biliary colic	
Mesenteric infarct	
Diverticulitis	
Penetrating peptic ulcer	
Proximal small intestine obstruction	
Gradual onset (hours)	
Appendicitis	Cystitis
Strangulated hernia	Pyelonephritis
Distal small bowel intestinal obstruction	Salpingitis
Cholecystitis	Prostatitis
Pancreatitis	Threatened abortion
Gastritis	Urinary retention
Peptic ulcer	Pneumonitis
Diverticulitis	Pericarditis
Flare of Crohn's disease	Herpes zoster
Mesenteric lymphadenitis	Tabes dorsalis
Abscess (i.e., hepatic)	Tubo-ovarian abscess
Intestinal infarct	
Inflamed Meckel's diverticulum	
Sickle cell crisis	
Narcotic withdrawal	
Acute porphyria	

Table 4.1 Differential diagnosis of acute abdominal pain based on onset of symptoms

If a perforated viscus is considered, an abdominal radiograph can be used as the initial imaging study to look for free air in the abdomen. In this patient's case, CT scans of the abdomen and pelvis were available immediately and were therefore the initial study performed. Given the broad differential diagnosis, a CT scan with intravenous contrast is efficient, because it can evaluate the bowel wall, other abdominal organs, major blood vessels, and the abdominal wall. As shown in Figure 4.1, Lorraine's CT scan was significant for a circumferentially thickened colon from the splenic flexure through the sigmoid colon. Of

note, the aorta, pancreas, uterus, and ovaries appeared normal, and no intra-abdominal fluid collections were identified. This information, combined with her clinical history, narrows the differential diagnosis to either an infectious or an ischemic insult to the colon.

Given the abrupt onset of Lorraine's symptoms, the presence of atrial fibrillation, hypotension, increasing pain, and tachycardia, as well as her radiological and lab studies, an acute ischemic event to the colon seemed the most likely diagnosis; she was taken urgently to the operating room. During exploratory

Box 4.1 Pertinent laboratory values for Case 1

WBC: 19.4×10^3

Hemoglobin: 13 g/dL

Platelets: 210×10^3

L-lactate: 7 mmol/L

Na^+: 137 mmol/L

K^+: 4.6 mmol/L

Cl^-: 103 mmol/L

CO_2: 20 mmol/L

BUN: 24 mg/dL

Creatinine: 1.2 mg/dL

Lipase: 18 U/L

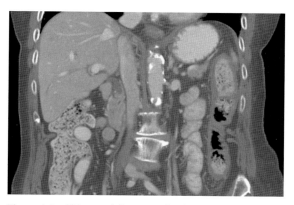

Figure 4.1 CT scan abdomen and pelvis with contrast. Note diffuse colonic wall thickening from the splenic flexure to the sigmoid colon.

laparoscopy, she was found to have an infarcted segment of colon in the distribution of the inferior mesenteric artery (IMA); she underwent a left hemicolectomy. Lorraine's final diagnosis was determined to be acute mesenteric arterial embolism to the IMA.

Patient management

Acute mesenteric ischemia (AMI) occurs when the blood supply to the mesenteric circulation is abruptly disrupted, leading to ischemia of the bowel. This may ultimately progress to infarction. This condition can be categorized as either arterial or venous, with arterial causes further subdivided into occlusive and non-occlusive ischemia. Arterial occlusion typically develops due to an embolic source, with 50% of all cases of arterial AMI occurring secondary to embolization to the superior mesenteric artery (SMA). Another 25% of cases occur secondary to thrombosis of a pre-existing atherosclerotic vessel. Non-occlusive arterial hypoperfusion accounts for the remaining 25% of cases of arterial AMI, with common mechanisms including vasospasm, or severe atherosclerosis in the setting of low cardiac output [4,5]. Venous occlusion is typically due to thrombosis or vascular strangulation and is less common than arterial occlusion [4].

AMI is associated with a mortality rate of around 60%, with some reports as high as 93% in the setting of embolic occlusion of the SMA [6]. Mortality increases dramatically once bowel infarction has occurred. Associated risk factors for AMI include advanced age, arrhythmias, coronary artery disease, valvular lesions, abdominal malignancies, or hypercoaguable states [7]. There does not seem to be a preference for race or sex for the development of AMI, but, as advanced age is a risk factor, it is likely that the prevalence of this disease will increase as the population ages.

Our patient demonstrated AMI as a consequence of mesenteric arterial embolization to the IMA, which is uncommon due to its small caliber. More frequently, the site of embolization is the SMA due to its larger size, as well as its less acute angle of origin from the aorta [8]. Most thrombi originate from the left atrium or ventricle, but may also arise from a valvular site, so it is logical to conclude that this patient's untreated atrial fibrillation played a role in her disease process.

The diagnosis of AMI largely depends on the clinical history, with careful attention to the character and timing of symptoms as well as the age of the patient. For instance, our patient had known risk factors for a cardiac arrhythmia and advanced age, along with a history of characteristic symptoms including the acute onset of abdominal pain, progression of pain, GI bleeding, nausea, and vomiting. A timely diagnosis is critical to maximize the patient's likelihood of survival because mortality increases significantly once bowel infarction has occurred [9].

A diagnostic approach suggested by the American Gastroenterological Association (AGA) includes initial resuscitation with intravenous fluids, followed by initial imaging with either a CT scan or an abdominal plain film. If physical exam findings and history are convincing for AMI, the patient should go directly to angiography, which is considered the diagnostic gold standard. If these tests are normal and the patient has persistent worrisome clinical findings, laparotomy may be required [10].

The therapeutic goal in the management of AMI is to quickly restore blood supply to the affected segment of bowel. Initial medical therapy should focus on fluid resuscitation and hemodynamic support, bowel rest, correction of electrolyte and acid–base disorders, empiric broad-spectrum antibiotic therapy, and possibly anticoagulant therapy, if the patient does not have any evidence of GI bleeding [11]. In this patient who demonstrated signs of either perforation or infarction (peritoneal signs, elevated serum lactate, leukocytosis, fever), emergency surgical exploration was warranted. If the bowel appears viable intraoperatively, embolectomy or revascularization can be performed surgically. If gangrenous bowel is seen, resection is indicated [12]. In patients who do not require emergent surgical intervention, other options include angiographic interventions (embolectomy, thrombolysis, vasodilator therapy) [13].

Case 2: recurrent abdominal pain

Case presentation

Sophia is a 48-year-old mortgage broker who presents for the evaluation of recurrent abdominal pain. She developed this pain 1 day ago and, since its onset, her symptoms have both worsened and changed in quality. Initially, the pain was dull, mild in intensity, and located throughout the upper abdomen. The intensity of her pain has increased steadily over the last 24 hours and is now severe, sharp, and localized to the epigastrium, with radiation to her back. Sophia notes that eating and drinking make her pain considerably worse. She recently developed nausea and vomiting; the vomitus consisted of recently ingested food and bile.

On review of systems, Sophia feels constipated and has not had a bowel movement for 2 days. She denies fever and chills, and states that her weight has been stable over the last year. She admits to having similar symptoms in the past. Sophia notes a worsening of her symptoms with the consumption of fatty foods, but cannot recall any other inciting event.

Sophia experienced the same symptoms 1 year ago and was told by a local emergency department physician that she had acute pancreatitis at that time, based on her symptoms and an elevated serum amylase and lipase. As part of her evaluation, she reports that an ultrasound scan of her abdomen demonstrated several small gallstones, but no evidence of choledocholithiasis or biliary obstruction. She improved clinically over 2 days with bowel rest and supportive therapy, and then underwent an elective cholecystectomy several weeks later. She felt well for several months but then developed similar symptoms 6 months ago. Evaluation at that time was consistent with another episode of acute pancreatitis. She recovered quickly with supportive therapy over the course of 3 days. During that admission, Sophia admitted to consuming five glasses of wine per week. She was advised to stop all alcohol use, and has been compliant since that time. She does not take any medications or herbal supplements, has never consumed illicit drugs, and has no known medication allergies. Sophia's only other surgery was an appendectomy at age 10. She does not have any other chronic medical problems, and denies any known family history of pancreatitis.

On physical examination, Sophia appears distressed with her hands clutched to her right upper abdomen. Her vitals signs reveal a temperature of 101°F, a heart rate of 118 beats/min, a blood pressure of 116/70 mmHg, and a respiratory rate of 22/min. On physical examination, her head, ears, eyes, nose, and throat are normal. Examination of the heart reveals tachycardia, but no rubs, murmurs, or gallops. Her lungs are clear to auscultation. Her abdomen is not distended; bowel sounds are decreased. She is very tender to light pressure in the right upper quadrant of her abdomen with guarding, but no evidence of rebound tenderness. Her abdomen is mildly tympanitic, without ascites or hepatomegaly; Murphy's sign is not present. Examination of the extremities is normal.

Questions

The clinical questions that need to be answered when evaluating this patient's case include:

- What is the next step in diagnosing the cause of her symptoms?
- What treatment options are available?
- Is there a way to prevent future episodes of pain?

Differential diagnosis

This case is a challenge for the clinician who is presented with a patient returning with symptoms similar to a previous diagnosis of acute pancreatitis. Although her clinical history supports a diagnosis of recurrent acute pancreatitis, it is the responsibility of the clinician to consider competing diagnoses and not to be overly influenced by the previous diagnosis. The initial step involves distinguishing organic from functional disorders.

According to the International Foundation for Functional Gastrointestinal Disorders (IFFGD), a functional disorder is characterized by an alteration in GI motility, intestinal nerve sensitivity, or abnormal central nervous system control of either of these functions. Functional bowel disorders are classified using a symptom-based approach because an organic or structural lesion cannot be identified by radiological or biochemical studies. There are a total of 28 adult functional GI disorders (FGID), which are classified into six major categories including esophageal, gastroduodenal, bowel (small and large intestine), functional abdominal pain syndromes (FAPSs), biliary, and anorectal [14].

Reviewing this case, functional bowel disorders that should be considered in the differential diagnosis include the irritable bowel syndrome (IBS), functional dyspepsia, functional abdominal pain syndrome, and a functional biliary syndrome (either functional gallbladder or sphincter of Oddi disorder). Characteristics that make a functional disease less likely include the infrequency of her pain episodes (this is her third acute episode of pain in 1 year, with spontaneous resolution and long asymptomatic periods), and the presence of objective findings such as fever and tachycardia. Additional data obtained during the course of her evaluation will help to distinguish a functional from an organic process.

Organic causes of acute-onset, recurrent, abdominal pain are abundant and may originate from any number of different organ systems, including gastrointestinal, hepatobiliary, genitourinary, cardiopulmonary, and musculoskeletal. Table 4.1 lists the differential diagnoses with regard to acute abdominal pain of gradual onset.

To elucidate the correct diagnosis, the clinician must first narrow the differential diagnosis using the location and quality of her pain, while considering the results of previous investigations. The patient describes right upper quadrant pain with radiation to her back. Anatomic structures that correlate with right upper quadrant pain include the pancreas, stomach, gallbladder, liver, small bowel, right hemidiaphragm, right lung, and right kidney. Specific disease processes that occur in each of these organs should be reviewed and associated with the acute onset of pain. Diseases that fit these criteria include pancreatitis, cholecystitis (although not in this specific patient), cholangitis, small bowel obstruction or infarction, peptic ulcer disease, Meckel's diverticulitis, acute hepatitis, pneumonia, pericarditis, pyelonephritis, and renal colic.

The physician evaluating Sophia ordered several studies including a plain film of the abdomen to exclude a perforation or obstructive process, chest radiograph, ECG, a panel of lab tests including a CBC, complete metabolic profile, serum amylase, lipase, and triglycerides, and urinalysis.

Diagnostic findings and final diagnosis

Sophia's physical examination revealed a tender right upper quadrant; palpation caused pain to radiate to her back. Although not pathognomonic, a complaint of boring right upper quadrant pain radiating in a band-like pattern to the back is seen in nearly half of those with acute pancreatitis, and should prompt the evaluating physician to consider this diagnosis. Objective findings of a fever and tachycardia suggest an acute inflammatory process, and speak against a functional cause of her pain. Diminished bowel sounds may represent a small bowel or colonic ileus, which can occur with an acute inflammatory process in the abdomen. The absence of a rigid abdomen is evidence against visceral perforation.

The ECG, chest radiograph, and urinalysis were normal. Leukocytosis further supports an acute inflammatory process (Box 4.2).

The patient's serum amylase and lipase were both significantly elevated. Although amylase is routinely ordered in the evaluation of acute pancreatitis, its specificity is low because a variety of other conditions

Box 4.2 Pertinent laboratory values for Case 2

WBC: 14.2×10^3

Hemoglobin: 14 g/dL

Platelets: 255×10^3

L-Lactate: 1 mmol/L

Na^+: 138 mmol/L

K^+: 4.4 mmol/L

Cl^-: 109 mmol/L

CO_2: 22 mmol/L

BUN: 18 mg/dL

Creatinine: 1.1 mg/dL

Lipase: 3442 U/L

Amylase: 5422 U/L

Triglyceride: 124 mg/dL

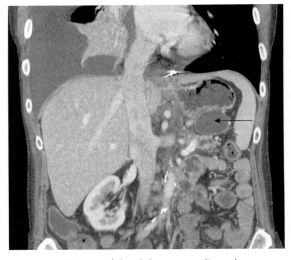

Figure 4.2 CT scan of the abdomen revealing a large cyst in the tail of the pancreas(arrow).

can cause hyperamylasemia. Serum lipase is more sensitive and specific for the diagnosis of acute pancreatitis, especially when levels are three times higher than the upper limits of normal. For this reason, serum lipase has replaced amylase testing in many centers [15]. Combined testing of amylase and lipase has not been shown to help in diagnostic accuracy [16]. Newer tests that are more specific for acute pancreatitis include trypsinogen-activated peptide or trypsinogen 2, although these are not widely available [17,18]. Hypertriglyceridemia is likely not the cause of her pancreatitis, as her serum triglycerides were normal.

An abdominal radiograph was normal, without evidence of free air or calcifications in the pancreas; the latter can be seen in some patients with chronic pancreatitis. An ileus was also not seen on this film, although findings can be delayed after the clinical presentation. A CT scan is typically not indicated in the initial presentation of acute pancreatitis; it is usually reserved for patients suspected of developing a complication associated with pancreatitis, such as pseudocyst formation or pancreatic necrosis. A CT scan was performed in this patient because of recurrent symptoms of upper abdominal pain without an obvious etiology. This demonstrated a large fluid collection in the pancreatic tail consistent with pseudo-

cyst formation, in addition to inflammatory changes in the peripancreatic fat consistent with acute pancreatitis (Figure 4.2).

Based on Sophia's clinical presentation of acute-onset abdominal pain with radiation to her back, nausea, and vomiting, along with objective findings of fever, elevated serum amylase, and lipase, and a CT scan confirming inflammatory changes in the pancreas with formation of a pseudocyst, the diagnosis was recurrent acute pancreatitis.

Patient management

Acute pancreatitis refers to acute inflammation of the pancreas which develops secondary to an inappropriate activation of trypsinogen (to trypsin) within the pancreas, leading to autodigestion of the acinar cells [19]. This condition is quite prevalent, accounting for more than 220 000 hospital admissions in the USA in 2003 [20]. The two most common risk factors are alcohol and gallstones, which together account for up to 80% of cases [21]. Other less common risk factors are listed in Box 4.3. This patient presented with a third episode of pancreatic inflammation after a cholecystectomy and cessation of alcohol. It is, therefore, important to evaluate her for other, less common etiologies of recurrent pancreatitis.

Box 4.3 Causes of acute pancreatitis (% of cases)

Gallstones (45%)

Alcohol (35%)

Other (10%):

Medications
- azathioprine
- thiazides
- estrogens
- didanosine

Hypercalcemia

Hypertriglyceridemia

Obstructive:
- tumor

Post-ERCP

Hereditary

Trauma

Viral:
- mumps
- Epstein–Barr virus
- Coxsackie viruses
- echoviruses
- measles

Vascular:
- vasculitis

Post-cardiac bypass

Toxins:
- organophosphate insecticides
- venom of scorpion *Tityus trinitatis*

Developmental abnormalities:
- annular pancreas
- pancreas divisum

Idiopathic (10%)

Medications known to be associated with acute pancreatitis are listed in Box 4.3. However, this patient was not taking any medications. The diagnosis of familial pancreatitis is unlikely given the absence of similarly afflicted family members and the late age of onset. Laboratory studies excluded hypertriglyceridemia and hypercalcemia, and there is no history of trauma or previous invasive interventions. Infectious causes of acute pancreatitis are rare and include the mumps and Coxsackie virus, among others [22]. The

patient had no signs or symptoms consistent with these infections. A vasculitic process such as that seen with systemic lupus erythematosus (SLE) is unlikely given the lack of other associated symptoms. Developmental abnormalities of the pancreas and microlithiasis warrant further investigation.

The next step in the evaluation involves further imaging of the pancreas and biliary system. Endoscopic ultrasonography (EUS) and endoscopic retrograde cholangiopancreatography (ERCP) are two imaging modalities appropriate at this time. EUS is capable of identifying small stones (microcrystals) and sludge in the biliary tree, as well as anatomic anomalies of the pancreas that may have been missed by less sensitive, external imaging techniques. ERCP allows for evaluation of the biliary tree and pancreatic ductal system, and any appropriate therapeutic intervention (e.g. stone removal).

The management of acute pancreatitis focuses on identifying and treating the underlying cause and providing supportive therapy. The mainstays of supportive therapy include an initial period of pancreatic rest by limiting oral intake, pain management, and, most importantly, aggressive volume resuscitation with intravenous crystalloid solution to prevent hemoconcentration [23]. Severe pancreatitis can be fatal in up to 10–30% of patients, making it important to identify those patients at high risk for the development of severe disease so that they can be appropriately triaged to a more intensive level of care. This is accomplished by monitoring the patient using laboratory data and scoring systems that can potentially identify organ failure. Severity scoring systems such as Ranson's score (validated only for alcoholic pancreatitis) or the Acute Physiology and Chronic Health Evaluation (APACHE) are commonly used to predict complications and mortality.

Complications of acute pancreatitis include pseudocyst formation and pancreatic necrosis. Fluid collections are common, and can occur in up to 60% of patients hospitalized with acute pancreatitis [24]. Typically, these collections are ill defined and most will resolve spontaneously. If organized and symptomatic, they can be drained endoscopically. Pancreatic necrosis is associated with a high mortality if the necrosed parenchyma becomes secondarily infected. Management includes early initiation of broad-spectrum antibiotics, and surgical intervention if the necrotic tissue is infected.

Case 3: lower abdominal pain

Case presentation

Hank is a 37-year-old truck driver referred for the evaluation of a 2-year history of lower abdominal pain. He describes a near daily ache or discomfort in the left lower abdomen. He occasionally feels bloated but denies significant abdominal distension. The pain does not radiate into his back, groin, epigastrium, or thighs, and he cannot reproduce the pain with movement. His lower abdominal discomfort temporarily resolves after having a bowel movement, which occurs no more than twice a week.

On review of systems, his pain is not associated with fevers, chills, or night sweats. He denies dysuria and hematuria. His weight has been stable for the past 5 years. He cannot recall any precipitating event associated with the onset of his pain and denies trauma to his back, pelvis, or abdomen. He does not have odynophagia, dysphagia, nausea, upper abdominal pain, or vomiting. He has no past medical history of note. He states that for the last 2 years he has had to strain in order to have a bowel movement and his stools are typically very hard and pellet like. He has not seen any blood in his stool and denies melena. He last saw a physician 3 years ago; he had a normal blood count at that time. He does not take any medications on a routine basis and denies any medication allergies. He had a tonsillectomy at age 5. He does not smoke and drinks 2–3 beers each weekend. He has no family history of note.

Hank treated his pain with acetaminophen, aspirin, and several anti-inflammatory agents without relief. Milk of magnesia, magnesium citrate, docusate sodium, senna, and cascara were only partially effective at relieving his constipation and did not help his abdominal pain.

Physical examination reveals a well-appearing, appropriate and interactive, young-looking man. Vital signs are within normal limits and his BMI is 23 kg/m^2. Examination of the head, neck, heart, lungs, back, and extremities is normal. His abdomen is soft and flat, and no scars are present. Bowel sounds are normal; no bruit or succussion splash is heard. The liver is not enlarged, the spleen cannot be palpated, and no masses are felt. He has some discomfort with palpation in the left lower quadrant, but no rebound or guarding. There is no evidence of a hernia with cough or straining. Rectal examination is normal and the prostate is neither tender nor enlarged.

Questions

The clinical questions that need to be answered when evaluating this patient's case include:
- What is the differential diagnosis for his pain and constipation?
- What diagnostic studies, if any, should be performed?
- What treatment options are available?

Differential diagnosis

The most efficient and most accurate approach would be to evaluate this patient using three distinct pathways. The first pathway involves differentiating acute from chronic abdominal pain. The second involves reviewing the differential diagnosis of chronic constipation. The third consists of determining whether this patient's symptoms represent an organic disorder or an FGID.

Acute abdominal pain is defined as the onset of new abdominal pain less than 24 hours in duration, whereas chronic abdominal pain is defined as the presence of pain for more than 2 months [25]. A differential diagnosis for acute and chronic abdominal pain is provided in Table 4.1 and Box 4.4.

Chronic constipation can be defined using either the Rome III criteria [26] (Box 4.5) or the more clinically oriented American College of Gastroenterology (ACG) definition [27]. The latter definition states that a patient meets criteria for chronic constipation if he or she has unsatisfactory defecation characterized by infrequent stools, difficult stool passage, or both, for at least 3 months out of the last 12 (which need not be consecutive). A differential diagnosis for chronic constipation is provided in Box 4.6.

Finally, the clinician needs to determine whether the patient's symptoms represent an organic or a functional gastrointestinal disorder. Functional bowel disorders are characterized by symptoms of GI tract dysfunction in the absence of any known biochemical, mechanical, or radiographic findings that could explain the symptoms [27].

Returning to the patient, the evaluating physician ordered a CBC, serum electrolytes, BUN/creatinine,

Box 4.4 Differential diagnosis of chronic abdominal pain

Complications from surgery

Functional dyspepsia

Gastroparesis

Chronic functional abdominal pain

Chronic pancreatitis

Sphincter of Oddi dysfunction

Irritable bowel syndrome

Scar tissue/adhesions

Autoimmune disorders (systemic lupus erythematosus, polyarteritis nodosa)

Chronic intestinal pseudo-obstruction (CIP)

Infiltrative disorders (lymphoma)

Chronic mesenteric ischemia

Inflammatory bowel disease

Lead toxicity

Neuropathies (autonomic, diabetic)

Box 4.5 Rome III criteria for chronic constipation (modified from American College of Gastroenterology Chronic Constipation Task Force [27])

Symptom onset at least 6 months before diagnosis

Presence of symptoms for the last 3 months (see below)

Insufficient criteria for IBS

Loose stools are rarely present without the use of laxatives

Symptoms include two or more of the following during at least 25% of defecations:

Straining

Lumpy or hard stools

Sensation of incomplete evacuation

Sensation of anorectal obstruction or blockade

Manual maneuvers to facilitate evacuation

Fewer than three bowel movements per week

Box 4.6 Differential diagnosis of chronic constipation

Primary causes

Normal transit constipation

Slow transit (colonic inertia) constipation

Irritable bowel syndrome with constipation

Evacuation disorders (i.e., pelvic floor dyssynergia).

Secondary causes

Mechanical obstruction (masses, strictures)

Neurological disorders (Parkinson's disease, multiple sclerosis)

Metabolic disorders (hypercalcemia, diabetes, hypothyroidism)

Medications (narcotics, high-dose tricyclic antidepressants, some selective serotonin reuptake inhibitors)

Anorectal disorders (prolapse, descending perineum syndrome)

Psychogenic (anorexia, depression)

Dietary/lifestyle (low fiber intake)

Iatrogenic (prior surgery)

glucose, thyroid-stimulating hormone (TSH), abdominal radiograph, and flexible sigmoidoscopy.

Diagnostic findings and final diagnosis

The patient's physical examination was essentially normal, except for mild tenderness in the left lower quadrant. The chronicity of symptoms (2 years), combined with the absence of warning signs, should reassure both the patient and the clinician. The presence of mild left lower abdominal discomfort on examination is non-specific and could represent a process involving the sigmoid colon, the abdominal wall, the iliopsoas muscle, or referred pain from elsewhere in the abdominal cavity. To help distinguish abdominal muscle wall pain from visceral pain, the patient should be asked to cross his arms, and sit half-way up while the abdominal examination is repeated (Carnett's test). Contraction of the abdominal wall muscles should reduce pain produced during palpation of an inflamed viscus, in contrast to muscle wall pain (or pain from nerve entrapment, an abdominal wall hernia, or a rectus sheath hematoma) which fails to improve. The *obturator test* and the *reverse psoas maneuver* can be used to identify obturator and psoas inflammation due to appendicitis or a pelvic abscess or hematoma. Careful examination of the groin, testicles, and scrotum can diagnose a hernia (either femoral or inguinal), which was not found in this patient.

The normal CBC strongly argues against both an inflammatory process and an infiltrative disorder especially given the 2-year history of symptoms. Abdominal radiograph was normal. Flexible sigmoidoscopy is safe, easy to perform, and an excellent test to exclude mechanical obstruction of the lower GI tract. In a young patient (age < 40) without anemia, unintentional weight loss, rectal bleeding, or a family history of colorectal cancer, the likelihood of finding a sinister process in the right colon is exceedingly low, which is why a flexible sigmoidoscopy was recommended, rather than a full colonoscopy. In a patient over 50, or with anemia or a family history of colorectal cancer, colonoscopy would be more appropriate.

This patient has a constellation of symptoms including lower abdominal pain and discomfort, bloating, and constipation. The chronicity of symptoms, coupled with the absence of warning signs, should lead the astute clinician to the confident diagnosis of IBS with constipation. Although an overlap exists in the current definitions of chronic constipation and IBS, the fact that this patient's abdominal discomfort was temporally related to having a bowel movement defined him as having IBS with constipation rather than chronic constipation [26]. The normal results of the diagnostic studies described above support the clinical diagnosis of IBS.

Patient management

IBS is one of the most common medical conditions seen in primary care and accounts for nearly a third of referrals to gastroenterologists [28]. The peak prevalence occurs in the third and fourth decades of life, although most patients develop typical symptoms in their late teenage years or early 20s. Symptoms are frequently present for years before being properly

> ### Box 4.7 Rome III criteria for irritable bowel syndrome (IBS) (modified from Longstreth et al. [26])
>
> Symptom onset at least 6 months before diagnosis
>
> Recurrent abdominal pain or discomfort for at least 3 days of the month in the last 3 months associated with at least two of the following:
>
> Improvement with defecation
>
> Onset associated with change in stool frequency
>
> Onset associated with change in stool form

diagnosed; a typical IBS patient may see three doctors over 3 years before a definitive diagnosis is made [29]. IBS is twice as common in women as in men; differences in hormone levels, greater routine healthcare for women and increased healthcare-seeking behavior may account for this disparity. For most patients IBS is a chronic disorder; once diagnosed, nearly 75% of patients still carry the diagnosis 5 years later [30].

The Rome III criteria for IBS are shown in Box 4.7. The ACG defines IBS as abdominal discomfort in association with altered bowel habits (either constipation or diarrhea) [31].

Pathophysiologically, symptoms of IBS arise due to abnormalities in intestinal motility, alterations in visceral sensory function, and changes in central nervous system processing of sensory information [32]. This intimate, bidirectional connection between the brain and the GI tract has been labeled the brain–gut axis.

Diagnosing IBS need not be difficult or prohibitively expensive. After a thorough interview and careful physical examination, if warning features (anemia, unintentional weight loss, evidence of GI bleeding, family history of colorectal cancer or IBD) are absent, and the patient meets Rome III criteria, the diagnosis can be made at the time of the first office visit. Routinely evaluating *all* IBS patients with a battery of tests is neither required nor cost-effective [33]. In fact routine testing (CBC, TSH, lactose breath test, flexible sigmoidoscopy, and barium enema or colonoscopy) in patients with IBS was not found to yield any greater number of significant abnormalities than when these same tests were performed in healthy volunteers [33]. However, patients with IBS, especially those with diarrhea predominance, may be at an increased risk for celiac disease, and it is worthwhile to check for this, especially in a patient who has failed to respond to initial therapy [34]. Using these simple guidelines, the accuracy of making a diagnosis of IBS in clinical practice has been shown to be very high [35,36].

At present, the treatment of IBS should focus on the most predominant symptom, which will vary from patient to patient. It is important to note that the only medication currently approved for the treatment of constipation-predominant IBS in the USA is lubiprostone; this is approved for adult women with IBS and constipation [37]. Long-term outcome studies will be required to properly evaluate the efficacy of lubiprostone, a chloride channel activator, for the treatment of global IBS symptoms [38]. Fiber products, polyethylene glycol, lactulose, and lubiprostone can be used to treat constipation, while loperamide, diphenoxylate atropine, cholestyramine, probiotics, and antibiotics may be used to treat diarrhea [39]. Low-dose tricyclic antidepressants are often helpful for chronic functional abdominal pain, whereas episodic abdominal pain due to cramps and spasms may improve with smooth muscle antispasmodics such as hyoscyamine or dicyclomine [40,41].

Discussion

Physicians need to be adept at evaluating and treating abdominal pain, since it is one of the most common symptoms reported by patients. The first step is to distinguish acute (onset within 24 hours) from chronic abdominal pain (present > 2 months). Acute abdominal pain almost always reflects an organic process. Chronic abdominal pain may reflect an ongoing organic process, although it more commonly reflects visceral hypersensitivity, changes in central or peripheral sensory processing, the presence of scar tissue or adhesions, or a learned behavior with secondary rewards. In the following sections the evaluation, diagnosis, and management of both acute and chronic abdominal pain will be discussed.

Initial approach to the patient with abdominal pain

Evaluating abdominal pain is similar to solving a puzzle. The history, physical examination, and results of specialized tests are all individual pieces that must fit precisely together to arrive at a diagnosis. It is uncommon for any single symptom or physical examination finding to have enough information to accurately diagnose the cause of abdominal pain. It is also important to remember that abdominal pain is a very subjective experience, and that no currently available test can accurately, reliably, and consistently quantify abdominal pain. This means that the physician will likely need to explore the background and life experiences of the patient in order to understand how these factors might influence symptom expression.

The evaluation of abdominal pain begins with a thorough history to help identify the underlying cause and to guide the examiner in performing a focused physical examination. It is important to take into account the patient's intelligence level and ability to communicate because these factors will greatly influence the history. Points of interest that need to be addressed during the history include:
- the onset and timing of pain
- the associated symptoms and signs
- the intensity, duration, location, and radiation (if any) of the pain
- the chronology and progression of symptoms
- the character of the pain
- precipitating events
- exacerbating and alleviating factors
- prior treatments employed to relieve the pain.

The age of the patient is obviously important because some disorders are more prevalent in very young patients (e.g. intussusception), some are more common in children and teenagers (e.g. appendicitis), whereas others are more common in older patients (e.g. diverticulitis). These questions are in addition to the usual questions about travel, previous surgery, family history, medications, prior trauma or accidents, sexual and menstrual history, and acute and chronic medical problems. In the evaluation of patients with chronic pain, it is also important to determine why the patient is undergoing evaluation at this time.

The onset and timing of acute abdominal pain can provide an important clue to the diagnosis. An *abrupt* onset may represent a perforated ulcer, a ruptured abscess, or an intestinal infarct. Pain that develops *rapidly* (over minutes) may represent volvulus, a perforated viscus, or biliary colic. Pain that develops *gradually* (over hours) may represent appendicitis, pancreatitis, or distal small bowel obstruction (see Table 4.1).

Serious episodes of abdominal pain are occasionally characterized by a period of symptom quiescence after the initial presentation. For example, patients with a perforated viscus or intestinal infarction may note resolution of their intense initial pain for several hours after perforation or infarction first occurs, only to suffer a recurrence of pain when peritonitis develops. Objective testing is required in all patients with acute abdominal pain (see below) and, if normal, close surveillance in a supervised setting for several hours is imperative to monitor for progression of a serious disorder.

When the onset of pain is more gradual, the differential diagnosis is much larger and the clinician has significant latitude in deciding about the urgency and direction of the evaluation. Guiding factors include the patient's history, the nature and location of the pain, and the physical examination. In all cases, a follow-up appointment within 24–72 hours is warranted, even if just a telephone call, so that any important new symptom will not be missed. It is best for the physician to initiate this follow-up because it will obviate the need for the patient to decide whether a change in symptoms warrants repeat evaluation.

Some patients with chronic abdominal pain recall a preceding event (e.g. abdominal trauma, surgery, an infectious gastroenteritis) that seemed to cause the chronic abdominal pain. More commonly, however, chronic symptoms cannot be attributed to a specific event and may develop insidiously. Chronic abdominal pain that cannot be attributed to an underlying organic process is commonly due to a functional disorder such as IBS or functional dyspepsia.

Associated symptoms and signs can be helpful in the diagnosis of abdominal pain (Table 4.2). The presence of fever may represent acute gastroenteritis, diverticulitis in an older patient, cholecystitis, or ascending cholangitis. Associated nausea and vomiting are common in patients with pancreatitis, cholecystitis, hepatitis, and bowel obstructions. Concurrent bloody diarrhea may signal the onset of intestinal ischemia, ulcerative colitis, or an infection with an enteroinvasive organism (e.g. *Salmonella*, *Shigella*, *Escherichia coli* O157.H7). Non-bloody diarrhea in conjunction with abdominal pain most commonly represents acute gastroenteritis, but it can also be associated with IBS or Crohn's disease.

Physicians almost always question their patients about the intensity of abdominal pain, and many use a scale of 1–10 to help the patient determine the severity of the pain. Unfortunately, given the subjective nature of pain, trying to determine the intensity of pain for a specific organic process as a measure for all patients is not useful. However, the intensity of pain can be used to follow the progression or resolution of an underlying organic process in individual patients. Serial examinations, with repeated questioning about the intensity of the pain, should be performed. In addition, the patient's demeanor, along with vital signs, should be checked during episodes of pain. Some processes characteristically have more intense pain than others; perforated viscus, acute volvulus, intussusception, ruptured aneurysm, and mesenteric thrombosis all usually produce severe abdominal pain. Pain that is more moderate in nature may reflect early pancreatitis, cholecystitis, diverticulitis, chronic volvulus, or early small bowel obstruction.

The patient should be questioned about the duration of each episode of pain, and the amount of time between episodes. As appendicitis progresses, the period of time between episodes of pain diminishes. Patients with a large bowel obstruction may have pain-free intervals of 10–20 min, whereas those with small bowel obstruction generally have shorter pain-free intervals.

The location of the pain can provide an important clue to the underlying pathophysiology. Periumbilical pain usually reflects a small intestinal process, whereas pain in the right upper quadrant may be due to cholecystitis, biliary colic, liver abscess, or peptic ulcer. Epigastric pain may be due to peptic ulcer, pancreatitis, mesenteric ischemia, and even appendicitis. Left lower quadrant pain usually reflects ureteral colic, or inflammation or spasm of the descending or sigmoid colon. Suprapubic pain may occur due to appendicitis or rectosigmoid disorders, whereas pain in the right lower quadrant may reflect appendicitis or terminal ileum involvement in Crohn's disease (Table 4.2).

The character of abdominal pain can provide an important clue to the diagnosis, and is discussed more fully below. Identifying events that precipitate abdominal pain may also help uncover the cause. Pain that arises in response to movement (e.g. twisting or turning of the trunk or pelvis) usually indicates referred pain from an adjacent area, such as the hip or lower back, rather than pain from an abdominal viscus. Cyclical pain in young women may be

Table 4.2 Characteristics of common causes of abdominal pain

Disorder	Character	Location
Peptic ulcer	Gnawing hunger; burning sensation	Epigastrium; may radiate to the back
Penetrating ulcer	Severe, steady boring pain	Epigastrium with radiation to the back
Perforated ulcer	Abrupt, severe pain; may be followed by pain-free period before symptoms worsen and intensify	Initially epigastric with radiation to back; then right lower quadrant
Small bowel obstruction	Crampy severe pain with partial obstruction; may come in waves; constant severe pain with complete obstruction	Periumbilical area
Large bowel obstruction	Crampy pain; less severe than small bowel obstruction; less sudden than more proximal obstruction	Localized over area of obstruction or more generalized
Intestinal infarct	Severe, excruciating, abrupt onset	Generalized
Intussusception	Sudden onset; severe crampy pain	Periumbilical
Cholecystitis	Constant severe pain; accompanied by nausea and vomiting	Right upper quadrant pain that may radiate to the infrascapular region
Biliary colic	Pain free periods interspersed with sharp pain	Epigastric radiating to the right upper quadrant and to the subscapular region
Pancreatitis	Severe constant pain associated with nausea and vomiting	Epigastric pain that may radiate to the back
Appendicitis	Pain that may wax and wane in intensity; often begins as a dull ache and increases in intensity	Often begins in the periumbilical area and then localizes in the right lower quadrant (McBurney's point); rarely radiates to the epigastrium or scrotum
Diverticulitis	Crampy, severe pain	Usually in the left lower quadrant
Ulcerative colitis	Crampy pain	Usually left lower quadrant or may be generalized with toxic megacolon
Crohn's disease	Crampy pain	Periumbilical or right lower quadrant

a sign of endometriosis, whereas pain that consistently develops after eating may represent mesenteric ischemia.

Elderly patients with abdominal pain require special attention because serious underlying conditions may produce only minimal symptoms. For example, the diagnosis of appendicitis or diverticulitis can be easily missed because pain may not be severe, and fever and leukocytosis may be minimal or absent. Therefore, careful follow-up of abdominal pain in elderly people warrants repeated abdominal examinations and serial measurements of vital signs and appropriate laboratory tests.

Types of abdominal pain

Pain involving the digestive system can be visceral, parietal, referred, neurogenic, or psychogenic. Pain caused by metabolic disease is ordinarily visceral or neurogenic.

Visceral pain

This can result from spasm or stretching of the muscle wall of a hollow organ, from distension of the capsule of a solid organ such as the liver, or from inflammation or ischemia of a visceral structure. Tenderness (including rebound tenderness) associated with visceral pain is often felt directly over the part of the digestive system that is involved, although small bowel tenderness is usually not well localized (except for the terminal ileum). Note that the visceral peritoneum is supplied by slowly conducting C-fibers which produce a large receptive field, accounting for the diffuse, non-specific nature of visceral pain. Abdominal viscera are insensitive to cutting, tearing, crushing, and burning.

Parietal pain

The parietal peritoneum is supplied by rapidly conducting A-type nerve fibers which produce a small, but well-localized receptive field. Parietal tenderness is more localized than visceral tenderness, and rebound tenderness from peritonitis is generally experienced directly over the involved area. A rigid abdomen associated with pain means that the inflammation is severe.

Referred pain

Both visceral and parietal pain may be referred to a remote site along shared dermatomes. Gallbladder pain, for example, typically radiates to the infrascapular area, whereas right diaphragmatic pain radiates to the right shoulder. Esophageal pain can be confused with the pain of myocardial ischemia because the pain may radiate to identical sites (e.g. neck, left arm). The more severe the visceral pain, the more likely it is to be referred to the back, as, for example, with esophageal spasm or cholecystitis. The skin overlying the dermatome to which the pain is referred may be hypersensitive. Deep palpation of the primary site of the painful organ may intensify the pain, not only locally, but also at the referred site, whereas the reverse is not true; deep palpation over the referred site does not enhance pain over the primary site.

Abdominal pain caused by metabolic disease

Metabolic disease may produce intestinal pain by a direct effect on the alimentary tract, e.g. in hereditary angioneurotic edema, C1 esterase deficiency may produce intestinal swelling, which can result in pain due to partial obstruction or intestinal spasm. Metabolic disorders may also produce gastrointestinal pain by a secondary effect, e.g. hyperparathyroidism may produce peptic ulcer or pancreatitis.

Neurogenic pain

Neurogenic abdominal pain is experienced by the patient as a burning sensation along the route of distribution of the nerve and is sometimes associated with hyperesthesia. Usually the spinal root is involved as a result of herpes zoster, carcinoma, or arthritis; however, peripheral neuropathies due to operative trauma or diabetes mellitus may also produce neurogenic abdominal pain. Neurogenic pain is not exacerbated or improved with eating or defecating.

Psychogenic pain

This may represent a conversion reaction that results in the perception of pain when no organic dysfunction exists. Alternatively it may represent a physiological response to psychological stress. For example, emotional stress can lead to painful intestinal spasm in patients with IBS. Pain or tenderness that represents a conversion reaction (emotions converted into somatic complaints) may disappear during periods of distraction. This type of pain is not explained by any known anatomic or physiological pathway.

Nature and location of pain

Esophageal pain

This is generally described as a pressure or a substernal squeezing or burning sensation; when severe it may radiate through to the back. Pain from the lower esophageal region may be referred more proximally, although processes in the upper esophagus rarely cause pain more distally.

Gastric pain

This is usually experienced in the subxiphoid area or the left upper quadrant. The pain of peptic ulcer may be described as a gnawing discomfort or a hunger sensation rather than pain. The temporal relationship of eating to symptoms of pain was previously used to distinguish gastric from duodenal ulcer; however, this is neither sensitive nor specific. A change in the character of the pain from a gnawing discomfort to a burning, boring, or knife-like pain with radiation to the back may indicate a penetrating ulcer. Pain that is precipitated by meals can be seen in patients with gastric outlet obstruction or proximal intestinal obstruction.

Duodenal pain

This is felt in the epigastric area or right upper quadrant and may radiate through to the back. When an ulcer perforates, the pain typically appears abruptly in the epigastric region and later settles into the right lower quadrant as gastric contents are spilled into the right paracolic gutter.

Small intestinal pain

This is generally diffuse and poorly localized. It is often described as crampy, sharp, or aching, and experienced in the periumbilical area; when severe, it also radiates through to the back. Pain arising from the terminal ileum may be localized to the right lower quadrant. Bloating, distension, and a dull ache are associated with prolonged mechanical obstruction or ileus.

Colonic pain

This is better localized, often to the lower abdomen. Sigmoid pain is felt in the left lower quadrant, and rectal pain is often described as being located over the rectum, usually in the midline. Gas pockets in the splenic flexure of the colon (seen most commonly in patients with IBS) produce left upper quadrant or left chest pain that may be confused with the pain of myocardial ischemia. Temporary relief is obtained by passing flatus. Colonic pain generally is crampy or of an aching quality unless perforation occurs, and then it is severe and constant. Associated fever and chills may suggest diverticulitis, a diverticular abscess, or ulcerative, infectious, or ischemic colitis.

Appendicitis

This often begins as diffuse abdominal pain that intensifies over a period of hours as it settles in the right lower quadrant. The pain of appendicitis is frequently aggravated by hyperextension of the right hip (reverse psoas maneuver).

Pancreatic pain

This is excruciating and constant and usually located in the upper abdomen, with radiation through to the back because of its retroperitoneal location. Chronic pancreatic pain (due to inflammation, pseudocyst, or carcinoma) is similar in nature and location to acute pancreatic pain but usually less severe. Acute pancreatitis is almost invariably associated with nausea and vomiting.

Gallbladder pain

This generally begins in the right upper quadrant or epigastrium and radiates to the interscapular or the right infrascapular area. It is excruciatingly severe, may be aggravated by deep inspiration, and is replaced by a dull, aching sensation that persists for hours after the severe pain subsides. Tenderness can be elicited by deep palpation under the rib in the area of the gallbladder, especially during deep inspiration. A midinspiratory halt (Murphy's sign) is frequently seen in patients with cholecystitis. Gallbladder pain frequently develops late at night after a heavy dinner. Associated fever, chills, and an elevated white cell count suggest ascending cholangitis or cholecystitis.

Hepatic pain

This is generally described as a dull ache and is localized to the right upper quadrant. The liver itself is insensitive to pain; hepatic pain develops due to stretching of Glisson's capsule. A tender liver can be demonstrated by palpating the edge during deep inspiration or by percussion over the lower right rib cage anteriorly.

Lastly, it is important to note that colicky pain is a widely used term that has widely different meanings to patients and physicians. Colicky pain is a nonspecific term that is used to describe a wave-like build-up of pain culminating in intense pain; it is often associated with nausea, vomiting, and diaphoresis. Symptoms are due to peristaltic contractions with an increase in intraluminal pressure.

Physical examination

The patient's position and general appearance can provide clues about the severity, duration, and frequently the cause of the underlying condition. A position of truncal flexure may be seen in patients with pancreatitis, whereas patients with gallbladder colic or a bowel obstruction are often very restless as they attempt to find a comfortable position. This is in sharp contrast to patients with peritonitis who attempt to avoid even the slightest movement.

59

Inspection of the abdomen should take place with adequate lighting in order to assess abdominal asymmetry and outline masses and pulsations. In thin patients with a partial bowel obstruction, peristaltic waves may be seen through the abdominal wall, and churning peristalsis may coincide with reports of crampy abdominal pain. Flank discoloration (Turner's sign) or periumbilical discoloration (Cullen's sign) result from retroperitoneal or intraperitoneal hemorrhage dissecting into the subcutaneous tissues and may indicate hemorrhagic pancreatitis. A strangulated hernia may protrude visibly from ventral defects, the inguinal area, or into the scrotum where peristaltic contractions may occasionally be appreciated. Patients with a subphrenic abscess or gallbladder disease may have inspiratory pain that results in splinting and avoidance of deep inspiration.

Auscultation should always be performed before palpation so that abdominal sounds may be evaluated before they are altered by palpation. Bowel sounds should not be reported as "absent" until after at least 2 minutes of careful listening. At times borborygmi will be audible without the stethoscope. Specifically one should search for hyperperistaltic or hypoperistaltic sounds, for the high tinkling sounds of obstruction, and for bruits suggesting vascular distortion from aneurysms, compression of blood vessels, or invasion of blood vessels (e.g. invasion of the splenic artery in advanced pancreatic carcinoma). Although a silent abdomen implies ileus, bowel sounds may also be quiet or markedly diminished late in the course of mechanical obstruction. If gastric outlet obstruction is suspected, the clinician should attempt to elicit a succussion splash. This is done by placing the stethoscope over the epigastrium and shaking the patient gently but abruptly. A sloshing sound indicates the presence of air and fluid. If a succussion splash is present 3 or more hours after eating, this indicates either gastric outlet obstruction or gastroparesis.

Gentle percussion should precede palpation and is an excellent means for detecting rebound tenderness, masses, and tympany (either generalized or localized) over an area of ileus or obstruction. As air will rise to the area between the liver and the abdominal wall, the absence of liver dullness with the patient in a recumbent position is an important finding because it indicates the presence of free air in the abdominal cavity.

Before palpation, it is wise to ask the patient to point to the site of maximum pain. Gentle palpation should at first avoid that site to minimize the chances that muscle guarding will interfere with the remainder of the examination. The patient should be lying perfectly supine with knees flexed to relax the abdominal wall muscles. Guarding may be localized over specific lesions (often inflammatory). Rebound tenderness usually indicates peritoneal irritation; board-like rigidity indicates an intra-abdominal catastrophe such as perforation or infarction. Pulsatile masses should be differentiated from laterally expansile masses because the former can represent a mass overlying an artery, whereas the latter implies aneurysmal dilation.

A rectal examination can localize areas of tenderness (prostatitis), and identify a mass or abscess. A genital and pelvic examination, similar to the rectal examination, should be performed in all patients with abdominal pain because it can detect hernias as well as genitourinary and other pelvic problems.

As mentioned earlier, repeated examinations are critical to assess progression of disease. In addition, repeated examinations help the examiner learn to correlate symptoms with pathology. Finally, if analgesic drugs have been administered, it is useful to re-examine the patient after the pain has been relieved to identify masses or localized tenderness that may have been obscured by guarding and rigidity.

Laboratory tests

A CBC, urinalysis, and test for occult blood in the stool are required in every person with serious acute abdominal pain, as are a chest radiograph and plain and upright films of the abdomen. However, it is important to note that fecal occult blood is a highly non-specific finding. Other laboratory tests should be ordered as indicated by the specific findings.

Radiology
Plain and upright films of the abdomen are helpful in delineating gas patterns, which may demonstrate displacement of the intestine by intra-abdominal masses or may show localized loops of ileus such as with pancreatitis or pyelonephritis. Air is distributed more widely in the small bowel in an ileus and intestinal obstruction. In the latter the typical stepladder pattern is often encountered, with slight separation of the loops due to edema of the wall of the small bowel; an upright film demonstrates air–fluid levels in the

dilated loops. Absence of air distal to a specific point (transition point) suggests obstruction at that point. Volvulus can be seen on a plain film as a sausage-shaped, air-filled or air-fluid filled viscus coming to an apex. In gastric volvulus the greater curvature is seen above the lesser curve, and a double air–fluid level is a classic finding. Free air under the diaphragm on the upright film indicates a perforated viscus unless the patient has had recent surgery (at which time air was introduced) or has pneumatosis cystoides intestinalis, in which case a large amount of air may appear sub-diaphragmatically from ruptured pseudocysts. The important clue to pneumatosis cystoides intestinalis is the presence of free air in the absence of signs and symptoms of perforation or peritonitis. Radiopaque gallbladder or kidney stones, or pancreatic calcifica-tions seen on an abdominal flat plate may help to corroborate a suspected diagnosis or point attention toward one of these organs.

Contrast studies have been largely replaced by endoscopic procedures in the evaluation of patients with abdominal pain. Endoscopy is both more sensi-tive and more specific than contrast radiology of the bowel, although considerably more expensive. An upper GI series is useful if there is a suspicion of extrinsic compression of the stomach or duodenum or partial gastric outlet obstruction at endoscopy. Barium enema can be useful in demonstrating a low site of obstruction and also in reducing an intussus-ception. A barium enema should always be preceded by digital examination of the rectum and by proctos-copy to be certain that the rectum is normal (e.g. that there is not a rectal carcinoma). A Tc-labeled HIDA radioisotopic study may demonstrate obstruction of the common bile duct or cystic duct and is most useful for evaluating a patient with suspected cholecystitis. This study requires injection of isotope and serial views for 1 hour.

Ultrasonography is an excellent means of demon-strating stones in the gallbladder but is not reliable in detecting ductal stones. Ultrasonography is also useful in evaluating a suspected abdominal aortic aneurysm; it is less commonly used now to image the pancreas, having been supplanted by CT. Sonography is often unsatisfactory in obese people and those with metal abdominal staples or sutures because adipose tissue and metal reflect sound.

CT is a sensitive means of demonstrating masses, obstruction, inflammatory processes, infarcted tissue,

and cysts but is expensive and exposes the patient to radiation.

Magnetic resonance imaging (MRI) is not routinely used as the initial imaging study of the abdomen but rather is used selectively to define mass lesions – especially in the liver, kidneys, or adrenal glands. In addition, magnetic resonance angiography (MRA) can be used to look for vascular abnormalities, such as hemangiomas or renal or hepatic vein throm-bosis. Magnetic resonance cholangiopancreatography (MRCP) is a non-invasive method that can accurately diagnose gallstones in the biliary tree, bile duct stric-tures, and tumors in the pancreas and biliary tree. MR technology is generally more expensive than CT.

Selective mesenteric angiography should be per-formed in patients suspected of having mesenteric vascular ischemia (particularly in elderly people with postprandial abdominal pain) or mesenteric vascular occlusion. This is particularly helpful in older patients, as normal arteriographic findings rule out mesenteric vascular disease; on the other hand, occlusion of even two of the three major aortic branches may occur without symptoms of mesenteric vascular disease.

Endoscopy

Upper gastrointestinal endoscopy is the ambulatory procedure of choice to diagnose upper GI disease and to obtain tissue for diagnosis. Endoscopy should be performed promptly when abdominal pain is associ-ated with upper GI bleeding.

Colonoscopy and flexible sigmoidoscopy may be appropriate for patients with abdominal pain who have occult rectal bleeding, in those suspected of diffuse colonic inflammatory disease or suspected ischemic colitis, and in patients with polypoid lesions on barium enema who require biopsy or resection of the lesion.

Treatment – general principles

Management of any type of pain can be significantly improved by considering several simple principles, e.g. reassurance that pain can be relieved by medica-tion or surgery can significantly raise the threshold of tolerance. On the other hand, the existence of severe pain sensitizes patients to additional, less intense pain (such as lumbar puncture or venepunc-ture), and the patient's "overreaction" to the second pain should not be taken to imply that the primary pain is psychogenic. Another common misconception is that the alleviation of pain by placebo implies psychogenic origin; in fact, organic pain may be more readily relieved by placebo than psychogenic pain.

The treatment of patients with abdominal pain depends on the severity of the pain, its rapidity of onset, and the nature of the underlying condition, if known. Severe pain with an abrupt or rapid onset frequently reflects a GI disorder that will require surgical intervention (see Table 4.1). Hospitalization and consultation with a surgeon should be requested immediately in almost all cases. Less severe pain should not be treated aggressively with analgesic drugs until an attempt has been made to establish a diagnosis, because the pain will often abate spontaneously within minutes or hours and will not recur. In such circumstances, no further evaluation is indicated. If the pain recurs or persists, and the cause is not obvious, the screening tests described previously should be done.

As a general rule, analgesic drugs may be prescribed to patients with persistent pain, but large doses of opiates should be avoided because they may aggravate some underlying conditions, e.g. opiates or anticholinergics may produce toxic megacolon in patients with active ulcerative colitis. Furthermore, there is the significant risk of opiate addiction in any patient where pain is likely to be of prolonged duration.

The reader is referred to the appropriate chapters to review the management of specific disorders.

References

1 Jones R, Lydeard S. Irritable bowel syndrome in the general population. *BMJ* 1999;**304**:87.

2 Yamamoto W, Kono H, Maekawa H, Fukuki T. The relationship between abdominal pain regions and specific diseases: An epidemiologic approach to clinical practice. *J Epidemiol* 1997;**7**:27.

3 Lange H, Jackel R. Usefulness of plasma lactate concentration in the diagnosis of acute abdominal disease. *Eur J Surg* 1994;**160**:381.

4 Mckinsey JF, Graham A, Gewertz BL. Diseases of the vascular system. In: Lawrence PF, Bell MR, Dayton MT (eds), *Essentials of General Surgery*, 3rd edn. Philadelphia: Lippincott Williams & Wilkins, 2000: 450.

5 Wilcox MG, Howard TJ, Plaskon LA. Current theories of pathogenesis and treatment of non-occlusive mesenteric ischemia. *Dig Dis Sci* 1995;**40**:709.

6 Acosta S, Ogren M, Sternby NH, et al. Incidence of acute thrombo-embolic occlusion of the superior mesenteric artery – a population-based study. *Eur J Vasc Endovasc Surg* 2004;**27**:145–50.

7 Mckinsey JF, Gewertz BL. Acute mesenteric ischemia. *Surg Clin North Am* 1997;**77**:307–18.

8 Cappell MS. Intestinal (mesenteric) vasculopathy. I. Acute superior mesenteric arteriopathy and venography. *Gastroenterol Clin North Am* 1998;**72**:65.

9 Kougias P, Lau D, El Sayed HF, et al. Determinants of mortality and treatment outcome following surgical interventions for acute mesenteric ischemia. *J Vasc Surg* 2007;**46**:467.

10 Brandt LJ, Boley SJ. AGA technical review on intestinal ischemia. American Gastrointestinal Association. *Gastroenterology* 2000;**118**:151.

11 Reinus JF, Brandt LJ, Boley SJ. Ischemic diseases of the bowel. *Gastroenterol Clin North Am* 1990;**19**:319.

12 Mansour MA. Management of acute mesenteric ischemia. *Arch Surg* 1999;**134**:328–30.

13 Yamaguchi T, Saeki M, Iwasaki Y, et al. Local thrombolytic therapy for superior mesenteric artery embolism: complications and long-term clinical follow-up. *Radiat Med* 1999;**17**:27–33.

14 Drossman DA. The Functional Gastrointestinal Disorders and the Rome III Process. *Gastroenterology* 2006;**130**:1377–90.

15 Treacy J, Williams A, Bais R et al. Evaluation of amylase and lipase in the diagnosis of acute pancreatitis *ANZ J Surg* 2001;**71**:577.

16 Werner M, Steinberg WM, Pauley C. Strategic use of individual and combined enzyme indicators for acute pancreatitis in patients with abdominal pain. *Clin Chem* 1989;**35**:967.

17 Neoptolemos JP, Kemppainen EA, Mayer JM, et al. Early prediction of severity in acute pancreatitis by urinary trypsinogen activation peptide: a multicentre study. *Lancet* 2000;**355**:1955–60.

18 Kemppainen E, Hedstrom J, Puolakkainen P, et al. Increased serum trypsinogen 2 and trypsin 2-alpha 1 antitrypsin complex values identify endoscopic retrograde cholangiopancreatography induced pancreatitis with high accuracy. *Gut* 1997;**41**:690–5.

19 DeFrances CJ, Hall MJ, Podgornik MN. 2003 National Hospital Discharge Survey. *Advance data from vital and health statistics*. No. 359. Hyattsville, MD: National Center for Health Statistics, 2005.

20 Conwell DL. Acute and chronic pancreatitis. *Clin Gastroenterol* 2001;**1**:47–52.

21 Whitcomb DC. Value of genetic testing in the evaluation of pancreatitis. *Gut* 2004;**53**:1710.

22 Parenti DM, Steinberg W, Kang P. Infectious causes of acute pancreatitis. *Pancreas* 1996;**13**:356–71.

23 Whitcomb DC. Clinical practice. Acute pancreatitis. *N Engl J Med* 2006;**354**:2142–50.

24 Robert JH, Frossard JL, Mermillod B, et al. Early prediction of acute pancreatitis: prospective study comparing computed tomography scans, Ranson, Glasgow, Acute Physiology and Chronic Health Evaluation II scores, and various serum markers. *World J Surg* 2002;**26**:612–19.

25 Silen W. *Cope's Early Diagnosis of the Acute Abdomen*, 18th edn. Oxford: Oxford University Press, 1991.

26 Longstreth GF, Thompson WG, Chey WD, et al. Functional bowel disorders. *Gastroenterology* 2006;**130**:1480–91.

27 American College of Gastroenterology Chronic Constipation Task Force. An Evidence based approach to the management of chronic constipation in North America. *Am J Gastroenterol* 2005;**100**:S1–4.

28 Lacy BE, Rosemore J, Corbin D, et al. Physicians' attitudes and practices in the evaluation and treatment of irritable bowel syndrome. *Scand J Gastroenterol* 2006;**41**:892–902.

29 Heitkemper M, Carter E, Ameen V, Olden K, Chang L. Women with irritable bowel syndrome: differences in patients' and physicians' perceptions. *Gastroenterol Nurs* 2002;**25**:192–200.

30 Drossman DA, Camilleri M, Mayer EA, Whitehead WE. AGA technical review on irritable bowel syndrome. *Gastroenterology* 2002;**123**:2108–31.

31 Brandt LJ, Bjorkman D, Fennerty MB, et al. Systematic review on the management of irritable bowel syndrome in North America. *Am J Gastroenterol* 2002;**97**:S7–26.

32 Camilleri M. Management of the irritable bowel syndrome. *Gastroenterology* 2001;**120**:652–68.

33 Cash BD, Schoenfeld P, Chey WD. The utility of diagnostic tests in irritable bowel syndrome patients: a systematic review. *Am J Gastroenterol* 2002;**97**:2812–19.

34 Sanders DS, Carter MJ, Hurlstone DP, et al. Association of adult coeliac disease with irritable bowel syndrome: a case-control study in patients fulfilling Rome II criteria referred to secondary care. *Lancet* 2001;**358**:1604–8.

35 Owens DM, Nelson DK, Talley NJ. The irritable bowel syndrome: long-term prognosis and the patient-physician interaction. *Ann Intern Med* 1995;**122**:107–12.

36 Vanner SJ, Depew WT, Paterson WG, et al. Predictive value of the Rome criteria for diagnosing the irritable bowel syndrome. *Am J Gastroenterol* 1999;**94**:2912–17.

37 www.fda.gov/medwatch/how.htm (accessed May 2, 2008).

38 Lacy BE, Levy LC. Lubiprostone: A novel treatment for chronic constipation. *Clin Int Aging* 2008;**3**:1–8.

39 Cash BD, Lacy BE. Systematic review: FDA-approved medications for adults with constipation. *Gastroenterol Hepatol* 2006;**2**:736–49.

40 Drossman DA, Toner BB, Whitehead WE, et al. Cognitive-behavioral therapy versus education and desipramine versus placebo for moderate to severe functional bowel disorders. *Gastroenterology* 2003;**125**: 19–31.

41 Lacy BE, De Lee R. Irritable bowel syndrome: A syndrome in evolution. *J Clin Gastroenterol* 2005;**39**: S230–42.

General reading

Handbook of Differential Diagnosis, vol 2. Part I, *The Abdomen*. Nutley, NJ: Rocom Press, 1974.

Ridge JA, Way LW. Abdominal pain. In: Sleisenger MH, Fordtran JS (eds), *Gastrointestinal Disease*, 5th edn. Philadelphia, PA: WB Saunders, 1993.

Sapira JD. *The Art and Science of Bedside Diagnosis*. Baltimore, MD: Urban & Schwarzenberg, 1990.

Silen W. *Cope's Early Diagnosis of the Acute Abdomen*, 18th edn. New York: Oxford University Press, 1991.

5

Hematemesis, Melena, and Occult Bleeding/Anemia

Grigorios I. Leontiadis[1] and Virender K. Sharma[2]

[1]University Department of Medicine, Division of Gastroenterology, Health Sciences Centre, Hamilton, ON, Canada

[2]Arizona Center for Digestive Health, Gilbert AZ, USA

Case 1: hematemesis, melena

Grigorios I. Leontiadis

Case presentation

A 48-year-old white woman presented to the emergency room with hematemesis. She had one episode of vomiting of half a cupful of dark red material 30 min before her visit. She had been feeling nauseated and lightheaded for the preceding 2 hours.

She had been taking 500 mg naproxen two or three times a week for regular tension headaches. She had also been taking over-the-counter (OTC) ranitidine (fewer than five 75-mg tablets per month) and antacids for an occasional slight burning sensation in her epigastrium. She had never sought medical advice for her dyspetic symptoms. She had nothing else of significance in her past medical history. She was a non-smoker, and drank fewer than 7 units of alcohol per week. The patient's father had had a perforated duodenal ulcer at the age of 35.

On examination the heart rate was 108 beats/min and the blood pressure was 115/75 mmHg. Physical examination was unremarkable. Rectal examination was normal; there was no melena. There were no signs of chronic liver disease.

The hemoglobin was 106 mg/L, with normal erythrocyte indices, white cell count, and platelet count. Liver function tests were also normal.

The patient was resuscitated with intravenous 0.9% NaCl. She was given an intravenous bolus of 80 mg pantoprazole and an intravenous infusion of pantoprazole was started at a rate of 8 mg/h. After 1 hour, her heart rate was 90/min and her blood pressure was 125/80 mmHg. She reported feeling much better. By this time, it was 10.00pm. As out-of-hours endoscopy had to be negotiated on a case-by-case basis, the on-call team decided to defer endoscopy until the next morning, provided that the patient remained hemodynamically stable. She was kept nil by mouth. Early next morning, she had an episode of melena which was witnessed by a nurse. Overnight her hemoglobin had fallen to 102 mg/L.

Questions

• What is the most likely cause of bleeding in this patient and why?

• Had a nasogastric tube been placed in the emergency room and had the aspirate contained bile but no blood, might you have discharged the patient home on a proton pump inhibitor and an appointment for an outpatient endoscopy?

Differential diagnosis

This patient had been bleeding from the upper gastrointestinal (GI) tract. Peptic ulcer is the leading cause of upper GI bleeding, representing around 50% of cases (62% in a US study [1], 35% in a UK study [2]). Our patient had been having occasional dyspep-

Problem-based Approach to Gastroenterology and Hepatology, First Edition. Edited by John N. Plevris, Colin W. Howden.
© 2012 Blackwell Publishing Ltd. Published 2012 by Blackwell Publishing Ltd.

tic symptoms, compatible with peptic ulcer disease. Furthermore, she had been using a non-steroidal anti-inflammatory drug (NSAID). She also had a family history of duodenal ulcer, which increased her likelihood of having *Helicobacter pylori* infection. The antacids and the low OTC doses of ranitidine that she had been taking could not have protected her from peptic ulcer bleeding.

Gastric and duodenal erosions, also possible in this patient because of her NSAID use, account for 11% of cases of upper GI bleeding [2].

Ruptured esophageal or gastric varices are a less common cause of upper GI bleeding (4–6% of cases) [1,2]. However, this diagnosis should always be carefully considered because it is requires specific management and has the highest mortality among treatable causes of upper GI bleeding (mortality rate of 23% versus 12% for peptic ulcer bleeding) [2]. Variceal bleeding was unlikely in this patient because there was no clinical or laboratory evidence of chronic liver disease or portal hypertension. For the same reason, portal hypertensive gastropathy (an even less common cause of upper GI bleeding) was not among the expected diagnoses.

The patient's history did not point towards any of the following causes of upper GI bleeding: esophagitis (4–10% of cases); Mallory–Weiss syndrome (4–5%); neoplasms (2–4%); or rarer causes such as telangiectasias, Dieulafoy's lesion, hemobilia, or Crohn's disease [1,2].

Diagnostic findings and final diagnosis

The patient underwent an emergency esophago-gastroduodenoscopy in the morning after admission. This demonstrated a normal esophagus and stomach, with no blood in the lumen. The duodenal bulb was edematous, and there was a large clot with a diameter of at least 30 mm attached to the anterior wall of the duodenal bulb (Figure 5.1). There was no active bleeding. The underlying lesion could not be viewed. The clot could not be removed by vigorous washing with water. The underlying duodenal wall was injected with 10 mL epinephrine 1:10 000 in 0.9% NaCl. The first injection caused some oozing of blood from beneath the clot, but this stopped after further injections. A polypectomy snare was used to "cheese-wire" the clot. However, during the manipulations with the polypectomy snare, the clot was completely detached

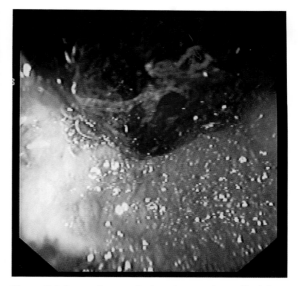

Figure 5.1 Large clot attached to the anterior wall of the duodenal bulb.

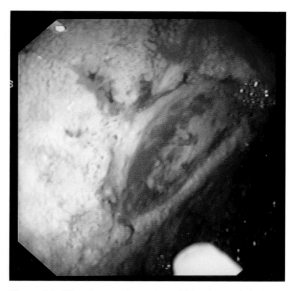

Figure 5.2 Ulcer base with oozing of blood revealed after removing the clot.

in a single piece and revealed a shallow but large oval-shaped ulcer with a maximum diameter of 20 mm. The base of the ulcer was clear with no visible vessels or other lesions, but there was mild oozing of blood from the edge of the ulcer (Figure 5.2). The bleeding was controlled with injection of a further 10 mL epinephrine 1:10 000 in 0.9% NaCl and 3 pulses of heater probe thermocoagulation (HPT) (30 J/pulse through a 2.4 mm probe). Two mucosal biopsies were taken, one from the antrum and one from the body of the stomach, in order to perform a rapid urease test for determination of *H. pylori* status.

The Rockall risk assessment score was 4 [3]. The patient returned to the ward and kept on intravenous infusion of 8 mg pantoprazole/h. The patient's hemodynamic status and hemoglobin concentration remained stable 24 hours after the endoscopy, and she had no further hematemesis or melena; the intravenous administration of pantoprazole was discontinued 72 h after endoscopy. The patient resumed oral feeding and was started on oral pantoprazole 40 mg twice a day. The following morning, she was discharged home. As the rapid urease test performed at endoscopy had been positive, she was prescribed a triple regimen for *H. pylori* infection consisting of 500 mg clarithromycin, 1 g amoxicillin, and 40 mg pantoprazole, all twice daily for 10 days, and a further 3 weeks of oral 40 mg pantoprazole once a day. She was advised to use paracetamol (acetaminophen) for headaches and to avoid further use of NSAIDs.

The patient remained asymptomatic apart from her usual headaches. A urea breath test was negative 3 weeks after the end of her pantoprazole course.

Patient management

Fundamental to the management of patients with upper GI bleeding is immediate evaluation and – if the patient is hemodynamically unstable – prompt resuscitation and restoration of intravascular volume and blood pressure [4,5]. However, it should be noted that recent evidence from retrospective studies suggests that over-transfusion can actually increase mortality [8].

Risk stratification of patients with respect to mortality and re-bleeding is also important for appropriate management [4,5]. Among several proposed risk scores, the Rockall risk score is the best validated and the most widely implemented (Table 1) [3,6].

Administration of a proton pump inhibitor (PPI) in patients with upper GI bleeding prior to endoscopy is a controversial issue. A Cochrane Collaboration meta-analysis of six randomized controlled trials

(RCTs) found that pre-endoscopic treatment with a PPI, compared with an H_2-receptor antagonist or placebo significantly reduced the proportion of patients with endoscopic signs of recent bleeding at index endoscopy and reduced the need for endoscopic therapy at index endoscopy. However, there was no effect on clinically important outcomes including mortality, re-bleeding, and the need for surgery [7]. These results have led to diverse recommendations. An international consensus concluded that "Pre-endoscopic PPI therapy may be considered to downstage the endoscopic lesion and decrease the need for endoscopic intervention but should not delay endoscopy" especially when endoscopy is expected to be delayed [4]. On the other hand, the UK guidelines stated that PPIs should not be used prior to endoscopy since "there is no evidence that it alters important clinical outcomes" [5].

Early endoscopy provides the diagnosis, improves risk classification, and allows for early discharge of low-risk patients. If the endoscopy demonstrates an ulcer with high-risk signs for re-bleeding (active bleeding or a non-bleeding visible vessel), endoscopic hemostatic treatment should be applied. This has been shown to reduce mortality, re-bleeding, and the need for surgery [9]. The preferable mode of endoscopic therapy is a combination of injection therapy with 1:10,000 solution of adrenaline with either thermocoagulation or clipping [4,5]. The management of ulcers with non-bleeding adherent clots is less clear. The current standard of practice consists of injecting epinephrine around the base of the clot, cold guillotining the clot with a polypectomy snare, and appropriately treating any underlying lesion [10].

There is strong evidence supporting the administration of PPIs following endoscopic diagnosis of peptic ulcer bleeding. A Cochrane Collaboration meta-analysis of RCTs has shown that this practice, compared to treatment with an H_2RA or placebo, reduced re-bleeding and the need for surgery and repeat endoscopic haemostatic treatment. Post-endoscopic PPI treatment also improved mortality among patients with active bleeding or a non-bleeding visible vessel especially when appropriate endoscopic haemostatic treatment had been applied [11]. High-dose intravenous PPI treatment is currently recommended in patients with peptic ulcer bleeding exhibiting high-risk endoscopic signs (active bleeding, non-bleeding visible vessel, or adherent clot) following endoscopic

Table 5.1 Rockall score

Variable	Score			
	0	1	2	3
Age (years)	<60	60–79	≥80	
Shock	"No shock"	"Tachycardia only"	"Hypotension"	–
Pulse rate (bpm):	<100	≥100	–	
SBP (mmHg):	≥100	≥100	<100	
Comorbidity	No major comorbidity	–	• Cardiac failure, • ischaemic heart disease, or • any major comorbidity	• Renal failure, • liver failure, or • disseminated malignancy
Diagnosis	• Mallory Weiss lesion, or • no lesion and no SRH"	All other diagnoses	Malignant lesions of gastrointestinal tract	–
Major SRH	• none, or • dark spot only	–	• Blood in upper gastrointestinal tract, • adherent clot, or • visible or spurting vessel	–

bpm: beats per minute; SBP: systolic blood pressure; SRH: stigmata of recent haemorrhage

haemostatic treatment [4, 5]. In patients with low-risk endoscopic lesions, high-dose oral PPI seems to be sufficient [11].

NSAIDs, aspirin, clopidogrel and anticoagulants should be discontinued in patients presenting with upper gastrointestinal bleeding, and should be restarted only if a strong indication is documented. NSAIDs can usually be withheld without problems until the ulcer has been healed. The timing for re-administration of aspirin, clopidogrel and/or anticoagulants should be individualized; these agents should be restarted as soon as the gradually decreasing risk for rebleeding is outweighed by the risk for cardiovascular complications for the individual patient, usually in less than 5 days [4,5].

Once the initial bleeding episode has been dealt with, continuation of PPI treatment for a further 4 weeks to ensure complete healing of the ulcer is recommended. All patients with bleeding ulcers should also be tested for *H. pylori* infection and treated appropriately if found to be infected [12,13]. Those requiring long-term treatment with aspirin or an NSAID should be offered co-therapy with either a PPI

or misoprostol to reduce the risks of recurrent ulceration and further episodes of bleeding [14].

Case 2: occult bleeding/anemia

Case presentation

A 72-year-old man presented to his primary care physician complaining of shortness of breath and fatigue. He was found to have hemoglobin of 7g% and microcytosis (mean corpuscular volume (MCV) of 76 fL). He denied any bright red blood per rectum or melena. He had a low serum iron (15 µg/dL), high total iron-binding capacity (436 µg/dL), and low ferritin (8 ng/mL), indicating iron deficiency anemia. He was transfused 2 units of packed red blood cells (RBCs) and his shortness of breath and fatigue improved. His post-transfusion hemoglobin was 9.8 g%. He was started on oral ferrous sulfate and scheduled for outpatient evaluation.

Upper endoscopy demonstrated a small hiatal hernia; small intestinal biopsies were negative for celiac disease. At colonoscopy, he had two small (<5 mm) polyps that were resected and found to be tubular adenomas. He was continued on oral iron and scheduled for a follow-up visit in 6 weeks; at follow-up, his hemoglobin was 8.5 g% with persistent features of iron deficiency.

Questions

• What is the most likely cause of this patient's iron deficiency anemia/obscure occult gastrointestinal bleeding?
• What are the next appropriate diagnostic tests?
• What is the management of this patient?

Differential diagnosis

Iron deficiency anemia is a common finding in elderly people. Even in the absence of GI symptoms, both upper endoscopy and colonoscopy should be performed to look for causes of iron deficiency anemia. Peptic ulcer disease is the most common cause, followed by colon cancer. However, erosive esophagitis has lately been reported as a common cause of both upper GI bleeding and iron deficiency anemia [15]. In the absence of any lesion on endoscopy and no evidence of celiac disease on small bowel biopsies, patients are routinely treated with oral iron therapy to see if the anemia resolves. However, if anemia does not resolve with oral iron therapy, small bowel evaluation is recommended [16].

Obscure GI bleeding (OGIB) comprises approximately 5% of all patients with GI bleeding; most lesions are located in the small intestine. The small bowel lesions causing anemia or occult bleeding can be broadly classified into vascular lesions such as angioectasia (Figure 5.3), inflammatory lesions (Figure 5.4) from Crohn's disease, NSAID enteropathy or celiac disease, and tumors (Figure 5.5). Common small bowel tumors include small bowel adenocarcinoma, lymphoma, carcinoids, and GI stromal tumors [16]. This patient had an absence of celiac disease on duodenal biopsies. The absence of diarrhea and the relatively late age of presentation counter the diagnosis of Crohn's disease – but do not, of course, rule it out. Although he did not present a history of NSAID use, the surreptitious use of NSAIDs – or even low-dose aspirin use for cardiovascular prophylaxis – may cause small bowel enteropathy. The most likely diagnoses in this patient were angioectasia or a small bowel tumor. Angioectasia are the most common cause of blood loss in elderly

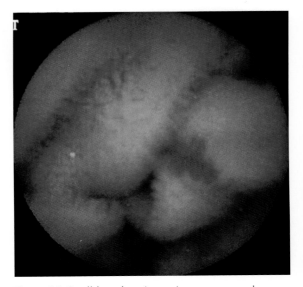

Figure 5.3 Small bowel angioectasia seen on capsule endoscopy.

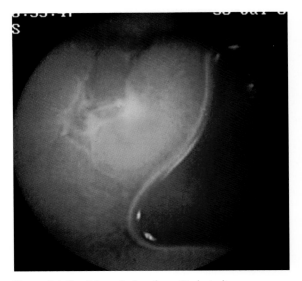

Figure 5.4 Small bowel ulcer from Crohn's disease seen on capsule endoscopy.

people, whereas inflammatory lesions and tumors are more common cause of small intestinal bleeding in younger patients. Although small bowel tumors are more likely to present with overt GI bleeding, they can present with iron deficiency anemia or occult bleeding – especially in elderly people.

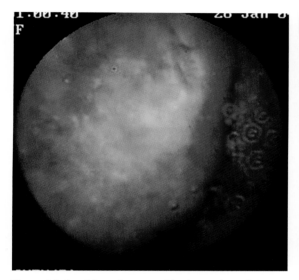

Figure 5.5 Small bowel tumor with ulcerated overlying mucosa seen on capsule endoscopy.

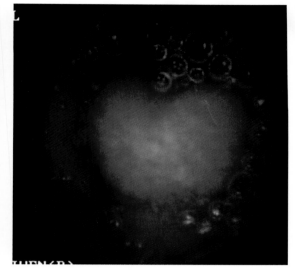

Figure 5.6 Small bowel polypoidal lesion with umblication on capsule endoscopy.

Diagnostic findings and final diagnosis

The patient was referred for a capsule endoscopy which revealed an ulcerated mass lesion in the mid small bowel (Figure 5.6); this was subsequently confirmed on computed tomography enterography (CTE) (Figure 5.7) which found no additional extraintestinal lesions. He underwent surgical resection of the small intestinal mass; histopathology revealed a carcinoid tumor with ulceration (Figure 5.8). He was kept on oral iron therapy postoperatively; his anemia resolved over the next 3 months.

Discussion on patient management

OGIB is defined as bleeding of unknown etiology that persists or recurs after an initial negative colonoscopy and upper endoscopy. OGIB is classified as either overt OGIB, which manifests as recurrent melena or hematochezia, or occult OGIB, which manifests as recurrent or persistent iron deficiency anemia despite iron therapy. Up to10% of all GI bleeding, and almost 90% of obscure GI bleeding is thought to be secondary to a small bowel pathology. Angioectasias are the most common cause of OGIB in elderly people, accounting for 30–40% of bleeding, whereas tumors are the predominant cause in patients aged 30–50 years. NSAID use and small bowel Crohn's disease can both cause ulcers and erosions in the small bowel

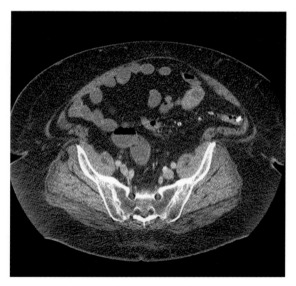

Figure 5.7 Computed tomography enterography shows thickened small bowel wall.

which can lead to GI blood loss. The management of OGIB has evolved significantly since the advent of capsule endoscopy [16].

There are currently three different capsule endoscopy (CE) systems available for clinical use: PillCam (Given Imaging Ltd, Yoqneam, Israel), EndoCam

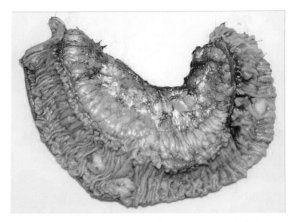

Figure 5.8 Resected small bowel specimen revealed three small bowel carcinoids, two with central umblication and ulceration.

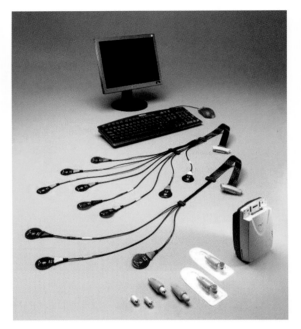

Figure 5.9 The capsule imaging system comprising the capsule endoscope, a data recording device, and a computer workstation.

(Olympus, Tokyo, Japan), and MiroCam (Intromedic, Seoul, Korea). The capsule imaging system comprises three main components: the capsule endoscope, a data-recording device, and a computer workstation (Figure 5.9). The small bowel capsule endoscope measures 11×26 mm. It contains light-emitting diodes as a light source, a lens, a color camera chip, two batteries, a radiofrequency transmitter, and an antenna. The small bowel capsule obtains two or more images/second as it travels passively through the small bowel and transmits these images wirelessly to the data recording device. At the conclusion of the examination, the images are downloaded on to the computer workstation and analyzed by a medical professional [17].

A meta-analysis by Triester et al. evaluated 21 prospective comparative studies of CE in OGIB and found it to have a significantly higher yield than push enteroscopy (54% vs 24%) and small bowel radiography (42% vs 6%) for the diagnosis of a small bowel source of GI bleeding. CE had a higher yield for detection of vascular and inflammatory lesions and tumors compared with other diagnostic modalities [18].

Based on CE findings, further endoscopic evaluation with push or balloon-assisted enteroscopy (BAE) can obtain tissue for histology or be used for endoscopic therapy. Push enteroscopy utilizes a longer endoscope that can be advanced into the jejunum and allows for evaluation of the proximal small bowel beyond the reach of a standard upper endoscope. It can be used to perform diagnostic biopsies and thera-

peutic procedures such as hemostatic therapy and polyp resection in the proximal small bowel. The diagnostic yield of push enteroscopy in patients with OGIB and negative bidirectional endoscopy is approximately 40–65%, resulting in a change in the management of 40–73% of patients. It may also improve clinical outcomes by reducing bleeding and transfusion requirements [17]. BAE is a new endoscopic technology that offers the potential for complete small bowel examination with a bidirectional approach and treatment of previously inaccessible lesions. A meta-analysis comparing BAE and CE reported comparable yield between these two technologies, although BAE afforded the advantages of obtaining biopsies and performing therapy. BAE is complementary to CE for patients with OGIB. As BAE is invasive and less acceptable to patients, it is mostly used as a diagnostic and therapeutic tool after initial CE either finds a lesion or is unrevealing [19]. Prospective large-scale studies are being performed to better define the exact role of BAE in patients with OGIB. Intraoperative enteroscopy is another modality for the evaluation of the small bowel and is performed during open laparotomy or with laparoscopic assistance. Intraoperative enteroscopy is considered the gold standard for complete small bowel evaluation. Its diagnostic yield for identifying a bleeding source is reported to be 70–82%, with therapeutic efficacy in about half of those with a lesion. However, due to its significant morbidity and occasional mortality, intraoperative enteroscopy is the tool of last resort [17].

CTE and magnetic resonance enterography (MRE) are relatively new radiological imaging techniques that can evaluate the small bowel in more detail. Both CTE and MRE can detect small bowel dilation, wall thickening and increased enhancement due to tumor or inflammation. They may also detect extraintestinal lesions and are considered complementary to CE. In particular, these techniques may have a role in the diagnosis, staging, and management of inflammatory bowel disease and small bowel tumors [17].

Conclusion

CE has become the gold standard for the evaluation of the small bowel mucosa in patients with obscure occult GI bleeding or iron deficiency anemia. CE allows for the non-invasive inspection of the entire small bowel and has the highest diagnostic yield for small bowel lesions in patients with OGIB. Based on the results of CE, further diagnostic testing or therapeutic interventions can be recommended.

References

1 Longstreth GF. Epidemiology of hospitalization for acute upper gastrointestinal hemorrhage: a population-based study. *Am J Gastroenterol* 1995;**90**:206–210.
2 Rockall TA, Logan RF, Devlin HB et al. Incidence of and mortality from acute upper gastrointestinal haemorrhage in the United Kingdom. *BMJ* 1995;**311**:222–6.
3 Rockall TA, Logan RF, Devlin HB et al. Risk assessment after acute upper gastrointestinal haemorrhage. *Gut* 1996;**38**:316–21.
4 Barkun AN, Bardou M, Kuipers EJ, et al. International consensus recommendations on the management of patients with nonvariceal upper gastrointestinal bleeding. *Ann Intern Med* 2010;**152**:101–13.
5 Palmer K, Balfour R, Cairns C, et al. Management of acute upper and lower gastrointestinal bleeding. A national clinical guideline. Scottish Intercollegiate Guidelines Network 2008. http://www.sign.ac.uk/pdf/sign105.pdf Assessed Aug 9, 2011.
6 Das A, Wong RC. Prediction of outcome of acute GI hemorrhage: a review of risk scores and predictive models. *Gastrointest Endosc* 2004;**60**:85–93.
7 Sreedharan A, Martin J, Leontiadis GI, et al. Proton pump inhibitor treatment initiated prior to endoscopic diagnosis in upper gastrointestinal bleeding. *Cochrane Database Syst Rev* 2010; (7):CD005415.
8 Hearnshaw SA, Logan RF, Palmer KR, et al. Outcomes following early red blood cell transfusion in acute upper gastrointestinal bleeding. *Aliment Pharmacol Ther* 2010;**32**:215–24.
9 Cook DJ, Guyatt GH, Salena BJ, et al. Endoscopic therapy for acute nonvariceal upper gastrointestinal haemorrhage: a meta-analysis. *Gastroenterology* 1992;**102**:139–48.
10 Kovacs TO, Jensen DM. Endoscopic treatment of ulcer bleeding. *Curr Treat Options Gastroenterol* 2007;**10**:143–8.
11 Leontiadis GI, Sharma VK, Howden CW. Proton pump inhibitor therapy for peptic ulcer bleeding: Cochrane collaboration meta-analysis of randomized controlled trials. *Mayo Clin Proc* 2007;**82**:286–96.
12 Malfertheiner P, Megraud F, O'Morain C, et al. Current concepts in the management of *Helicobacter pylori* infection: the Maastricht III Consensus Report. *Gut* 2007;**56**:772–81.
13 Chey WD, Wong BC, Practice Parameters Committee of the American College of Gastroenterology. American College of Gastroenterology guideline on the management of *Helicobacter pylori* infection. *Am J Gastroenterol* 2007;**102**:1808–25.
14 Leontiadis GI, Sreedharan A, Dorward S, et al. Systematic reviews of the clinical effectiveness and cost-effectiveness of proton pump inhibitors in acute upper gastrointestinal bleeding. *Health Technol Assess* 2007;**11**:iii–iv, 1–164.
15 Rockey DC, Cello JP. Evaluation of the gastrointestinal tract in patients with iron-deficiency anemia. *N Engl J Med* 1993;**329**:1691–5.
16 Leighton JA, Goldstein J, Hirota W, et al. Obscure gastrointestinal bleeding. *Gastrointest Endosc* 2003;**58**:650–55.
17 Li F, Leighton JA, Sharma VK. Capsule endoscopy: a comprehensive review. *Minerva Gastroenterol Dietol* 2007;**53**:257–72.
18 Triester SL, Leighton JA, Leontiadis GI, et al. A meta-analysis of the yield of capsule endoscopy compared to other diagnostic modalities in patients with obscure gastrointestinal bleeding. *Am J Gastroenterol* 2005;**100**:2407–18.
19 Pasha SF, Leighton JA, Das A, et al. Double-balloon enteroscopy and capsule endoscopy have comparable diagnostic yield in small-bowel disease: a meta-analysis. *Clin Gastroenterol Hepatol* 2008;**6**:671–6.

6 Acute Diarrhea and Vomiting

John P. Flaherty and Michael P. Angarone

Division of Infectious Diseases, Northwestern University Feinberg School of Medicine, Chicago, Illinois, USA

Case 1: patient with nausea, vomiting, and diarrhea

Case presentation

A 52-year-old woman presents with diarrhea, nausea, vomiting, and low-grade fever (38.2°C). She is having bowel movements every 30 min. She describes the diarrhea as watery with some mucus, but no blood. She reports rectal urgency and cramping abdominal pain with bowel movements. She works as a nurse in an emergency department observation unit and has had contact with patients with acute gastroenteritis. She denies any recent travel.

Past medical history
Type 1 diabetes; received a pancreas transplant 3 years ago
Chronic anemia
Gastroesophageal reflux disease (GERD)
Dyslipidemia
Hypothyroidism
Previous cholecystectomy

Medications
Mycophenolate mofetil 1 g twice daily
Tacrolimus 2 mg twice daily
Esomeprazole 40 mg orally daily
Levothyroxine 100 μg daily
Aspirin 325 mg daily
Atorvastatin 10 mg daily

Social history
She has no pets
She denies tobacco, alcohol, or illicit drug use

Family history
Irritable bowel syndrome in two of her sisters

Physical examination
Temperature 36.6°C
Blood pressure 130/80 mmHg
Pulse 66 beats/min
Respiratory rate 18/min
O_2 saturation 99% on room air
Alert, oriented; in no acute distress
Heart exam showed a 2/6 systolic flow murmur
Lung exam was clear
Abdominal exam was soft, non-tender, with normal bowel sounds, and no costovertebral angle tenderness
Extremity exam showed no edema

Laboratory results (normal values in brackets)
WBC 1.8 (4–11) × 10^9/L (Neutrophils 52%)
Hemoglobin 9.3 (11.5–16.5) g/dL
Hematocrit 27.9% (38–46)
MCV 87 (78–98) fL
Platelet count 419 (150–400) × 10^9/L
Urinalysis negative
Na^+ 137 (135–145) mmol/L
K^+ 4.0 (3.5–5) mmol/L

Problem-based Approach to Gastroenterology and Hepatology, First Edition. Edited by John N. Plevris, Colin W. Howden.
© 2012 Blackwell Publishing Ltd. Published 2012 by Blackwell Publishing Ltd.

Cl⁻ 111 (98–108) mmol/L
HCO₃⁻ 15 (22–30) mmol/L
Blood urea nitrogen (BUN) 23 (6–21) mg/dL
Creatinine 1.7 (0.5–1.2) µmol/L

She improves clinically with intravenous fluids. Stool samples are obtained for culture, ova and parasites, *Clostridium difficile* toxin assay, and fecal leukocytes; all are negative.

She is readmitted 1 week later with persistent diarrhea – up to 50 watery stools per day and 15 lb (8.3 kg) weight loss. Her nausea, vomiting, and fever have resolved.

Stool culture (x3) ova and parasite exam (x3), giardia and cryptosporidia antigen (x3), microsporidia exam (x3), isospora exam (x3) *C. difficile* toxin assay (x3), *C. difficile* culture, and fecal leukocytes are all negative. Epstein–Barr virus PCR (polymerase chain reaction) and cytomegalovirus PCR assays are negative. Tacrolimus level is 11.1 ng/mL (normal range 6 to 15 ng/ml). EGD and colonoscopy are unremarkable. Random biopsies of the duodenum and stomach are unremarkable. Biopsy of the colon shows edema of the lamina propria and no viral inclusions. Biopsy of the terminal ileum shows focal crypt atrophy.

Norovirus real time (RT)-PCR is positive for subtype G II.

Her immunosuppressive medication dosages are reduced. She is treated with tincture of opium.

Questions

• In patients with acute gastroenteritis, when are additional diagnostic and therapeutic interventions indicated?
• What epidemiological clues suggest particular etiological agents in cases of acute diarrhea?
• Why is norovirus such a common cause of gastroenteritis?
• What diagnostic tests confirm the diagnosis of norovirus gastroenteritis and when are they indicated?
• What is the usual clinical course of norovirus gastroenteritis?

Acute diarrhea and vomiting

Diarrheal illness is a significant cause of morbidity and mortality worldwide. The World Health Organization (WHO) estimated that diarrheal diseases were the fifth leading cause of death worldwide, responsible for 2.2 million deaths (or 3.7% of all deaths) in 2004 [1]. Diarrhea remains the second leading cause of death among children aged <5 globally, causing 1.5 million deaths each year [2]. In the developed world, acute gastroenteritis is a major cause of physician visits and absence from school or work. The Centers for Disease Control and Prevention (CDC) estimated that food-borne illnesses, most of which are associated with acute diarrheal disease, account for 76 million illnesses, 325 000 hospitalizations, and 5000 deaths each year in the USA [3].

Most cases of acute diarrhea are mild and self-limited and do not justify the cost or potential morbidity of diagnostic or therapeutic interventions. Certain indications should prompt further evaluation or treatment, including [4]:
• profuse diarrhea with dehydration
• grossly bloody stools
• high fever
• persistent symptoms >48 h without improvement
• recent antibiotic therapy
• associated severe abdominal pain – especially in older patients – age >70 years
• immune compromise
• new community outbreak of illness.

For patients with acute diarrheal illnesses, it is important to adequately assess the patient's level of hydration and to replace volume losses. Important clues to the level of dehydration include the duration of illness, alertness, skin turgor, mucous membrane dryness, sunken eyes, and postural hypotension. Empiric antimicrobial therapy might be warranted in several settings:
• Severe inflammatory diarrhea (bloody stools, high fever) – except cases of suspected or confirmed enterohemorrhagic *Escherichia coli* (EHEC) in which antibiotic therapy has no established impact on the duration of illness but probably does not increase the risk of hemolytic–uremic syndrome (HUS) [5].
• Moderate or severe diarrhea and a history of recent travel
• In elderly or immunocompromised individuals after recent antimicrobial use [6].

Etiology of acute diarrhea and vomiting

There are a number of epidemiological and clinical clues that may suggest a likely infectious agent.

Epidemiological factors that should be considered include food consumption (e.g. raw, undercooked meats, raw seafood), antibiotic administration (antibiotic-associated diarrhea or *C. difficile* infection), and recent travel (bacterial pathogens such as enterotoxigenic *E, coli*, *Salmonella*, *Shigella*, and *Campylobacter* spp., and protozoa such as *Giardia* sp.). Acute diarrhea in hospitalized patients may be associated with medications or tube feedings, but, in the absence of an outbreak of norovirus infection, *C. difficile* is the only enteric pathogen that merits serious initial consideration. Day care exposure may be associated with outbreaks of norovirus or rotavirus disease, *Shigella*, and *Giardia* spp. Other epidemiological clues include immune deficiency:

- IgA deficiency predisposes to giardiasis
- HIV/AIDS may be associated with *Mycobacterium avium* complex and protozoal (*Cryptosporidium* and *Microsporidium* spp.) infection
- Solid organ transplantation predisposes to cytomegalovirus (CMV) colitis.

Clinical features can also be used to identify the infectious agent. Bloody diarrhea is associated with shiga toxin-producing *E. coli*, *Shigella*, and *Entamoeba histolytica* infections. Dysentery is associated with *Shigella* and *Campylobacter* infection. Malabsorption and weight loss are associated with Giardia infection.

Stool cultures should be obtained on initial presentation in immunocompromised patients (HIV-infected, elderly, patients with comorbidities or underlying inflammatory bowel disease), those with severe or bloody diarrhea, and food handlers. Sending stool samples for ova and parasites is not cost-effective for most patients with acute diarrhea; consider testing those with persistent diarrhea, men who have sex with men, during a community waterborne outbreaks (associated with *Giardia* and *Cryptosporidium* spp.), or those with bloody diarrhea and a history of travel to an area endemic for *Entamoeba histolytica*.

Norovirus gastroenteritis

Norovirus is a leading cause of gastroenteritis – responsible for 23–60% of the illness burden caused by known enteric pathogens and half of all gastroenteritis outbreaks [7–9]. Norovirus has been estimated to cause 23 million infections annually in the USA [3].

The success of norovirus as a human pathogen may be credited to:
- A low infectious dose
- Prolonged asymptomatic shedding after recovery from the acute illness
- The virus's ability to persist in the environment
- Tremendous genotypic and phenotypic diversity and limited immunological cross-protection.

Norovirus is spread easily – 10–100 virions are enough to infect a healthy adult [10]. Secondary attack rates among close contacts and family members are up to 30%. Most transmission occurs via fecal–oral spread but airborne dispersion is an important route of dissemination in some cases – particularly when an index case is vomiting nearby [11,12]. Virus can be shed in low titers for up to 8 weeks in healthy people – long after clinical recovery [13,14] – and for more than a year in immunocompromised individuals [15]. Norovirus persists in the environment – on surfaces, in water, and on food over a range of temperatures (0–60°C) – for 3–4 weeks, and is relatively resistant to many commonly used disinfectants [16]. The lay term "gastric flu" has often been applied to norovirus gastroenteritis and, although considered a misnomer by physicians, there is an important parallel between influenza virus and norovirus. Both are single-stranded RNA viruses that undergo frequent mutation, resulting in antigenic shift and recurring epidemics, and periodic recombination events, resulting in the evolution of new strains and occasional pandemics. This evolution is driven by immune selective pressure [17–19].

Acute infection with noroviruses produces a reversible histopathological lesion in the jejunum characterized by blunting of the villi and monocytic and neutrophilic infiltrates in the lamina propria [20–22]. On electron microscopy, the epithelial cells are intact, microvilli shortened, and the intercellular spaces widened. Norovirus gastroenteritis is associated with transient malabsorption of D-xylose and fat and decreased activity of brush-border enzymes including alkaline phosphatase and trehalase, but the precise mechanisms of the norovirus diarrhea remain unknown [23].

Norovirus infection is generally mild and self-limited but can be severe and sometimes fatal in vulnerable populations, including young children and elderly people. The availability of more reliable diagnostic testing has confirmed that norovirus may be a cause of significant morbidity in highly immunosuppressed individuals [15,24,25]. In a case series of 12 allogeneic hemopoietic stem cell transplant recipients, norovirus was associated with persistent diarrhea and weight loss [24]. In 10 patients, diarrhea persisted for a median of 3 months.

Severe consequences including acute renal failure, arrhythmias and acute graft rejection have been reported in 8.3% of transplant recipients with norovirus infection [26]. Traditionally, norovirus gastroenteritis has been diagnosed clinically:

• Vomiting in most cases
• An incubation period of 24–48 hours
• A median illness of 12–60 hours
• Negative stool culture [27].

However, the signs and symptoms of illness are not sufficiently characteristic to enable a diagnosis to be made on clinical grounds alone. Laboratory testing for norovirus is not routinely available to most clinicians and electron microscopy and ELISA (enzyme-linked immunosorbent assay) tests have been relatively insensitive. RT-PCR has significantly improved the sensitivity of testing but availability remains limited [28,29]. The indications for diagnostic testing with RT-PCR will expand as the test becomes more widely available and less costly. Unfortunately, there is no specific antiviral therapy for norovirus infection and treatment is limited to supportive care, particularly replacement of volume losses.

Case 2: patient with fever, vomiting and diarrhea post-chemotherapy

Case presentation

A 51-year-old woman with a history of colorectal cancer presents with complaints of fevers, nausea, vomiting, and diarrhea. She recently completed a cycle of chemotherapy comprising folinic acid, oxaliplatin, and 5-fluorouracil 2 days before presentation and had received a dose of 5-fluorouracil on the afternoon of presentation. She reports multiple episodes of watery diarrhea, at least 10 bowel movements in the past 6 hours. She denies any blood in the stool or any melena. She reports diffuse, cramping abdominal pain relieved with bowel movements, nausea, and three episodes of non-bloody, bilious emesis. Fevers developed on the morning of presentation. Other associated symptoms are fatigue, lightheadedness without loss of consciousness, anorexia, and weak-

ness. She was last treated with an antibiotic (moxifloxacin) 6 weeks ago for a possible pneumonia. She has had episodes of diarrhea and nausea with prior cycles of chemotherapy, lasting 12–24 h.

Past medical history
Hypertension, hyperlipidemia, GERD, colorectal cancer with liver metastases

Medications
Metoprolol, lorazepam, tolterodine, lansoprazole, vitamin B complex

Social history
Former employee at a nuclear power plant
Quit tobacco 4 years ago, has a 20 pack-year history
She does not drink alcohol or use illicit drugs

Physical examination
Temperature 38.4°C
Blood pressure 126/78 mmHg
Heart rate 126 beats/min
Somnolent, thin female (150–420)
Oral cavity with dry mucous membranes
Heart with tachycardia, regular rhythm, no murmurs
Lungs clear to auscultation
Abdomen diffusely tender throughout, no guarding, no distension, hyperactive bowel sounds, no masses, no hepatomegaly
Extremities without edema or cyanosis

Laboratory results (normal values in brackets)
WBC 17.4 (4–11) $\times 10^9$/L
Hemoglobin 12.3 (11.5–16.5) g/dL
Platelets 57 (150–420) $\times 10^9$/L
BUN 12 (6–21) mg/dL
Creatinine 1.0 (0.5–1.2) μmol/L
CT scan of the abdomen and pelvis shows colonic wall thickening and edema extending from the hepatic flexure to the rectum. Multiple liver metastases are stable in appearance.

Microbiology
Stool culture, ova and parasite exam are negative; C. *difficile* toxin assay is positive.

Treatment
Treatment is initiated with metronidazole 500 mg orally four times a day for 14 days. Over the next 3

days the diarrhea and nausea resolve. Approximately 2 weeks after completion of the metronidazole, the diarrhea and fevers recur. Stool testing is again positive for C. difficile toxin. A second course of metronidazole is started and her diarrhea resolves. One week after completing the metronidazole, diarrhea recurs again and stool assay is once more positive for C. difficile toxin. She is treated with oral vancomycin 125 mg every 6 h for 14 days, followed by a prolonged dose taper. Following completion of the vancomycin taper, her diarrhea does not recur.

Questions

1. What are the current epidemiology and pathophysiology of C. difficile infection?
2. What are the risk factors for C. difficile infection?
3. What diagnostic tests are indicated for C. difficile infection?
4. What are the most effective available therapies for C. difficile infection?
5. What are the risk factors for recurrent C. difficile infection?
6. What treatment is appropriate for recurrent C. difficile infection?

Epidemiology and pathophysiology of C. difficile infection

C. difficile infection is currently the most common cause of hospital-acquired infectious diarrhea in North America and Europe. Since 2000 there has been a 25% increase in the incidence of C. difficile infection every year [30–35]. Furthermore, the severity of illness related to C. difficile infection has increased substantially in the past decade. C. difficile infection has transformed from a nuisance to a potentially life-threatening illness with an attributable mortality rate of up to 16.7% [35]. This change is largely the result of the emergence of a hypervirulent stain of C. difficile: the restriction-endonuclease analysis group BI, North American pulsed-field gel electrophoresis type 1 (BI/NAP-1) strain. C. difficile produces diarrhea through the actions of two toxins (toxins A and B), which cause colonic cell death and inflammation [36,37]. The BI/NAP-1 strain of C. difficile produces >10-fold more toxin in vitro than historical control strains, which may explain the increased severity of illness [38,39]. The diarrhea that results from infection ranges from mild, watery diarrhea to fulminant colitis with toxic megacolon [30].

C. difficile infection accounts for 15–25% of all cases of antibiotic-associated diarrhea (AAD) [40]. Other causes of AAD have been linked to infection with other enteric pathogens (e.g. C. perfringens and Staphylococcus aureus), drug effects on gastrointestinal motility (e.g. erythromycin and amoxicillin–clavulanate), and reduction of the normal anaerobic microflora resulting in decreased absorption of carbohydrates [40]. The diarrhea of C. difficile infection typically occurs during or shortly after receipt of an antibiotic, but may be delayed by weeks. In mild-to-moderate disease the only symptom is watery, foul-smelling stools. Patients may experience up to 10 or more bowel movements a day. Other clinical findings include fever, abdominal cramps, and leukocytosis [41,42]. Severe disease is signified by the presence of nausea and vomiting, dehydration, and lethargy. The lack of stool passage may be a sign of paralytic ileus which may progress to toxic megacolon [30,41]. Endoscopic examination of the colon may reveal pseudomembranous colitis [41].

Risk factors for C. difficile infection

The risk of developing C. difficile infection depends on acquisition of a toxigenic strain of C. difficile and antibiotic exposure, and is further influenced by particular host factors such as age and immune status. Hospitalization is a prime risk factor for the development of C. difficile infection. The prevalence of C. difficile spores in the hospital environment is relatively high and higher rates of colonization have been found in hospitalized individuals (10–25%) when compared with the general population (2–3%) [43–45]. Elderly patients and those with impaired immune responses are at substantially higher risk for developing C. difficile infection [30,46]. Other factors that may contribute to the development of C. difficile infection include underlying comorbidity, non-surgical gastrointestinal (GI) procedures, the use of acid-suppressing medicines (especially proton pump inhibitors), and admission to an intensive care unit (ICU) [47,48].

The most significant risk factor for the development of C. difficile infection is exposure to antibiotics or other agents that disrupt the normal colonic micro-flora. The indigenous microflora of the colon provides an important defense against *C. difficile* and other intestinal pathogens, providing so-called "coloniza-tion resistance," which can be disrupted by antibiot-ics, inflammation, or cytotoxic chemotherapy [36]. Essentially every antibiotic has been associated with *C. difficile* infection [47]. The intrinsic resistance of *C. difficile* to a broad range of antibiotic agents gives the organism a unique survival advantage. Fluoroquinolones have become a major risk factor for *C. difficile* infection, especially the BI/NAP-1 epi-demic strain which shows a much higher rate of resistance to these agents [38].

Cytotoxic chemotherapeutic agents may lead to infection with *C. difficile* in the absence of antibio-tic exposure. Most chemotherapeutic agents cause mitotic arrest of colonic epithelial cells, which results in necrosis, inflammation, and desquamation of mucous membranes [49]. This damage to the colonic surface may lead to an environment that is suitable for the growth of *C. difficile*. These agents may also alter the colonic microflora, in a manner similar to antibiotics, which may enhance the growth of *C. dif-ficile* [49]. The chemotherapy agents that are most frequently associated with *C. difficile* infection are cisplatin, 5-fluorouracil, and doxorubicin [49].

Diagnostic tests for *C. difficile* infection

The clinical diagnosis of *C. difficile* infection is based on the findings of diarrhea, fever, abdominal pain, and leukocytosis during or after treatment with antibiotics. Confirmation of the diagnosis is based on the identification of *C. difficile* toxin in stool or the recovery of a toxin-producing strain of *C. dif-ficile* from stool [36]. Culture for *C. difficile* is highly sensitive, but cannot distinguish between toxigenic and non-toxigenic strains [30]. The gold standard for *C. difficile* infection testing has been the cell cyto-toxicity assay which can detect picogram levels of toxin and is very specific, with a moderate sensitiv-ity (about 85%) [50,51]. The long turnaround time of at least 24 h is the limiting factor for this testing method.

Direct testing for *C. difficile* toxin is available through the use of enzyme immunoassay (EIA). Most current EIAs test for both toxin A and toxin B. These tests have the advantage of a rapid turnaround time (between 1 and 2 h) and high specificity, but typically have low sensitivity [30]. The sensitivity and the nega-tive predictive value of these tests can be increased with testing of multiple stool specimens, with one study demonstrating an increase in sensitivity from 72% with the first stool to 84% with the second stool [52].

Newer testing methods aim at improving sensitivity of toxin detection, shortening turnaround time, and limiting laboratory resources. The common antigen, or glutamate dehydrogenase (GDH), is an enzyme that is produced by *C. difficile* and is easily detectable by EIA with a sensitivity ranging from 96% to 100% [53,54]. Testing for GDH quickly identifies the presence of *C. difficile* with accuracy similar to stool culture. However, similar to culture, it cannot distinguish toxigenic from non-toxigenic strains [53,54]. The GDH assay is commonly paired with either the cytotoxic assay or the toxin EIA to detect *C. difficile* toxin. In this two-step protocol, stool specimens that are positive for GDH are further tested with a cytotoxic assay or toxin EIA; GDH-negative stools are considered *C. difficile* negative [30]. This approach reduces the number of specimens tested, reduces total cost, and increases the diagnostic accuracy of the specific toxin assays [53,54].

The future of *C. difficile* diagnosis lies in the use of RT-PCR amplification of *C. difficile* specific genes. Currently available commercial assays utilize the toxin B gene (*tcdB*) to identify the presence of toxi-genic *C. difficile* in stool specimens [55–59]. RT-PCR of the *tcdB* gene has been compared with standard testing methods and has demonstrated a higher sen-sitivity, faster turnaround time, and specificity equal to cell culture cytotoxin assays [55]. Widespread use of the RT-PCR is limited by availability and expense. The RT-PCR assay may be combined with the screen-ing GDH assay to limit cost [56]. RT-PCR testing can provide early confirmation of *C. difficile* infection which can facilitate early and appropriate patient management.

Treatment of *C. difficile* infection

Treatment of *C. difficile* infection involves the discon-tinuation, if possible, of the offending antimicrobial agent and initiating therapy directed at *C. difficile* once the diagnosis is suspected. The most frequently used and studied agents for therapy of *C. difficile* infection are oral vancomycin and metronidazole. Metronidazole is considered the initial treatment of choice for mild-to-moderate *C. difficile* infection and achieves bactericidal levels in the colon. However, as diarrhea improves, the colonic levels of metronidazole decrease [60]. The standard dose of metronidazole therapy is 500 mg orally given three times a day or 250 mg orally four times a day for 10–14 days [61] (Table 6.1). Clinical trial data comparing metronidazole and vancomycin have typically demonstrated equivalent efficacy [62–64]. However, recent reports have described increased failure rates of metronidazole compared with vancomycin in the treatment of *C. difficile* infection [65,66].

Oral vancomycin was until recently the only US Food and Drug Administration (FDA)-approved treatment for *C. difficile* infection [61]. Oral vancomycin achieves high concentrations within the lumen of the colon with minimal systemic absorption [67]. Standard dosing of vancomycin is 125 mg orally four times a day for 10–14 days [61]. The efficacy of oral vancomycin has been demonstrated in multiple trials, with a cure rate of 94–100% and relapse rate of 6–11% [62–64]. In a recent randomized clinical trial, treatment with vancomycin was superior to metronidazole in the treatment of severe *C. difficile* infection, with cure rates of 97% and 76% respectively (*P* = 0.02) [64].

In 2011, the US FDA approved the macrocyclic antibiotic fidaxomicin for the treatment of *C. difficile* infection. Fidaxomicin is more active against *C. difficile* than vancomycin (by a factor of 8), has a prolonged postantibiotic effect, and demonstrates minimal systemic absorption and minimal impact on the colonic microbiota. Fidaxomicin has been shown to be non-inferior to vancomycin for the treatment of *C. difficile* infection with a significantly lower rate of recurrence [68]. The role of fidaxomicin in the treatment of *C. difficile* infection is undefined, but this agent appears promising and merits consideration, particularly in patients with recurrent disease.

A growing subset of patients with *C. difficile* infection may progress to fulminant disease characterized by sepsis, septic shock, and toxic megacolon [69]. Emergency colectomy may be lifesaving in this situation. A retrospective, cohort study of 165 cases of *C. difficile* infection who required ICU admission or prolongation of ICU stay reported that 87 (53%) cases

Table 6.1 Suggested treatment for *Clostridium difficile* Infection

Disease severity	Therapy
Mild to-moderate disease[a]	Metronidazole 500 mg every 8 h, 10–14 days, or
	Metronidazole 250 mg every 6 h, 10–14 days, or
	Vancomycin 125 mg every 6 h, 10–14 days
	Fidaxomicin 200 mg every 12 h, 10 days
Severe disease[b]	Vancomycin 125–250 mg every 6 h, 10–14 days
Fulminant colitis or toxic megacolon	Vancomycin 125–250 mg every 6 h orally +
	Metronidazole 500 mg every 6 h intravenously
	Consider IVIG
	Consider emergency colectomy
First recurrence	Repeat initial regimen as above (metronidazole or vancomycin)
Second recurrence	Oral vancomycin taper and/or pulsed dose
	125 mg every 6 h for 14 days, then 125 mg twice a day for 1 week, then 125 mg daily for 1 week, then 125 mg every 2 days for 8 days, then 125 mg every 3 days for 15 days
Third (or more) recurrence	Vancomycin 125 mg every 6 h for 14 days, followed by:
	Rifaximin 400 mg twice daily for 14 days, or
	Nitazoxanide 500 mg twice a day for 10 days, or
	IVIG, or
	Fecal reconstitution therapy
	Probiotics (*S. boulardii*, *Lactobacillus* species)

[a]Mild-to-moderate disease defined as not meeting the definition of severe disease.
[b]Severe disease defined as two or more of the following: age >60 years, temperature >101°F (38.3°C), albumin level <2.5 mg/dL or peripheral WBC count >15 000 cells/mm^3. (From Zar [64].)

resulted in death within 30 days of ICU admission, 44% within 48 h. Independent predictors of 30-day mortality were [70]:

- leukocytosis $\geq 50\,000/mm^3$
- lactate $\geq 5\,mmol/L$
- age ≥ 75 years
- immunosuppression
- shock requiring vasopressors.

After adjustment for these confounders, patients who had emergency colectomy were less likely to die than those treated medically. Patients with *C. difficile* infection and marked leukocytosis or early septic shock should be considered for emergent colectomy.

Risks for recurrent *C. difficile* infection

Recurrent *C. difficile* infection results from relapse of endogenous infection or re-infection with a new strain of *C. difficile* [71]. Recurrence typically occurs within 2 weeks of discontinuing therapy, but may occur as long as 3 months after stopping therapy [36]. Symptomatic recurrence is seen in approximately 20% of those treated with vancomycin or metronidazole [72]. Given the high rate of recurrence, recurrent disease should be presumed when a patient with recently treated *C. difficile* infection presents with diarrhea.

The major risk factors for recurrent *C. difficile* infection are similar to the risk factors for a first episode of *C. difficile* infection and include [73]:

- continued use of a non-*C. difficile* active antibiotic
- age ≥ 65 years
- the use of acid-suppressing medicines.

Impaired immunity against *C. difficile* toxins and persistent disruption of the colonic microflora may also play a role in recurrent *C. difficile* infection. Patients with recurrent *C. difficile* infection have been found to have lower levels of toxin A-specific IgG and IgA [39,46.] This poor immune response may allow for their delayed clearance and continued activity of the toxins. The fecal microflora in individuals with recurrent *C. difficile* infection has been shown to have decreased diversity, altered variability of bacterial phylotypes, and a predominance of *C. difficile* in the microbial community [74]. This decreased diversity of the colonic microflora may allow for the continued propagation of *C. difficile*.

Treatment of recurrent *C. difficile* infection

Despite the high frequency of recurrent *C. difficile* infection, treatment remains a challenge. There are no controlled trials comparing treatment strategies and recommendations are based on case series and expert opinion. The first recurrence of *C. difficile* infection can be treated with a repeat course of vancomycin or metronidazole for 10–14 days and discontinuation when possible of any potentially inciting antibiotics [71,75]. Subsequent recurrences are more difficult to treat and often require prolonged therapy. A third recurrence is often treated with vancomycin, given as a taper, as pulsed dose or a combination of taper and pulsed dose (see Table 6.1) [71,75]. Most treatment recommendations favor some combination of vancomycin taper and/or pulsed dose treatment for a third (or more) recurrence, but these recommendations are based on clinical experience rather than controlled clinical trials [36,61,71,75].

Alternative treatment options for recurrence have included rifaximin, nitazoxanide, probiotics, fecal reconstitution, and intravenous immune globulin (IVIG) (see Table 6.1). Rifaximin has been shown to reduce subsequent recurrences in *C. difficile* infection in a small observational study when given after completion of vancomycin therapy [76]. A limiting factor to rifaximin use has been the rapid development of resistance [50]. The anti-anaerobic antibiotic nitazoxanide has also been effective in the treatment of recurrent *C. difficile* infection after metronidazole therapy [77]. Probiotics, such as *Saccharomyces boulardii* and *Lactobacillus* spp., are postulated to repopulate the colonic microflora and help restore colonization resistance. Placebo-controlled trials of *S. boulardii* combined with vancomycin have demonstrated inconsistent efficacy in recurrent *C. difficile* infection [78,79]. Clinical data are similarly variable for *Lactobacillus* supplementation. However, recent studies have demonstrated a significant decrease in the incidence of first occurrence of *C. difficile* infection with the prophylactic use of a *Lactobacillus* probiotic in patients on antibiotic therapy [80].

A more radical approach to reconstitution of colonic microflora is the use of fecal reconstitution therapy, or fecal transplantation. Feces collected from a healthy donor are homogenized and filtered and the filtrate is then instilled via a nasogastric tube or enema into the GI tract of the recipient [81,82]. In a case series of 16 patients with two or more episodes of C. difficile infection treated with fecal reconstitution, only one recurrence was noted after a single treatment [80]. Self-administered fecal transplantation via an enema was 100% effective in preventing recurrent C. difficile infection in one clinical trial [82].

Passive immunization with IVIG has been used to enhance the immune clearance of C. difficile toxins. A retrospective review of severe, refractory, recurrent C. difficile infection reported that 9 (64%) of 14 patients responded when IVIG 150–400 mg/kg was added to vancomycin therapy [83]. A phase 2 trial of humanized monoclonal antibody to toxin A and toxin B demonstrated decreased recurrence rates when combined with vancomycin or metronidazole [84].

References

1 World Health Organization. *The Global Burden of Disease: 2004 Update.* Geneva: WHO, 2009.

2 World Health Organization/UNICEF. *WHO/UNICEF Joint Statement: Clinical management of acute diarrhoea.* New York: UNICEF, 2004. Available at: www.afro.who.int/cah/documents/intervention/acute_diarrhoea_joint_statement.pdf. accessed March 15, 2010.

3 Mead PS, Slutsker L, Dietz V, et al. Food-related illness and death in the United States. *Emerg Infect Dis* 1999;5:607–25.

4 Goodgame R. A Bayesian approach to acute infectious diarrhea in adults. *Gastroenterol Clin North Am* 2006;35:249–73.

5 Safdar N, Said A, Gangnon RE, Maki DG. Risk of hemolytic uremic syndrome after antibiotic treatment of *Escherichia coli* O157:H7 enteritis: a meta-analysis. *JAMA* 2002;288:996–1001.

6 Guerrant RL, Van Gilder T, Steiner TS, et al. Practice guidelines for the management of infectious diarrhea. *Clin Infect Dis* 2001;32:331–51.

7 Chia JW, Hsu LY, Chai LY, Tambyah PA. Epidemiology and outcomes of community-onset methicillin-susceptible *Staphylococcus aureus* bacteraemia in a university hospital in Singapore. *BMC Infect Dis* 2008;8:14.

8 Said MA, Perl TM, Sears CL. Healthcare epidemiology: gastrointestinal flu: norovirus in health care and long-term care facilities. *Clin Infect Dis* 2008;47:1202–8.

9 Fankhauser RL, Noel JS, Monroe SS, Ando T, Glass RI. Molecular epidemiology of "Norwalk-like viruses" in

outbreaks of gastroenteritis in the United States. *J Infect Dis* 1998;178:1571–8.

10 Teunis PF, Moe CL, Liu P, et al. Norwalk virus: how infectious is it? *J Med Virol* 2008;80:1468–76.

11 Sawyer LA, Murphy JJ, Kaplan JE, et al. 25- to 30-nm virus particle associated with a hospital outbreak of acute gastroenteritis with evidence for airborne transmission. *Am J Epidemiol* 1988;127:1261–71.

12 Marks PJ, Vipond IB, Carlisle D, Deakin D, Fey RE, Caul EO. Evidence for airborne transmission of Norwalk-like virus (NLV) in a hotel restaurant. *Epidemiol Infect* 2000;124:481–7.

13 Chan MC, Sung JJ, Lam RK, et al. Fecal viral load and norovirus-associated gastroenteritis. *Emerg Infect Dis* 2006;12:1278–80.

14 Patel MM, Widdowson MA, Glass RI, Akazawa K, Vinje J, Parashar UD. Systematic literature review of role of noroviruses in sporadic gastroenteritis. *Emerg Infect Dis* 2008;14:1224–31.

15 Kaufman SS, Chatterjee NK, Fuschino ME, et al. Characteristics of human calicivirus enteritis in intestinal transplant recipients. *J Pediatr Gastroenterol Nutr* 2005;40:328–33.

16 Johnston CP, Qiu H, Ticehurst JR, et al. Outbreak management and implications of a nosocomial norovirus outbreak. *Clin Infect Dis* 2007;45:534–40.

17 Ambert-Balay K, Bon F, Le Guyader F, Pothier P, Kohli E. Characterization of new recombinant noroviruses. *J Clin Microbiol* 2005;43:5179–86.

18 Nilsson M, Hedlund KO, Thorhagen M, et al. Evolution of human calicivirus RNA in vivo: accumulation of mutations in the protruding P2 domain of the capsid leads to structural changes and possibly a new phenotype. *J Virol* 2003;77:13117–24.

19 Etherington GJ, Dicks J, Roberts IN. High throughput sequence analysis reveals hitherto unreported recombination in the genus Norovirus. *Virology* 2006;345:88–95.

20 Agus SG, Dolin R, Wyatt RG, Tousimis AJ, Northrup RS. Acute infectious nonbacterial gastroenteritis: intestinal histopathology. Histologic and enzymatic alterations during illness produced by the Norwalk agent in man. *Ann Intern Med* 1973;79:18–25.

21 Schreiber DS, Blacklow NR, Trier JS. The small intestinal lesion induced by Hawaii agent acute infectious nonbacterial gastroenteritis. *J Infect Dis* 1974;129:705–8.

22 Schreiber DS, Blacklow NR, Trier JS. The mucosal lesion of the proximal small intestine in acute infectious nonbacterial gastroenteritis. *N Engl J Med* 1973;288:1318–23.

23 Navaneethan U, Giannella RA. Mechanisms of infectious diarrhea. *Nat Clin Pract Gastroenterol Hepatol* 2008;5:637–47.

24 Roddie C, Paul JP, Benjamin R, et al. Allogeneic hematopoietic stem cell transplantation and norovirus gastroenteritis: a previously unrecognized cause of morbidity. *Clin Infect Dis* 2009;**49**:1061–8.

25 Westhoff TH, Vergoulidou M, Loddenkemper C, et al. Chronic norovirus infection in renal transplant recipients. *Nephrol Dial Transplant* 2009;**24**:1051–3.

26 Mattner F, Sohr D, Heim A, Gastmeier P, Vennema H, Koopmans M. Risk groups for clinical complications of norovirus infections: an outbreak investigation. *Clin Microbiol Infect* 2006;**12**:69–74.

27 Kaplan JE, Feldman R, Campbell DS, Lookabaugh C, Gary GW. The frequency of a Norwalk-like pattern of illness in outbreaks of acute gastroenteritis. *Am J Public Health* 1982;**72**:1329–32.

28 Trujillo AA, McCaustland KA, Zheng DP, et al. Use of TaqMan real-time reverse transcription-PCR for rapid detection, quantification, and typing of norovirus. *J Clin Microbiol* 2006;**44**:1405–12.

29 Pang XL, Preiksaitis JK, Lee B. Multiplex real time RT-PCR for the detection and quantitation of norovirus genogroups I and II in patients with acute gastroenteritis. *J Clin Virol* 2005;**33**:168–71.

30 Bartlett JG, Gerding DN. Clinical recognition and diagnosis of *Clostridium difficile* infection. *Clin Infect Dis* 2008;**46**(suppl 1):S12–18.

31 Loo VG, Poirier L, Miller MA, et al. A predominantly clonal multi-institutional outbreak of *Clostridium difficile*-associated diarrhea with high morbidity and mortality. *N Engl J Med* 2005;**353**:2442–9.

32 Lyytikainen O, Turunen H, Sund R, et al. Hospitalizations and deaths associated with *Clostridium difficile* infection, Finland, 1996–2004. *Emerg Infect Dis* 2009;**15**:761–5.

33 McDonald LC, Owings M, Jernigan DB. *Clostridium difficile* infection in patients discharged from US short-stay hospitals, 1996–2003. *Emerg Infect Dis* 2006;**12**:409–15.

34 Pepin J, Saheb N, Coulombe MA, et al. Emergence of fluoroquinolones as the predominant risk factor for *Clostridium difficile*-associated diarrhea: a cohort study during an epidemic in Quebec. *Clin Infect Dis* 2005;**41**:1254–60.

35 Pepin J, Valiquette L, Cossette B. Mortality attributable to nosocomial *Clostridium difficile*-associated disease during an epidemic caused by a hypervirulent strain in Quebec. *Can Med Assoc J* 2005;**173**:1037–42.

36 Kelly CP. A 76-year-old man with recurrent *Clostridium difficile*-associated diarrhea: review of C. difficile infection. *JAMA* 2009;**301**:954–62.

37 Reineke J, Tenzer S, Rupnik M, et al. Autocatalytic cleavage of *Clostridium difficile* toxin B. *Nature* 2007;**446**:415–19.

38 McDonald LC, Killgore GE, Thompson A, et al. An epidemic, toxin gene-variant strain of *Clostridium difficile*. *N Engl J Med* 2005;**353**:2433–41.

39 Warny M, Pepin J, Fang A, et al. Toxin production by an emerging strain of *Clostridium difficile* associated with outbreaks of severe disease in North America and Europe. *Lancet* 2005;**366**:1079–84.

40 Bartlett JG. Clinical practice. Antibiotic-associated diarrhea. *N Engl J Med* 2002;**346**:334–9.

41 Mogg GA, Keighley MR, Burdon DW, et al. Antibiotic-associated colitis – a review of 66 cases. *Br J Surg* 1979;**66**:738–42.

42 Bartlett JG, Taylor NS, Chang T, Dzink J. Clinical and laboratory observations in *Clostridium difficile* colitis. *Am J Clin Nutr* 1980;**33**(11 suppl):2521–6.

43 Bartlett JG. *Clostridium difficile*: history of its role as an enteric pathogen and the current state of knowledge about the organism. *Clin Infect Dis* 1994;**18**(suppl 4):S265–72.

44 McFarland LV, Mulligan ME, Kwok RY, Stamm WE. Nosocomial acquisition of *Clostridium difficile* infection. *N Engl J Med* 1989;**320**:204–10.

45 Simor AE, Bradley SF, Strausbaugh LJ, Crossley K, Nicolle LE. *Clostridium difficile* in long-term-care facilities for the elderly. *Infect Control Hosp Epidemiol* 2002;**23**:696–703.

46 Kyne L, Warny M, Qamar A, Kelly CP. Asymptomatic carriage of *Clostridium difficile* and serum levels of IgG antibody against toxin A. *N Engl J Med* 2000;**342**:390–7.

47 Bignardi GE. Risk factors for Clostridium difficile infection. *J Hosp Infect* 1998;**40**:1–15.

48 Pant C, Madonia P, Minocha A. Does PPI therapy predispose to *Clostridium difficile* infection? Nat *Rev Gastroenterol Hepatol* 2009;**6**:555–7.

49 Kamthan AG, Bruckner HW, Hirschman SZ, Agus SG. *Clostridium difficile* diarrhea induced by cancer chemotherapy. *Arch Intern Med* 1992;**152**:1715–17.

50 O'Connor JR, Galang MA, Sambol SP, et al. Rifampin and rifaximin resistance in clinical isolates of *Clostridium difficile*. *Antimicrob Agents Chemother* 2008;**52**:2813–17.

51 Turgeon DK, Novicki TJ, Quick J, et al. Six rapid tests for direct detection of *Clostridium difficile* and its toxins in fecal samples compared with the fibroblast cytotoxicity assay. *J Clin Microbiol* 2003;**41**:667–70.

52 Manabe YC, Vinetz JM, Moore RD, Merz C, Charache P, Bartlett JG. *Clostridium difficile* colitis: an efficient clinical approach to diagnosis. *Ann Intern Med* 1995;**123**:835–40.

53 Crobach MJ, Dekkers OM, Wilcox MH, Kuijper EJ. European Society of Clinical Microbiology and Infectious Diseases (ESCMID): data review and recommendations

for diagnosing *Clostridium difficile*-infection (CDI). *Clin Microbiol Infect* 2009;**15**:1053–66.

54 Ticehurst JR, Aird DZ, Dam LM, Borek AP, Hargrove JT, Carroll KC. Effective detection of toxigenic *Clostridium difficile* by a two-step algorithm including tests for antigen and cytotoxin. *J Clin Microbiol* 2006;**44**:1145–9.

55 Eastwood K, Else P, Charlett A, Wilcox M. Comparison of nine commercially available Clostridium difficile toxin detection assays, a real-time PCR assay for *C. difficile* tcdB, and a glutamate dehydrogenase detection assay to cytotoxin testing and cytotoxigenic culture methods. *J Clin Microbiol* 2009;**47**:3211–17.

56 Goldenberg SD, Cliff PR, Smith S, Milner M, French GL. Two-step glutamate dehydrogenase antigen real-time polymerase chain reaction assay for detection of toxigenic *Clostridium difficile*. *J Hosp Infect* 2010;**74**:48–54.

57 Kvach EJ, Ferguson D, Riska PF, Landry ML. Comparison of BD GeneOhm Cdiff real-time PCR assay with a two-step algorithm and a toxin A/B enzyme-linked immunosorbent assay for diagnosis of toxigenic *Clostridium difficile* infection. *J Clin Microbiol* 2010;**48**:109–14.

58 Larson AM, Fung AM, Fang FC. Evaluation of tcdB real-time PCR in a three-step diagnostic algorithm for detection of toxigenic *Clostridium difficile*. *J Clin Microbiol* 2010;**48**:124–30.

59 Novak-Weekley SM, Marlowe EM, Miller JM, et al. *Clostridium difficile* testing in the clinical laboratory by use of multiple testing algorithms. *J Clin Microbiol* 2010;**48**:889–93.

60 Bolton RP, Culshaw MA. Faecal metronidazole concentrations during oral and intravenous therapy for antibiotic associated colitis due to *Clostridium difficile*. *Gut* 1986;**27**:1169–72.

61 Gerding DN, Muto CA, Owens RC Jr. Treatment of *Clostridium difficile* infection. *Clin Infect Dis* 2008;**46**(suppl 1):S32–42.

62 Teasley DG, Gerding DN, Olson MM, et al. Prospective randomised trial of metronidazole versus vancomycin for *Clostridium difficile*-associated diarrhoea and colitis. *Lancet* 1983;ii:1043–6.

63 Wenisch C, Parschalk B, Hasenhundl M, Hirschl AM, Graninger W. Comparison of vancomycin, teicoplanin, metronidazole, and fusidic acid for the treatment of *Clostridium difficile*-associated diarrhea. *Clin Infect Dis* 1996;**22**:813–18.

64 Zar FA, Bakkanagari SR, Moorthi KM, Davis MB. A comparison of vancomycin and metronidazole for the treatment of *Clostridium difficile*-associated diarrhea, stratified by disease severity. *Clin Infect Dis* 2007;**45**:302–7.

65 Musher DM, Aslam S, Logan N, et al. Relatively poor outcome after treatment of *Clostridium difficile* colitis with metronidazole. *Clin Infect Dis* 2005;**40**:1586–90.

66 Pepin J, Alary ME, Valiquette L, et al. Increasing risk of relapse after treatment of *Clostridium difficile* colitis in Quebec, Canada. *Clin Infect Dis* 2005;**40**:1591–7.

67 Young GP, Ward PB, Bayley N, et al. Antibiotic-associated colitis due to *Clostridium difficile*: double-blind comparison of vancomycin with bacitracin. *Gastroenterology* 1985;**89**:1038–45.

68 Louie TJ, Miller MA, Mullane KM, Weiss K, Lentnek A, Golan Y, Gorbach S, Sears P, Shue YK; OPT-80-003 Clinical Study Group. Fidaxomicin *versus* vancomycin for *Clostridium difficile* infection. *N Engl J Med.* 2011 Feb 3;**364**(5):422–31. PubMed PMID: 21288078.)

69 Dallal RM, Harbrecht BG, Boujoukas AJ, et al. Fulminant *Clostridium difficile*: an underappreciated and increasing cause of death and complications. *Ann Surg* 2002;**235**:363–72.

70 Lamontagne F, Labbe AC, Haeck O, et al. Impact of emergency colectomy on survival of patients with fulminant *Clostridium difficile* colitis during an epidemic caused by a hypervirulent strain. *Ann Surg* 2007;**245**:267–72.

71 Johnson S. Recurrent *Clostridium difficile* infection: a review of risk factors, treatments, and outcomes. *J Infect* 2009;**58**:403–10.

72 Aslam S, Hamill RJ, Musher DM. Treatment of *Clostridium difficile*-associated disease: old therapies and new strategies. *Lancet Infect Dis* 2005;**5**:549–57.

73 Garey KW, Sethi S, Yadav Y, DuPont HL. Meta-analysis to assess risk factors for recurrent *Clostridium difficile* infection. *J Hosp Infect* 2008;**70**:298–304.

74 Chang JY, Antonopoulos DA, Kalra A, et al. Decreased diversity of the fecal Microbiome in recurrent *Clostridium difficile*-associated diarrhea. *J Infect Dis* 2008;**197**:435–8.

75 Kelly CP, LaMont JT. Clostridium difficile – more difficult than ever. *N Engl J Med* 2008;**359**:1932–40.

76 Johnson S, Schriever C, Galang M, Kelly CP, Gerding DN. Interruption of recurrent *Clostridium difficile*-associated diarrhea episodes by serial therapy with vancomycin and rifaximin. *Clin Infect Dis* 2007;**44**:846–8.

77 Musher DM, Logan N, Hamill RJ, et al. Nitazoxanide for the treatment of *Clostridium difficile* colitis. *Clin Infect Dis* 2006;**43**:421–7.

78 McFarland LV, Surawicz CM, Greenberg RN, et al. A randomized placebo-controlled trial of Saccharomyces boulardii in combination with standard antibiotics for *Clostridium difficile* disease. *JAMA* 1994;**271**:1913–18.

79 Surawicz CM, McFarland LV, Greenberg RN, et al. The search for a better treatment for recurrent Clostridium difficile disease: use of high-dose vancomycin combined with *Saccharomyces boulardii*. *Clin Infect Dis* 2000;**31**:1012–17.

80 Gao XW, Mubasher M, Fang CY, Reifer C, Miller LE. Dose-response efficacy of a proprietary probiotic formula of *Lactobacillus acidophilus* CL1285 and *Lactobacillus casei* LBC80R for antibiotic-associated diarrhea and *Clostridium difficile*-associated diarrhea prophylaxis in adult patients. *Am J Gastroenterol* 2010;**105**:1636–41.

81 Aas J, Gessert CE, Bakken JS. Recurrent *Clostridium difficile* colitis: case series involving 18 patients treated with donor stool administered via a nasogastric tube. *Clin Infect Dis* 2003;**36**:580–5.

82 Silverman MS, Davis I, Pillai DR. Success of Self-administered home fecal transplantation for chronic *Clostridium difficile* infection. *Clin Gastroenterol Hepatol* 2010;**8**:471–3.

83 McPherson S, Rees CJ, Ellis R, Soo S, Panter SJ. Intravenous immunoglobulin for the treatment of severe, refractory, and recurrent *Clostridium difficile* diarrhea. *Dis Colon Rectum* 2006;**49**:640–5.

84 Lowy I, Molrine DC, Leav BA, et al. Treatment with monoclonal antibodies against Clostridium difficile toxins. *N Engl J Med* 2010;**362**:197–205.

7

Chronic Diarrhea and Malabsorption

Paul Beck, Remo Panaccione, and Subrata Ghosh

Division of Gastroenterology, University of Calgary, Alberta, Canada

Case 1: diarrhea and anemia

Case presentation

A 35-year-old woman presented with lethargy and increasing feeling of weakness. She had lost approximately 3 kg in weight over the past year. Her food intake was unchanged. She had no dyspeptic symptoms or vomiting. Her bowel habits were unchanged and she generally opened her bowels three to four times a day, with many of the bowel movements being somewhat loose. She felt bloated with some cramping abdominal pain, relieved by defecation. Five years ago she was diagnosed as having irritable bowel syndrome. She had recurrent mouth ulcerations. She described palpitations but no chest pain. She has a son aged 12 years, but had two miscarriages subsequently. Her menstrual periods were described as normal. One year ago she had to be treated with antibiotics for a lung infection. There was no relevant family history.

Examination

On examination she appeared somewhat pale, with a body mass index of 19. She also had angular stomatitis. Her pulse was irregular with a variable rate of around 112 beats/min. Her blood pressure was 154/82 mmHg. Abdominal examination was unremarkable and heart sounds suggested atrial fibrillation with no murmurs.

Laboratory investigations

Laboratory results showed (normal values in brackets):
Hb 9.1 (11.5–16.5) g/dL
Urea 3.8 (2.5–6.5) mmol/L
MCV 76 (78–98) fL
Creatinine 82 (50–120) mmol/L
WCC 4.8 (4–11) × 10^9/L
Platelets 310 (150–420) × 10^9/L
Sodium 139 (135–145) mmol/L
Potassium 4.8 (3.5–5.0) mmol/L
Albumin 34 (35–55) g/L
Calcium 2.14 (2.10–2.55) mmol/L
ESR 28 mm/h
CRP 0.6 (0.2–1.0) mg/dL
Ferritin: 12 (20–250) μg/L
Transferrin saturation 14 (22–40)%
Liver function tests – normal
Thyroid function tests – TSH 0.11 (0.17–3.2) mU/L
T_4 24.3 (11–22) pmol/L
Vitamin B_{12} 150 (155–800) pmol/L
Red cell folate 250 (360–1400) nmol/L
Vitamin (25-OH) D 74 (80–200) nmol/L

Questions

• What is the differential diagnosis of iron deficiency anemia?
• What is the optimal strategy to investigate her symptoms?

Problem-based Approach to Gastroenterology and Hepatology, First Edition. Edited by John N. Plevris, Colin W. Howden.
© 2012 Blackwell Publishing Ltd. Published 2012 by Blackwell Publishing Ltd.

Table 7.1 Common causes of iron deficiency anemia

Category	Causes	Investigation
Low iron intake	Poor appetite	Endoscopy
	Depression	Assessment for depression
	Strict vegan	Dietary assessment
Malabsorption	Celiac disease	Anti-TTG antibody
	Small bowel Crohn's disease	Colonoscopy + TI biopsy
		Small bowel radiology
		SBCE
		Deep enteroscopy + biopsy
Increased iron loss	Peptic ulcer Gastric/esophageal cancers	Endoscopy
	Colon cancer	Colonoscopy
	Menstrual blood loss	Gynecologic evaluation
	Inflammatory bowel disease	Colonoscopy + biopsy
		Small bowel radiology
		SBCE
		Deep enteroscopy + biopsy
	NSAID enteropathy	Small bowel radiology
		SBCE
	Intestinal vascular lesions	Colonoscopy ± SBCE
		Mesenteric angiography
		Deep enteroscopy (therapeutic)
	Hematuria	Abdominal/renal ultrasound
		Urologic evaluation

NSAID, non-steroidal anti-inflammatory drug; TTG, tissue transglutaminase; TI, terminal ileum; SBCE, small bowel capsule endoscopy.

• What is the explanation of associated symptoms such as palpitation?

Differential diagnosis

Iron deficiency anemia in a woman in her mid-30s may be caused by a number of different conditions [1]. These may be categorized as intestinal and extraintestinal causes (Table 7.1).

Chronic blood loss is the most common etiology of iron deficiency anemia, but may not be associated with a history of overt bleeding noticed by the patient. These patients are investigated by endoscopic examinations of the upper and lower intestinal tracts. Wireless capsule endoscopy has emerged as the best investigation of the small intestine for a cause of chronic blood loss. Intestinal vascular lesions may sometimes require selective mesenteric angiography. Malabsorption may be diagnosed by a combination of imaging and biochemical investigations such as 3-day fecal fat excretion, abnormal oral D-xylose test, small intestinal radiology (computed tomography [CT] enterography, magnetic resonance [MR] enterography, small bowel enteroclysis), IgA anti-tissue transglutaminase antibody, and IgA anti-endomysial antibody. Other organic causes of chronic blood loss such as gynecological causes and renal carcinoma may require abdominal and pelvic ultrasonography and a CT scan.

The association of diarrhea with iron deficiency anemia and vitamin and trace element deficiency would strongly suggest intestinal malabsorption. Malabsorption leads to an increased 3-day fecal fat if the patient is on an adequate fat intake. Other tests for fat malabsorption would include octanoic acid breath test. Malabsorption leads to osmotic diarrhea calculated as fecal osmolality being at least 50 mosmol/L greater than fecal $(Na^+ + K^+) \times 2$. The cause of malabsorption is detected by systematic investigation of the small intestine especially to exclude celiac disease and small intestinal Crohn's disease, the two most common causes in the west. Systemic effects of malabsorption may be detected by a DEXA (dual energy X-ray absorptiometry) bone scan showing osteopenia or osteoporosis (vitamin D and calcium malabsorption), abnormal coagulation tests (due to vitamin K malabsorption), abnormal nerve conduction studies confirming peripheral neuropathy (vitamin B_{12} deficiency), and megaloblasts in the bone marrow (due to folate and/or vitamin B_{12} malabsorption).

Palpitations may be associated with anemia or may be a manifestation of the irregularly irregular pulse of atrial fibrillation. The latter can be a manifestation of thyrotoxicosis. Autoimmune thyroid disease may be associated with celiac disease.

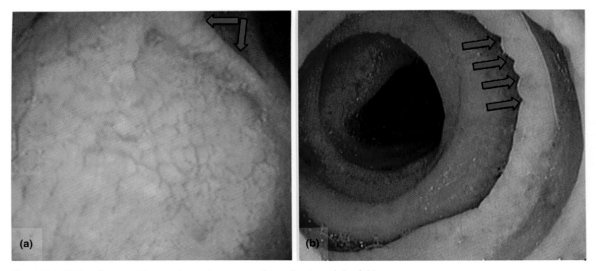

Figure 7.1 Celiac disease: (a) typical mosaic pattern; (b) scalloping of the folds.

Diagnosis

Her investigations demonstrated a raised IgA anti-tissue transglutaminase antibody. This has a specificity and sensitivity for detection of celiac disease of over 95%. This is negative in IgA deficiency, which may be associated with celiac disease. The diagnosis is confirmed by biopsy of the small intestine (duodenum, generally second part), showing villous atrophy, crypt hyperplasia, increased intraepithelial lymphocytes, and abnormal cuboidal appearance of intestinal epithelial cells (Figures 7.1 and 7.2). Some of the symptoms of irritable bowel syndrome such as bloating may be common in celiac disease [2].

Celiac disease is common in the west and increasingly diagnosed in other parts of the world such as north India and the Middle East. The prevalence may be as high as 1 in 100 to 1 in 250. It is rare in African–Caribbean, Japanese, or Chinese individuals [3].

A number of autoimmune disorders is associated with celiac disease and this association is genetic. This includes type 1 diabetes mellitus, autoimmune thyroid disease (as in this patient's case), and autoimmune liver disease. Her ECG showed atrial fibrillation, and she had folate deficiency as well as borderline vitamin B_{12} deficiency. In celiac disease folate and vitamin D deficiencies are common.

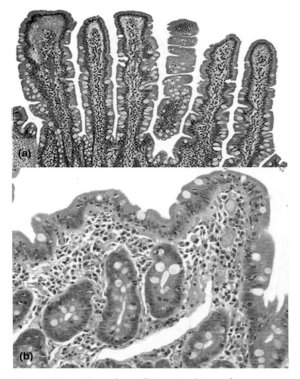

Figure 7.2 (a) Normal, small intestine biopsy for comparison; (b) celiac – subtotal villous atrophy: biopsy from patient (image courtesy of Dr B Langdale-Brown).

Management

The patient went on a strict gluten-free diet, as well as iron and folic acid supplementation. The key management strategies include consultation with a skilled dietician, education about the disease, and lifelong adherence to a gluten-free diet. Rarely, in refractory celiac disease, corticosteroids or immunosuppressive drugs such as azathioprine may be necessary [3]. Disease control may be assessed by repeating the IgA anti-tissue transglutaminase antibody. Her thyroid disease was controlled with β blockers for symptomatic control of atrial fibrillation followed by radio-iodine therapy.

Discussion

Celiac disease commonly presents as iron deficiency anemia. The prevalence of celiac disease in symptomatic iron deficiency anemia is 10–15% and in asymptomatic iron deficiency anemia 3–6% [4]. The classic presentation with malabsorption is now less common, but some biochemical evidence of malabsorption and diarrhea are often present. HLA-DQ2 and HLA-DQ8 haplotypes are strongly associated with celiac disease. Concordance for celiac disease in first-degree relatives ranges between 8% and 18% and may be as high as 70% in monozygotic twins. Clinical presentation may be strikingly variable and asymptomatic celiac disease detected by screening serology may be seven times more common than symptomatic disease. Apart from anemia, osteopenia, hyposplenism, elevated liver enzymes, amenorrhea, infertility, peripheral neuropathy, and muscle weakness may be present. More patients are diagnosed in adult life than in childhood. Celiac disease is a model for immunological disease with a defined environmental trigger. Gluten (prolamins and glutenins) from wheat, rye, barley, and wheat, rye and barley drive a gliadin-specific complex T-cell response; in addition an increase in intraepithelial T lymphocytes, crypt hyperplasia, and villous atrophy followed by total mucosal atrophy characterize stages of celiac disease pathology.

Abdominal discomfort and bloating are common symptoms often leading to a mistaken diagnosis of irritable bowel syndrome. Malabsorption is rarely investigated with fecal fat and D-xylose tests, which are relatively crude tests that are prone to errors. IgA anti-tissue transglutaminase and IgA anti-endomysial antibody tests are now widely available and used in patients presenting with anemia, diarrhea, or irritable bowel syndrome-like symptoms. Microscopic colitis and collagenous colitis may be associated and responsible for watery diarrhea. Down syndrome and a wide range of autoimmune diseases, such as dermatitis herpetiformis, type 1 diabetes mellitus, autoimmune thyroid disease, microscopic colitis, primary biliary cirrhosis, IgA mesangial nephropathy may be associated with celiac disease. Intestinal T-cell lymphoma, small intestinal adenocarcinoma and esophageal squamous cell carcinoma may be associated with celiac disease.

Case 2: abdominal pain, diarrhea and weight loss

Case presentation

A 29-year-old sales representative presented with a 3-month history of ill health, malaise, increasing abdominal pain and distension, diarrhea, and weight loss of approximately 4 kg over 6 months. His bowels opened seven to eight times a day with intermittent rectal bleeding. His appetite was poor. He felt nauseated but never vomited. He felt feverish and described joint pain and stiffness in his upper and lower limbs. His symptoms commenced a month after returning from a holiday in the Dominican Republic. However, he described that he had not been feeling well for the past year.

His past medical history included an appendectomy aged 14 years and a fracture of the forearm after a skiing accident aged 25 years. He smoked 10–15 cigarettes a day. His illness resulted in him losing his job because he was frequently absent.

There was no relevant family history. The patient was using loperamide intermittently to control the diarrhea and organic yogurts containing probiotics. He used naproxen for abdominal pain.

Examination

The patient appeared pale and unwell. His body mass index was 18.5. He had a few aphthous ulcers in his mouth. There was no evidence of joint swelling. His abdomen was tender to palpate, especially in the right lower quadrant. The abdomen was not distended and the bowel sounds were normal. No masses were palpable. The perianal area was normal on inspection.

His laboratory investigations showed (normal values in brackets):

Hb 12.1 (13.5–17.5) g/dL
Urea 3.0 (2.5–6.5) mmol/L
MCV 72 (76–98) fL
WCC 12.8 (4–11) × 10^9/L
Platelets 510 (150–420) × 10^9/L
Sodium 138 (135–145) mmol/L
Potassium 4.2 (3.5–5.0) mmol/L
Creatinine 86 (50–120) mmol/L
Albumin 32 (35–55) g/L
Calcium 2.12 (2.10–2.55) mmol/L
ESR 38 mm/h
CRP 12.8 (0.2–1.0) mg/dL
Ferritin 280 (20–250) μg/L
Transferrin saturation: 14 (22–40)%
Liver function tests – normal
Thyroid function tests – TSH 1.22 (0.17–3.2) mU/L
T_4 14.2 (11–22) pmol/L
Vitamin B_{12} 130 (155–800) pmol/L
Red cell folate 350 (360–1400) nmol/L
Vitamin (25-OH) D 92 (80–200) nmol/L

A plain abdominal radiograph was normal. Abdominal ultrasonography showed thickened loops of intestine in the right lower quadrant of abdomen. A colonoscopy showed patchy ulcerations in the sigmoid and transverse colon with longitudinal fissuring ulcerations (Figure 7.3). Biopsies showed chronic inflammatory infiltrate and non-caseating granulomas (Figure 7.4).

Questions

- What is the differential diagnosis?
- What further investigations will be useful?
- What initial treatment should be considered?
- What long-term management goals should be pursued?

Differential diagnosis

A history of 3 months' diarrhea and abdominal pain makes infection unlikely. Most enteric infections settle within 2 weeks. Box 7.1 shows infective causes of diarrhea and abdominal pain that may be protracted.

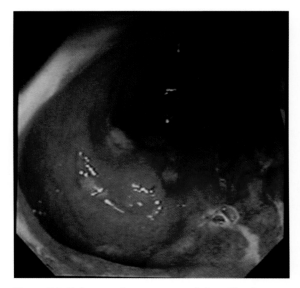

Figure 7.3 Colonoscopic appearance of sigmoid colon with deep fissuring ulceration, cobblestoning, and areas of normal looking mucosa.

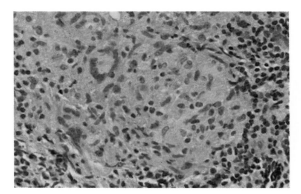

Figure 7.4 Non-caseating granuloma in biopsy.

Enteric infections may be associated with arthralgia and arthritis (Reiter's syndrome). Opportunistic infections with cryptosporidia, microsporidia, cryptococci, cyclospora, and cytomegalovirus occur in transplant recipients, patients on immunosuppressive drugs and in HIV/AIDS. Whipple's disease is a rare multisystem infection with *Tropheryma whipplei*. Apart from the above conditions, diarrhea and abdominal pain lasting for 3 months or more would generally exclude infective causes.

Box 7.1 Infective causes of long-standing diarrhea and abdominal pain

Chronic infections

Intestinal tuberculosis	History of travel or residence
Intestinal schistosomiasis	
Giardiasis	
Amebiasis	
Yersiniosis	

Opportunistic infections

Acquired immune deficiency syndrome	Sexual history, drug abuse
Immunosuppressive drugs	Immunosuppressive drugs

Antibiotic-associated diarrhea

Clostridium difficile	Antibiotic exposure

Whipple's disease

Tropheryma whipplei infection

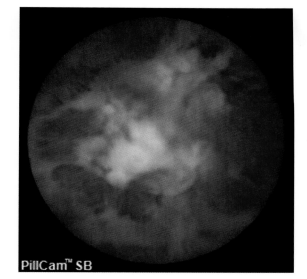
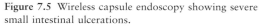

Figure 7.5 Wireless capsule endoscopy showing severe small intestinal ulcerations.

Celiac disease may present with diarrhea but significant abdominal pain is unusual. Inflammatory parameters are generally normal in celiac disease, although the platelet count may be raised due to hyposplenism. Inflammatory bowel disease (ulcerative colitis and Crohn's disease) may be associated with weight loss, diarrhea, abdominal pain, and arthralgia/arthritis. Neoplastic causes would be unusual at this age but include lymphoma, carcinoma, and metastatic disease affecting the small intestine.

The demonstration of patchy fissuring ulcerations and histological demonstration of non-caseating granuloma strongly suggest the diagnosis of Crohn's disease. It is therefore important to characterize the disease anatomically in detail. Therefore the patient should be considered for small intestinal radiology – barium follow-through/small bowel enteroclysis is increasingly replaced by cross-sectional imaging such as CT enterography or MR enterography. The latter investigations are more accurate at picking up intestinal wall thickening, local fistulae, abscess, or collection and activity of the disease. In some centers, contrast-enhanced abdominal ultrasonography may give similar information, but is more operator-dependent. Superficial mucosal ulcerations in the small intestine may be accurately demonstrated by wireless capsule endoscopy, although this is contraindicated in the presence of a history of intestinal obstructive symptoms.

Diagnosis

The diagnosis of Crohn's disease was further established by wireless capsule endoscopy which demonstrated extensive distal small intestinal ulceration in two segments of the ileum (Figure 7.5). MR enterography demonstrated a long (45 cm) ulcerated segment of distal ileum with local fistula tracts, as well as a skip lesion more proximally in the ileum affecting approximately 30 cm. The distal intestine was grossly thickened but no abscess cavity could be identified. The presence of extensive and patchy ulcerations of both small and large intestine, associated with mouth ulcers and arthralgia, granulomas in the biopsy from the colon, and raised systemic markers of inflammation make the diagnosis of Crohn's disease virtually certain, although, rarely, intestinal tuberculosis may mimic such a distribution of Crohn's disease.

Initial management

The patient was started on vitamin B_{12} supplementation and oral folate. 5-aminosalicylic acid (5-ASA) preparations are generally ineffective in Crohn's disease. The patient had several predictors of poor outcome including his smoking status, relatively young age of onset, extensive small and large intestinal involvement, and local fistula tracts from the small intestine. Therefore the patient was started on prednisolone 40 mg/day orally and azathioprine 2 mg/kg body weight. After 4 weeks of steroid therapy, the patient continued to feel unwell with abdominal pain and diarrheal stools five times a day. Repeat colonoscopy showed persistent ulceration in the colon which appeared more extensive than at initial colonoscopy. As induction therapy with prednisolone was considered a failure, alternative induction therapy with infliximab 5 mg/kg i.v. was given at 0, 2, and 6 weeks. This produced a dramatic response and prednisolone could be tapered off after 10 weeks. The patient continued on azathioprine 2 mg/kg daily orally and infliximab 5 mg/kg i.v. every 8 weeks as long-term therapy.

Patient management

Emerging evidence supports changing our current paradigm to reflect a more aggressive approach. This involves use of early immunosuppressive therapy with azathioprine, 6-mercaptopurine, or methotrexate immediately on diagnosis, combined with biologic treatment using anti-tumor necrosis factor (TNF) therapy. A key benefit of this earlier, aggressive therapy algorithm is increased rates of mucosal healing, with the potential for less complications and surgery along the disease course. Although, in the short term, mucosal healing does not appear to correspond closely with clinical remission as measured by the Crohn's disease activity index (CDAI) [5], it is gaining favor as a treatment goal because it has been associated with more durable long-term remission and reduced rates of surgery [6].

Beaugerie et al. performed a study to identify the factors that, when present at diagnosis, predicted a 5-year disabling disease course [7]. These factors are: age <40 years, the presence of perianal disease, and an initial requirement for steroids. The positive predictive value (PPV) of disabling disease in patients with two and three predictive factors of disabling disease was 91% and 93%, respectively, and the presence of even one high-risk factor had a PPV of approximately 60%. However, the definition of disabling disease in this study was not clearly focused on complications and surgery. In clinical practice several other features are often considered to indicate unfavorable disease course, such as complex perianal disease, extensive jejunoileal disease, severe extensive colitis, and continuing smoking.

The benefits of early immunosuppressive therapy were shown in a pediatric study [8]. In this pediatric study, patients received a tapering dose of corticosteroid and concomitant 6-mercaptopurine or placebo within 8 weeks of initial diagnosis. Only 9% of the remitters in the 6-mercaptopurine group relapsed compared with 47% of the placebo group during 18 months of treatment. This strategy was widely adopted by pediatric gastroenterologists.

The effects of very early intervention with anti-TNF therapy are evident in the results of the REACH trial of children with Crohn's disease with a mean disease duration of 1.6 years. Responders to induction therapy with infliximab were randomized to maintenance treatment every 8 or 12 weeks. At 54 weeks, remission was achieved in 56% of patients receiving infliximab every 8 weeks [9]. Although the populations are divergent in many respects, adults with a median disease duration of >7 years in the ACCENT I study had a much lower 54-week remission rate of 30% [6].

Similarly, early treatment benefits have been demonstrated with certolizumab in PRECiSE 2 and adalimumab in the CHARM study. Subanalyses of these studies confirmed that disease duration (<2 years) had a statistically significant effect on remission, such that the highest remission rates were observed in patients with the shortest disease duration ($P = 0.002$) [10,11].

The healing benefits of early anti-TNF treatment were demonstrated most dramatically in the "step-up top-down" (SUTD) study. Patients had newly diagnosed (<4 years), active Crohn's disease (CDAI >200) not previously treated with steroids or immunosuppressive agents. Most were included in the study at diagnosis. Investigators compared the standard step-up treatment from steroids with immunosuppressants and then infliximab, with a top-down treatment approach starting with infliximab plus immunosuppressive agents (azathioprine, methotrexate) for their ability to induce and maintain remission [12]. In this study infliximab was given as a three-dose induction therapy followed by episodic administration on relapse.

Symptom response was similar between the two groups at 2 years. However, an endoscopic substudy of 44 patients (24 top-down and 20 step-up treatment patients), performed at 2 years to compare with baseline findings, observed complete ulcer disappearance in 73% of the patients who received top-down treatment and in 30% of the patients who received step-up treatment ($P = 0.003$) [12]. Remission also occurred earlier in the top-down treatment group. The top-down group had fewer relapses over 2 years. Thus, early initiation of infliximab therapy was associated with higher rates of mucosal healing, which may permit improved long-term outcomes.

Biologic dual therapy is important and likely to provide the strongest form of induction therapy with the highest maintenance of remission. Immunosuppressive therapy along with a biologic not only prevents antibody formation and associated loss of efficacy, but may also enhance clinical efficacy via separate pathways. In the GETAID study, steroid-dependent patients achieved a higher rate of steroid-free remission with the combination of infliximab and azathioprine compared with azathioprine alone [13].

Biologic dual therapy is mandatory and indisputable if the biologic is taken intermittently (episodic) [6]. Given compliance and insurance issues, this may occur more often than physicians think. The use of biologic dual therapy if the biologic is taken on a regular basis (scheduled) is more controversial (see below). Subgroup analysis of the ACCENT I and II, CHARM, and PRECISE 1 and 2 studies have not shown dual therapy to be superior to anti-TNF monotherapy.

The removal of azathioprine concomitant treatment from infliximab-treated children because of the extremely rare hepatosplenic T-cell lymphoma [14] may have been counterproductive; any small gain in safety may have been completely counterbalanced by increased immunogenicity and decreased efficacy. In the IMID study, Van Assche et al. noted that continuation of immunosuppressants beyond 6 months offered no clear benefit over scheduled infliximab monotherapy [15]. Nevertheless, the study was too

underpowered and too short term to reach this conclusion. Infliximab monotherapy appeared to be as effective as infliximab plus a concomitant immunomodulator in maintaining remission in patients with Crohn's disease at 2 years. However, infliximab monotherapy was associated with lower median and trough serum infliximab levels and a higher incidence of antibodies to infliximab. The effects of long-term biologic monotherapy with infliximab have yet to be determined.

Biologic triple therapy – corticosteroid tapering off over 12 weeks plus an immunosuppressive agent plus infliximab for induction, then followed by biologic dual therapy – may result in higher induction of remission rates and higher maintenance of remission rates. The Canadian COMMIT trial incorporated such an approach in the initial induction phase. In this trial, patients with active Crohn's disease who required steroids due to a disease flare were randomized to treatment with infliximab plus methotrexate or infliximab alone. Patients were assessed at 1 year for the primary endpoint of treatment failure (failure to enter prednisone-free remission [CDAI < 150] at week 14 or failure to maintain remission through week 50). Induction and maintenance of remission and the ability to taper steroids was similar, with infliximab alone and infliximab combined with the immunomodulator [16]. It is important to note that this study design used biologic triple therapy for induction (steroids, infliximab in all plus methotrexate or placebo) followed by biologic dual therapy for maintenance. Remission rates at the end of 1 year were near 70%, a rate much higher than had ever been seen previously in biologic clinical trials.

In the international SONIC trial, patients with active Crohn's disease being placed on azathioprine treatment for the first time were randomized to receive infliximab alone or infliximab and azathioprine combination or azathioprine alone. The primary end point was corticosteroid-free remission at week 26. The patients in the combination arm of the study had a higher remission rate (57%) compared with the infliximab alone group (45%). Similar improvements were seen with mucosal healing [17]. Most importantly the azathioprine monotherapy arm fared the worst, with only a 17% mucosal healing rate at week 26 associated with a 31% clinical remission rate.

To summarize, based on current evidence, and until further research permits development of a new consensus, clinicians might consider the following approach to treating Crohn's disease.

• Patients at low risk could be treated with one tapering dose of corticosteroids, given that 40% will achieve a long-term sustained remission.

• Patients in the high-risk category, or low-risk patients with a second disease flare within a year should receive immunosuppressive therapy with the tapering corticosteroid at the time of "first diagnosis or second flare-up."

• Patients who cannot taper corticosteroids despite immunosuppressive therapy should be treated with a biologic to achieve remission. Increasingly monotherapy with azathioprine is considered inadequate and combination of azathioprine and anti-TNF considered optimum approach.

Patients should be reassessed regularly and at structured time intervals to determine whether a particular therapy has been effective and should be continued, or whether a therapy should be abandoned and new therapies implemented or added to meet the defined treatment goals in inflammatory bowel disease.

Certain patients, such as those with complex perianal disease, extensive jejunoileal Crohn's disease, and severe pediatric Crohn's disease with growth retardation, may be considered for top-down therapy with a biologic agent from presentation.

In addition, new data presented recently suggest that infliximab given postoperatively after ileal resection may be considerably superior to placebo in preventing significant endoscopic recurrence which may be associated with clinical recurrence [18]. This is another example of starting really early during the "natural" history of the disease with anti-TNF, in this case a defined start point of a disease-free state after ileal resection.

In summary, when infliximab became available for therapy, it was used as third line after corticosteroids and immunomodulator therapies, often in an episodic fashion. It soon became clear that this was a highly immunogenic and suboptimal regimen and scheduled maintenance therapy with anti-TNF became the standard. The GETAID trial and the SONIC trial have now clearly made the case for infliximab to be used as second-line therapy after failure of steroids in combination with immunomodulator drugs. In addition the COMMIT trial has also shown that combination induction therapy with infliximab and corticosteroids (with or without methotrexate) may result in very high induction efficacy, which may translate into better long-term efficacy than the initial pivotal trials such as ACCENT I trial. In addition, the SUTD study suggested that even earlier therapy with infliximab and azathioprine may provide the best mucosal healing with the potential for altering the disease course. These strategy studies now are defining better positioning of anti-TNF therapy and have led to the recognition of the limitations of azathioprine. In future, more precise identification of those with a more aggressive disease course may permit earlier intervention of biologic agents to alter the disease course long term. This will almost certainly require a panel of markers, genetic, serologic, inflammatory parameters, and phenotypic subclassification.

Case 3: diarrhea in a patient with type 1 diabetes

Case presentation

A 17-year-old girl diagnosed with type 1 diabetes mellitus a year ago presented with episodes of watery, non-bloody diarrhea and urgency for 6 months. She gave no history of abdominal pain and her weight had stabilized after commencement on insulin. Her diabetic control posed difficulties in the start with a few hypoglycemic episodes, but her glycemic control was more stable in the last few months.

Her physical examination was unremarkable. There was no evidence of peripheral neuropathy. Her blood pressure was 110/68 mmHg with no postural drop and a pulse rate of 74 beats/min. She herself had commenced a gluten-free diet which did not help her diarrhea.

Laboratory investigations were as follows (normal values in brackets):

Hb 14.2 (11.5–16.5) g/dL
Urea 4.2 (2.5–6.5) mmol/L
MCV 84 (76–98) fL
Creatinine 74 (50–120) mmol/L
WCC 10.8 (4–11) × 10^9/L
Platelets 324 (150–420) × 10^9/l
Sodium 140 (135–145) mmol/L
Potassium 3.8 (3.5–5.0) mmol/L
Albumin 38 (35–55) g/L

Calcium 2.18 (2.10–2.55) mmol/L
ESR 12 mm/h
CRP 1.1 (0.2–1.0) mg/dL
Ferritin 210 (20–250) µg/L
Hemoglobin A1c 6.6 (4.3–6.1)%
Transferrin saturation 26 (22–40)%
Magnesium 0.90 (0.65–1.05) mmol/L
Liver function tests – normal
Thyroid function tests – TSH 0.23 (0.17–3.2) mU/L
T_4 19.2 (11–22) pmol/L
Vitamin B_{12} 438 (155–800) pmol/L
Red cell folate 750 (360–1400) nmol/L
Vitamin (25-OH) D 102 (80–200) nmol/L

Questions

• What is the differential diagnosis of diarrhea in a diabetic patient?
• How should this patient be investigated?

Differential diagnosis

The principal causes of diarrhea associated with diabetes mellitus are shown in Table 7.2. In addition, concurrent diarrhea-predominant irritable bowel syndrome, thyrotoxicosis, bile acid malabsorption, laxative abuse, and microscopic colitis also need to be considered. Acute episodes of diarrhea may result from infections.

Diarrhea, defined as daily stool weight >200 g with loose consistency due to high water content, may have a multitude of causes.

Table 7.2 Causes of chronic diarrhea in diabetes mellitus

Cause	Diabetes type	Pathogenesis
Celiac disease	1	Shared autoimmunity
Pancreatic insufficiency	2	Chronic pancreatitis
Bacterial colonization	1 and 2	Autonomic neuropathy
Dietary	1 and 2	Sorbitol (sugar free)
Drugs	2	Metformin
Somatostatinoma	2	Inhibiting intestinal function

It is usual to consider chronic diarrhea as being either osmotic or secretory. This helps in defining investigative strategy. Some distinguishing features are shown in Table 7.3.

Systematic analysis is required to reach a diagnosis [19]. Preliminary screening tests would include celiac serology (IgA anti-tissue transglutaminase antibody), thyroid function tests, stool for ova, parasites, and cysts, fecal elastase, inflammatory parameters, flexible sigmoidoscopy or colonoscopy, and biopsies. Other tests may include glucose hydrogen breath test (to exclude bacterial colonization), SeHCAT (to exclude bile acid malabsorption), and small bowel radiology. Bacterial colonization is associated with autonomic neuropathy and intestinal dysmotility permitting bacterial overgrowth. Other diabetic end-organ damage is usually present. Large-volume secretory diarrhea requires further investigations to exclude hormone-secreting neuroendocrine tumors. These investigations are complex and expensive, and therefore prior establishment of secretory diarrhea by stool osmotic gap is useful.

Diagnosis

The patient did not have features of generalized malabsorption. Her celiac serology was negative. Colonoscopy and biopsies excluded microscopic colitis. Fecal elastase was normal making pancreatic insufficiency unlikely. Her glucose hydrogen breath test was normal excluding bacterial colonization. Her stool osmotic gap was 180 mosmol/kg and 174 mosmol/kg on two occasions, strongly suggesting

Table 7.3 Distinction between chronic osmotic and secretory diarrhea

Feature	Osmotic	Secretory
Fasting	Diarrhea ceases	Diarrhea continues
Stool osmotic gap[a] (mosmol/kg)	>100	<50
Typical causes	Malabsorption, osmotic laxatives	Neuroendocrine tumors, many laxatives

[a]Osmotic gap = $290 - (Na^+ + K^+) \times 2$ mosmol/kg.

osmotic diarrhea. Lactose hydrogen breath test was negative excluding lactose intolerance. Three-day fecal fat output on normal diet was 4 g/24 h (normal <7 g/24 h).

As she had osmotic diarrhea it indicated an osmotically active substance in her stool. Osmotic laxative abuse (lactulose, magnesium) was a possibility but appeared unlikely on questioning the patient and her parents. On further questioning, it emerged that she has been using quite large amounts of diabetic sweets, chewing gums, and mints [20]. These contain sorbitol which is osmotically active. On stopping sorbitol intake her diarrhea ceased promptly [21].

Diarrhea-predominant irritable bowel syndrome is relatively common at this age group and a diagnosis of IBS can be made based on clinical features if the Rome III criteria are fulfilled. In a diabetic patient, however alternative causes should be excluded first.

Discussion

Diarrhea may be acute or chronic, large volume or small volume, secretory or osmotic, watery or fatty, and bloody or non-bloody. Chronic diarrhea is generally non-infective; large-volume diarrhea often indicates a small bowel or right colonic cause. Fatty diarrhea indicates generalized malabsorption. Bloody diarrhea indicates an inflammatory or neoplastic cause. Drugs such as metformin, non-steroidal anti-inflammatory drugs (NSAIDs), colchicine, proton pump inhibitors, antibiotics, antineoplastic agents, and antacids containing magnesium are often incriminating causes of diarrhea. Generally osmotic diarrhea is easier to evaluate than secretory diarrhea.

Most individuals are unaware of sorbitol in their diet and as little as 10 g sorbitol may give rise to diarrhea in both healthy individuals and people with diabetes. It is especially likely to give rise to diarrhea when consumed separately from a composite meal, as in the case of chewing gums and diabetic sweeteners.

References

1 Goddard AF, McIntyre AS, Scott BB. Guidelines for the management of iron deficiency anaemia. British Society of Gastroenterology. *Gut* 2000;**46**(suppl 3–4):IV1–5.
2 Ford AC, Chey WD, Talley NJ, Malhotra A, Spiegel BM, Moayyedi P. Yield of diagnostic tests for celiac disease in individuals with symptoms suggestive of irritable bowel syndrome: a systematic review and meta-analysis. *Arch Intern Med* 2009;**169**:651–8.
3 Rostom A, Murray JA, Kagnoff MF. American Gastroenterological Association (AGA) technical review on the diagnosis and management of celiac disease. *Gastroenterology* 2006;**131**:1981–2002.
4 Dube C, Rostom S, Sy R, et al. The prevalence of celiac disease in average-risk and at-risk Western European populations: a systematic review. *Gastroenterology* 2005;**128**(4 suppl 1):S57–67.
5 Modigliani R, Mary JY, Simon JF, et al. Clinical, biological, and endoscopic picture of attacks of Crohn's disease. Evolution on prednisolone. Groupe d'Etude Therapeutique des Affections Inflammatoires Digestives. *Gastroenterology* 1990;**98**:811.8.
6 Rutgeerts P, Feagan BG, Lichtenstein GR, et al. Comparison of scheduled and episodic treatment strategies of infliximab in Crohn's disease. *Gastroenterology* 2004;**126**:402–13.
7 Beaugerie L, Seksik P, Nion-Larmurier I, Gendre JP, Cosnes J. Predictors of Crohn's disease. *Gastroenterology* 2006;**130**:650–6.
8 Grancher K, Kohn N, Lesser M, Daum F. A multicenter trial of 6-mercaptopurine and prednisolone in children with newly diagnosed Crohn's disease. *Gastroenterology* 2000;**119**:895–902.
9 Hyams J, Crandall W, Kugathasan S, et al. Induction and maintenance infliximab therapy for the treatment of moderate-to-severe Crohn's disease in children. *Gastroenterology* 2007;**132**:863–73.
10 Schreiber S, Hanauer SB, Lichtenstein GR, Sandborn WJ. Superior efficacy of certolizumab pegol in early Crohn's disease is independent of CRP status. *Gastroenterology* 2007;**132**(suppl 1):A510.1 (abstract T1298).
11 Schreiber S, Reinsich R, Colombel J, et al. Early Crohn's disease shows high levels of remission to therapy with adalimumab: Sub-analysis of charm. *Gastroenterology* 2007;**132**:A-147.
12 D'Haens G, Baert F, van Assche G, et al. Early combined immunosuppression or conventional management in patients with newly diagnosed Crohn's disease: an open randomised trial. *Lancet* 2008;**371**:660–7.
13 Lemann M, Mary JY, Duclos B, et al. Infliximab plus azathioprine for steroid dependant Crohn's disease patients: a randomized placebo-controlled trial. *Gastroenterology* 2006;**130**:1054–61.
14 Shale M, Kanfer E, Panaccione R, Ghosh S Hepatosplenic T cell lymphoma in inflammatory bowel disease *Gut* 2008;**57**:1639–41.
15 Van Assche G, Magelaine-Beuzelin C, D'Haens G, et al. Withdrawal of immunosuppression in Crohn's disease treated with scheduled infliximab maintenance:

a randomized trial. *Gastroenterology* 2008;**134**: 1861–8.

16 Feagan BG, McDonald JWD, Panaccione R, et al. A randomized trial of methotrexate in combination with infliximab for the treatment of Crohn's disease. Presented at Digestive Disease Week, May 17–22, 2008, San Diego, CA.

17 Colombel JF, Sandborn WJ, Reinisch W, et al. SONIC: Infliximab, azathioprine, or combination therapy for Crohn's disease. *N Engl J Med* 2010 Apr 15;**362**: 1383–95.

18 Regueiro M, Schraut W, Baidoo L, et al. Infliximab prevents Crohn's disease recurrence after ileal resection. *Gastroenterology* 2009;**136**:441–50.

19 Fernandez-Banares F, Esteve M, Salas A, Alaina M, Farre C. Systematic evaluation of the causes of chronic watery diarrhea with functional characteristics. *Am J Gastroenterology* 2007;**102**:2520–8.

20 Bauditz J, Norman K, Biering H, Lochs H, Pirlich M. Severe weight loss caused by chewing gum. *BMJ* 2008;**336**:96–7.

21 Bodiga MS, Jain NK, Casanova C, Pitchumoni CS. Diarrhea in diabetics –the role of sorbitol. *J Am Coll Nutr* 1990;**9**:578–82.

8

Rectal Bleeding

Matthew Shale,[1] Lotte Dinesen,[1] and Subrata Ghosh[2]

[1]Gastrointestinal Section, Imperial College London, Hammersmith Hospital, London, UK
[2]Division of Gastroenterology, Department of Medicine, University of Calgary, Alberta, Canada

Case 1: intermittent small amounts of rectal bleeding

Case presentation

A 56-year-old woman is referred by her primary care physician for evaluation of intermittent rectal bleeding. She reports a 6-month history of intermittent small volumes of fresh bright-red blood noted on wiping, and occasionally in the toilet bowl. She had experienced similar symptoms attributed to hemorrhoids while pregnant 30 years previously, but had no other history of rectal bleeding. She denies pain with defecation, change in bowel habit, or tenesmus. She has suffered from constipation for many years, managed with laxatives on an as-required basis, and a diagnosis of irritable bowel syndrome had been made 18 years previously.

On direct questioning she gives a history of 5 kg weight loss in the preceding 4 months, which she believes relates to stress associated with looking after a sick elderly relative, but is otherwise systemically well. She experiences chronic intermittent abdominal pain and attributes this to her diagnosis of irritable bowel syndrome by her primary care physician. There has been no recent change in this symptom.

There is no family history of colorectal cancer or intestinal disease. She smokes 20 cigarettes per day, and drinks alcohol infrequently.

Her comorbidities include stable angina, hypertension, hypothyroidism, and depression. She is treated with low-dose aspirin, atenolol, nicorandil, atorvastatin, thyroxine, and fluoxetine. Her examination was as follows: there was no evidence of clubbing, anemia, or jaundice. The patient was overweight with a BMI of 29.5 kg/m². Cardiorespiratory examination was unremarkable. The abdomen was soft and non-tender and there was no palpable organomegaly. Rectal examination revealed a small skin tag, but no other pathology was detected by digital rectal examination or proctoscopy. Soft brown stool was present on the glove, without evidence of blood.

Laboratory results include (normal values in brackets):
Hb 11.9 (11.5–16.5) g/dL
Urea 3.8 (2.5–6.5) mmol/L
MCV 92 (76–98) fL
WCC 4.8 (4–11) × 10⁹/L
Platelets 310 (150–420) × 10⁹/l
Sodium 139 (135–145) mmol/L
Potassium 4.8 (3.5–5.0) mmol/L
Albumin 40 (35–55) g/L
Creatinine 110 (50–120) mmol/L
ESR 28 mm/h
Liver function tests – normal
Thyroid function tests – normal

Questions

• What is the differential diagnosis of chronic intermittent rectal bleeding?

Problem-based Approach to Gastroenterology and Hepatology, First Edition. Edited by John N. Plevris, Colin W. Howden.
© 2012 Blackwell Publishing Ltd. Published 2012 by Blackwell Publishing Ltd.

• What is the optimal method to investigate her symptoms?

• What value are "alarm features" in triaging patients with lower gastrointestinal (GI) bleeding for investigation?

• What medications are associated with lower GI bleeding?

Differential diagnosis

In cross-sectional studies in Europe and North America, up to 20% of adults reported at least one episode of rectal bleeding (hematochezia) in the preceding 12 months [1,2]. The number of patients presenting to medical care is somewhat lower than this; however, chronic intermittent rectal bleeding represents a common scenario in primary and secondary care.

The differential diagnosis of rectal bleeding is shown in Box 8.1. In patients with chronic low volume blood loss, however, a number of specific causes can be focused on, primarily neoplasia, and anorectal lesions.

The most significant and serious diagnosis that merits consideration in this scenario is colorectal neoplasia, including advanced (malignant) polyps. Many lesions, including invasive malignancy, may be asymptomatic, particularly when right-sided. To assist in the identification and triage of patients requiring further invasive investigation, a number of clinical "alarm" features have been identified, based on age and the presence of weight loss, change of bowel habit, and evidence of chronic blood loss such as iron deficiency anemia. Although these features have been incorporated into many referral guidelines, such symptoms are common in patients without neoplasia, and individually have a poor positive predictive value [3]. Models incorporating multiple variables may not perform any better. In a recent systematic review and meta-analysis of the literature, the passage of dark blood per rectum and a palpable abdominal mass were the only features of use in predicting the diagnosis of colonic cancer, largely attributable to their infrequent occurrence [3].

Anorectal lesions are common causes of low-volume intermittent hematochezia. Hemorrhoids are very common, affecting up to 75% of the general population at some stage, and are associated with constipation [4]. Most commonly they result in pain-

Box 8.1 Causes of lower gastrointestinal (GI) bleeding

Common

Diverticular disease[a]

Vascular ectasia[a]

Ischemic colitis[a]

Less common

Hemorrhoids[a]

Colonic malignancy

Inflammatory bowel disease

Infective colitis

Radiation colitis

Small bowel bleeding

Upper GI bleeding[a]

Post-polypectomy[a]

NSAID colopathy

Rare

Colorectal ulceration[a]

Colonic Dieulafoy's lesion[a]

Meckel's diverticulum[a]

Rectal varices[a]

Aortoenteric fistula[a]

Hemangioma

[a]Causes of bleeding most likely to present with acute massive rectal bleeding.

less intermittent low-volume fresh blood noted on toilet tissue, but in some cases bleeding is more brisk and may drip into the toilet at the end of defecation, or pool up in the rectum, and later be passed as a clot. Similar low-volume bleeding is seen with anal fissures, but is usually accompanied by severe defecatory pain. The diagnosis of anal fissure can often be made by simple external inspection. In addition to the fissure itself, sentinel skin tags are common, as is profound anal spasm upon parting the buttocks. Fissures occurring other than in the 6 or 12 o'clock position should prompt consideration of underlying conditions including inflammatory bowel disease, tuberculosis, syphilis, and HIV infection. Solitary rectal ulcer syndrome is associated with digital evacuation of feces, excessive straining at defecation, and

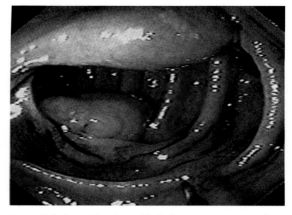

Figure 8.1 Sigmoid polyp with India ink tattoo to mark the site of the polyp.

rectal mucosal prolapse, and typically involves the anterior rectal wall. The condition is thought to occur as a result of localized ischemia, and has been linked to a variety of drugs including ergotamine derivatives, and possibly the potassium channel activator nicorandil [5].

Small-volume rectal bleeding may characterize distal colitis or proctitis proctitis; radiation proctopathy is an important differential in patients who have previously received pelvic radiotherapy [6].

Diagnosis

The patient underwent colonoscopic examination which demonstrated a 24 mm pedunculated polyp in the distal sigmoid colon, without evidence of recent hemorrhage (Figure 8.1). Full examination to the cecum revealed a further three small polyps all <10 mm. Retroflexion in the rectum did not reveal any hemorrhoids or alternate anorectal pathology. The polyp was snared and removed endoscopically without complication, and the site of removal was tattooed. Histological examination revealed villous morphology with a high-grade dysplasia, including a focus of carcinoma *in situ*, but no evidence of invasive malignancy. The other polyps were tubular adenomas.

The malignant potential of colonic polyps is related to features including size, histology, and the degree of dysplasia [7]. Histological characteristics include tubular or villous features, and the polyp is character-

ized based on the dominant morphology present. Tubulovillous adenomas demonstrate mixed features. Although polyps <10 mm are predominantly tubular and demonstrate low-grade dysplasia, the incidence of villous histology and high-grade dysplasia is much greater as polyp size increases to >10 mm. High-grade dysplasia encompasses severe dysplasia and carcinoma *in situ*, which does not breach the basement membrane. Polyps >10 mm, or with villous histology or high-grade dysplasia, may be termed 'adenomas with advanced pathology' (AAPs) in recognition of their greater malignant potential. The ultimate diagnosis in this patient is therefore an AAP.

Patient management

Colorectal neoplasia (including malignancy and advanced polyps) is responsible for approximately 10% of cases of rectal bleeding [1]. Polyps <10 mm very rarely bleed overtly, or indeed sufficiently to cause positive fecal occult blood testing. The importance of detecting such lesions mandates investigation of patients presenting with rectal bleeding to exclude the diagnosis.

The most appropriate endoscopic strategy to investigate intermittent rectal bleeding is flexible sigmoidoscopy in younger patients, who are less likely to have significant proximal pathology, and full colonoscopy in older patients [8]. This strategy is clinically practical and cost-effective. Definitions of the age at which colonoscopy becomes appropriate vary between guidelines, but 45–50 years of age is common. The significance of finding pathology such as hemorrhoids similarly changes with age. Although a patient aged 30 with hemorrhoids and an otherwise normal examination to the splenic flexure can be reassured, the presence of potentially responsible anorectal disease in an older patient with rectal bleeding should not preclude a full examination to exclude proximal neoplastic disease, which is significantly more common in this age group. Similarly, where an AAP is noted on limited examination in a young patient, a full colonoscopy is indicated to assess for further proximal pathology. Where a small distal polyp of low malignant potential is found, the need for full colonoscopy is more controversial, but studies suggest a three- to fourfold increased risk of proximal pathology even in this scenario [9].

The role of computed tomography (CT) in assessing the colon, particularly within a screening scenario, continues to be defined. At present is not considered a first-line investigation in patients with rectal bleeding. Patients with incomplete colonoscopy may be considered for CT colonography to ensure that the entire colon has been examined.

Large advanced polyps may generally be removed endoscopically or occasionally by surgical resection, with the optimal method depending on factors including its anatomic location, histology, gross morphological features, patient comorbidity or preference, and locally available expertise. The resection site should be tattooed to permit reliable identification in the future. Histological examination is focused on assessment for grade of dysphasia or carcinoma and, if the latter is present, for the degree of invasion within the polyp. Polyps with invasion beyond the muscularis mucosae into the submucosa are considered *malignant polyps*, and may warrant further surgical management.

Patients with colorectal polyps should be considered for further colonoscopic examination, at intervals related to the findings at the index examination. Where an AAP is sessile or has been removed in piecemeal fashion, limiting histological assessment of completeness of excision, a repeat procedure within 3 months should be undertaken to confirm full endoscopic removal [10]. This is often also true for sessile serrated lesions, which are attracting increasing attention. In the current case, the presence of more than three polyps with at least one >10 mm places this patient in a high-risk group for developing recurrent polyps in the future. The National Polyp Study showed that 10% of such patients will develop further advanced adenomas within 3 years, and 20% within 6 years [11]. Appropriate intervals for re-examination in this patient would be between 1 and 3 years after the index procedure, with European and North American consensus guidelines differing slightly in this regard [10,12]. The requirement for future procedures is then dictated by findings at each colonoscopy.

Undertaking colonoscopic polypectomy and surveillance has been prospectively demonstrated to result in around an 80% reduction in the subsequent incidence of colorectal malignancy, and improved survival in patients developing such malignancy [10–12]. It is important to stress optimum bowel preparation and technique of colonoscopy so as not to miss polyps or flat lesions, especially in the right side of the colon.

Case 2: acute severe lower GI bleeding

Case presentation

A 76-year-old man was admitted via the emergency room having presented with a 1-day history of passing fresh blood per rectum. While undergoing initial assessment in the department, he passed a large volume of bright red blood associated with the development of postural hypotension and tachycardia.

He denies abdominal pain, hematemesis, or previous rectal bleeding. He gives a history of chronic constipation but there has been no acute change in bowel habit. He also denies weight loss or systemic upset.

He has type 2 diabetes managed with dietary modification, dyslipidemia, and hypertension. He takes aspirin, ramipril, and simvastatin. He denies the use of non-steroidal anti-inflammatory drugs (NSAIDs).

He is a retired accountant, a life-long non-smoker, and consumes 8–10 units of alcohol per week.

Examination
Initial assessment reveals the patient to be alert and oriented, with a sinus tachycardia of 120 beats/min, and a BP of 110/56 mmHg with a postural systolic drop of >20 mmHg. He is afebrile, and there is no evidence of clubbing, jaundice, or stigmata of chronic liver disease. Cardiorespiratory examination is normal. His abdomen is soft and non-tender without any palpable organomegaly. Rectal examination reveals fresh bright red blood on the glove.

Laboratory results are as follows (normal values in brackets):
Hb 9.2 (13.5–16.5) g/dL
MCV 94 (78–98) fL
WCC 10 (4–11) × 10^9/L
Platelets 320 (150–420) × 10^9/L
Albumin 44 (35–55) g/L
Sodium 138 (135–145) mmol/L
Potassium 5.1 (3.5–5.0) mmol/L
Urea 4.0 (2.5–6.5) mmol/L
Creatinine 112 (50–120) mmol/L
Arterial blood sample (to exclude acidosis):
    pH 7.38 (7.35–7.45)
    PO_2 11.8 (>10.5) kPa
    PCO_2 3.8 (4.5–6) kPa
    Lactate 0.9 (<1) mmol/L
    Base excess −0.5 (−1 to +1)

Questions

- What are the initial management priorities in this situation?
- What is the likely anatomic site of acute severe rectal bleeding?
- What is the differential diagnosis of acute massive lower GI bleeding?
- What are the options for further investigation and treatment of this patient?

Differential diagnosis

Acute lower GI bleeding accounts for up to 20–24% of major GI bleeds, and is significantly more common in elderly people and men. Although many causes of lower GI bleeding are self-limiting, the mortality rate associated with this presentation is up to 4% [8].

Acute presentations with significant blood loss and evidence of hemodynamic compromise are less common than in upper GI bleeding (19 and 34%, respectively) [13]. When present, orthostatic hypotension, tachycardia, and delayed capillary refill reflect loss of >15% circulating volume. Initial assessment and management should therefore focus on resuscitation and stabilization of the patient to allow appropriate investigation and treatment to be undertaken.

The passage of fresh blood per rectum is most commonly due to bleeding distal to the ligament of Treitz, although a brisk bleed from an upper GI source may be responsible in up to 11% of cases [8,14]. The passage of a nasogastric tube and gastric lavage may aid in exclusion of an upper GI cause. Although a clear aspirate does not exclude the diagnosis, the presence of bile in the aspirate in the absence of blood makes such a source unlikely [15]. Similarly, an upper GI source may be more likely in a patient known to have significant upper GI tract pathology such as esophageal varices. In such patients, it may be appropriate to focus initial investigations on the upper GI tract.

In most cases of acute rectal bleeding, an anorectal or colonic cause is responsible (see Box 8.1). The most common etiologies are diverticular disease, ischemic colitis, and vascular ectasia [15,16].

Bleeding related to colonic diverticular disease accounts for up to 40% of all cases of acute severe rectal bleeding [15,16]. The incidence of diverticular bleeds increases with age, reflecting the increased prevalence of the underlying condition in elderly people. Bleeding occurs from arteries at the neck or dome of a diverticulum, and typically presents without pain.

Ischemic colitis is the cause of lower GI bleeding in up to 20% of cases, typically resulting from a sudden, often temporary, reduction in blood flow to the mesenteric vessels [16]. Patients commonly report a degree of abdominal pain before the passage of blood, and many have evidence of significant vascular disease or risk factors in their history. Such bleeding is usually of small volume and rarely requires transfusion.

Vascular ectasias are common in the elderly population, and account for 10–30% of lower GI bleeding, although they rarely cause acute severe hemorrhage [16].

Other causes of fresh rectal bleeding are less likely in this case. Bleeding from Meckel's diverticulum is a more common cause in younger patients, but is unlikely in a patient of this age. Hemorrhoids, polyps, and malignancy rarely present with acute severe bleeding. Similarly, the normocytic anemia in this case suggests acute bleeding in contrast to the chronic, often occult loss seen with neoplasms. The lack of altered bowel habit makes infective colitis or inflammatory bowel disease unlikely. The absence of a history of pelvic radiotherapy, recent colonoscopic polypectomy, NSAID use, or an aortic graft exclude other specific causes. Post-polypectomy hemorrhage is obviously associated with appropriate history of procedure.

Diagnosis

The patient was resuscitated with intravenous fluids and blood transfusion. The initial investigation was a selective mesenteric angiography which showed angiodysplasia in the right colon with no evidence of active bleeding (Figure 8.2). The gastroenterology and surgical teams jointly reviewed the patient, who was felt to be stable enough to undergo urgent colonoscopic evaluation. A nasogastric (NG) tube was inserted and revealed a bile-stained aspirate without any evidence of blood. He therefore underwent rapid bowel preparation using polyethylene glycol solution administered via the NG tube, and total colonoscopy was performed. Fresh blood was noted in the sigmoid colon on insertion, along with multiple diverticula (Figure 8.3); however, there was no obvious visible

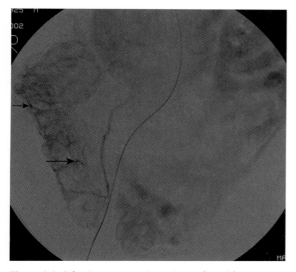

Figure 8.2 Selective mesenteric angiography with angiodysplasia of the right colon (arrows).

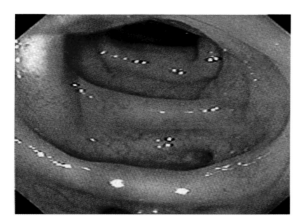

Figure 8.3 Diverticular disease in the sigmoid colon with recent hemorrhage.

vessel or source of bleeding. Full colonoscopy to the cecum was performed, and no other potential source of bleeding was seen, except non-bleeding vascular lesion in the cecum. Clear effluent was noted coming through the ileocecal valve. On withdrawal of the colonoscope through the sigmoid, fresh blood was seen to be coming from a diverticulum, with a visible vessel noted in the neck. Three metal endoscopic clips

were applied to the vessel and hemostasis achieved. The patient was returned to the ward and did not re-bleed.

Discussion

Diverticular disease is common, with the incidence increasing significantly with age to affect up to 75% of those aged >80 years [17]. Bleeding is typically painless, and occurs in 3–5% of patients with diverticular disease [18]. Such bleeds may be more common in NSAID users [18]. Bleeding is thought to occur due to penetration of an artery into the diverticulum, and it usually occurs in the absence of diverticulitis. In contrast to the predominant occurrence of diverticula in left colon, bleeding may be more common from right-sided diverticula. Although most cases settle spontaneously, recurrent bleeding occurs in up to 40% of patients, and may be more common in patients with a more severe initial bleed (as judged by transfusion requirements), although, in contrast to upper GI bleeding, validated prognostic scoring systems are not available. Many patients experience only minor or moderate bleeding, but some present as in this case, with acute massive hemorrhage. In such cases, the priority following initial resuscitation is to undertake investigation and management of the cause.

The initial examination should include digital rectal examination, and proctoscopy to rapidly exclude obvious anorectal sources of bleeding [15]. If this is negative, assessment of the colon is required, and can be achieved using endoscopic, radiological, or scintigraphic methods. The optimal approach remains controversial and is best tailored to locally available expertise.

Total colonoscopy is the preferred endoscopic approach, because pathology beyond the reach of the flexible sigmoidoscope is common. A rapid colonic purge with polyethylene glycol solution should be performed before the procedure, if necessary given via an NG tube. This both optimizes the diagnostic yield and decreases the risk of complications, including perforation, compared with the unprepared colon [15]. Colonoscopy has a diagnostic yield of 80–100% in acute severe rectal bleeding, and may be greatest when performed early (within 8 hours) rather than delayed up to 48 hours [19,20]. Early colonoscopy is associated with increased diagnostic yields and reduced length of hospital stay, although this has yet to be shown to translate into improvement in other clinical outcomes such as mortality, blood transfusion requirements, or rates of re-bleeding. Colonoscopic examination is focused on the identification of features that may point to a specific diagnosis such as the presence of diverticular disease, vascular ectasia, or ischemia (including hemorrhagic submucosal nodules, dusky cyanotic mucosa, or well-demarcated linear ulceration). The prognostic significance of endoscopic findings in the colon are less well defined than in the upper GI tract, but actively bleeding vessels, visible vessels, and overlying clot, particularly in the context of diverticular bleeds, may indicate a high risk of further bleeding. Options for endoscopic therapy include the use of metal clips, epinephrine injection, and thermal coagulative methods. The efficacy of such therapies is best defined in the treatment of diverticular hemorrhage, where a success rate of up to 100% has been reported by some authors [21]. In patients with suspected bleeding vascular ectasias, thermal and injection methods are available.

In patients judged too unstable to undergo colonoscopy, or where the source of bleeding is not established by an endoscopic approach, radiological or scintigraphic methods are invaluable. Options include labeled red cell scans, CT angiography, and digital subtraction angiography, with the last also providing the therapeutic option of superselective arterial embolization. Labeled red cell scintigraphy is able to demonstrate ongoing bleeding at rates as low as 0.1 mL/min, and is of primary use in localizing the bleeding site before intervention such as angiography, which is relatively insensitive to rates of blood loss <0.5–1 mL/min [18]. Where available, emergency angiography is an effective means of investigating and managing patients where colonoscopy is negative, and permits embolization of vessels feeding bleeding lesions using agents such as polyvinyl alcohol particles, sponges, or microcoils [22]. The sensitivity of angiography in acute lower GI bleeding is up to 80%, and associated therapies are highly effective (clinical success rate >80%); however, it may be associated with a risk of delayed rebleeding in up to 25% and colonic ischemia necessitating colectomy in around 10%. Important additional risks associated with angiography include contrast reactions and acute renal failure. CT angiography appears a promising diagnostic technique, particularly for the detection of vascular ectasia, but its place in the investigation and management of lower GI bleeding awaits clarification.

Direct comparative studies of these various modalities in investigating acute severe lower GI bleeding are limited, but generally suggest colonoscopy to be a safer technique with a greater diagnostic yield than angiography [14]. In an acute care scenario, the choice may depend on availability of expert intervention out of hours as well as support staff. In this case angiography picked up an incidental angiodysplasia.

Surgery represents the final option in the management of massive lower GI bleeding. Segmental resection is the preferred approach when preoperative localization of the bleeding source is possible. Such procedures may be associated with a mortality rate up to 30%, but this may represent selection bias, with the sickest patients receiving surgery. Indications for surgery for lower GI bleeding are not well defined, but American Society for Gastrointestinal Endoscopy (ASGE) guidance suggests consideration of surgery in patients with significant ongoing bleeding and a transfusion requirement of >6 units packed red cells in 24h [15]. The importance of pre-surgical localization of lesions is highlighted by reports of 1 year rebleed rates of up to 42% following "blind" segmental resection, versus 14% where preoperative angiographic localization is employed [23].

Barium enema is not of any diagnostic utility in acute lower GI bleeding, although intriguingly may represent a therapeutic technique in diverticular hemorrhage where a distinct bleeding point cannot be identified [24].

In cases where a colonic bleeding source cannot be identified despite such investigation, small bowel imaging may be appropriate. An estimated 1–9% of acute severe lower GI bleeds are due to small intestinal causes. In patients aged under 30 years, bleeding from a Meckel diverticulum is an important cause of acute severe bleeding, and can be diagnosed using technitium-99m-labeled pertechnate scanning, and treated by surgical resection. The role of small bowel imaging techniques including video capsule and double balloon enteroscopy in acute lower GI bleeding awaits definition, but they are increasingly employed if colonic investigations are negative.

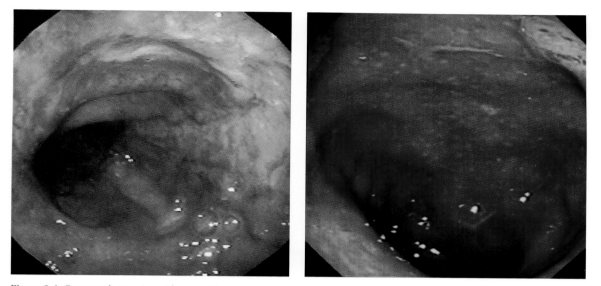

Figure 8.4 Congested rectosigmoid area with loss of vascular pattern and erythema with some granularity.

Case 3: recurrent rectal bleeding in an adolescent

Case presentation

A 19-year-old man has been attending pediatric and adult gastrointestinal departments for over 10 years with intermittent rectal bleeding. He describes mucus in his bowel movements and only occasional diarrhea. Some but not all of the bowel movements can be urgent. Generally he describes noticing streaks of rectal bleeding with his bowel movements, but occasionally the bleeding has been heavy. His parents remark having noticed rectal bleeding in him even as a baby. There is no relevant family history.

Examination showed a well looking young man with a BMI of 23 kg/m². He did not look pale, and abdominal examination was normal. Rectal examination showed blood on the gloves.

Laboratory investigations showed (normal values in brackets):

Hb 13.1 (13.5–17.5) g/dL
WCC 9.4 (4–11) × 10⁹/L
Platelets 340 (150–400) × 10⁹/L
Ferritin 46 (20–250) μg/L
Transferrin saturation 24 (22–40)%
CRP 0.8 (0.2–1.0) mg/dL
MCV 75 (75–98) fL

Liver function tests normal
Urea 3.5 (2.5–6.5) mmol/L
Creatinine 64 (50–120) mmol/L
Flexible sigmoidoscopy showed a congested, somewhat granular mucosa, which was erythematous, but did not show any ulcerations or friability (Figure 8.4). The mucosa was normal beyond 25 cm. Biopsies from affected area showed non-specific inflammation.

Questions

• What is the differential diagnosis of recurrent rectal bleeding in a young patient?
• What does the flexible sigmoidoscopic appearance indicate?
• What investigations might help reach a diagnosis?

Differential diagnosis

In a young patient with recurrent rectal bleeding, the differential diagnosis includes ulcerative proctitis, juvenile polyposis, familial adenomatous polyposis, vascular lesions, and anal fissures.

Inflammatory bowel disease affecting the rectum will be associated with ulcerations and friability and biopsies will show evidence of chronic inflammation. The polyposis syndromes include juvenile polyposis which may be familiar, as is familial adenomatous polyposis (FAP). Juvenile polyposis is associated with germline mutations of *BMPR1A* and *MADH4*, and these hamartomatous polyps may undergo malignant transformation. FAP is inherited as an autosomal dominant condition and associated with *APC* gene mutation. Isolated juvenile polyps, Peutz–Jeghers polyps, and intestinal lymphoma are considered in the differential diagnosis.

Juvenile polyps occur in children and present with painless hematochezia. These are generally solitary and benign and characterized by heavy eosinophilic infiltrate. Anal fissures in adolescents are generally associated with constipation and defecation is very painful. In a young patient with rectal bleeding a patient may sometimes require general anesthesia to permit flexible sigmoidoscopy or colonoscopy, but this is essential to diagnose a polyposis syndrome. Vascular lesions are often congenital such as cavernous hemangioma. Rectal varices are associated with portal hypertension. The flexible sigmoidoscopy showed congested hyperemic mucosa with loss of vascular pattern and some granularity, but no evidence of ulcerations or friability. This would be considered atypical for inflammatory bowel disease.

Diagnosis

As the biopsies only showed non-specific inflammation, further investigations were carried out. These included endoanal ultrasonography which showed submucosal dilated vascular lesions (Figure 8.5). A selective mesenteric angiography demonstrated a large vascular lesion in the pre-sacral area (Figure 8.6). Cavernous hemangioma of the rectum is typically associated with recurrent rectal bleeding and the diagnosis is often delayed due to erroneous diagnosis of hemorrhoids or inflammatory bowel disease [25]. Associated non-specific inflammation is common and may mislead clinicians to diagnose ulcerative proctitis. Treatment is generally by complete resection, either sphincter-preserving or abdominoperineal, depending on the extent of involvement.

Discussion

It is important to be aware of diseases that may mimic inflammatory bowel disease in the rectum. These include chronic infections such as tuberculosis and

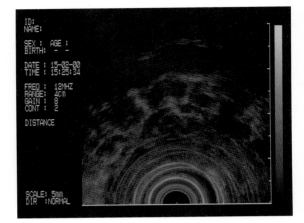

Figure 8.5 Endoanal ultrasonography showing numerous dilated blood vessels in the submucosa. (Figure courtesy of Dr Ian Penman.)

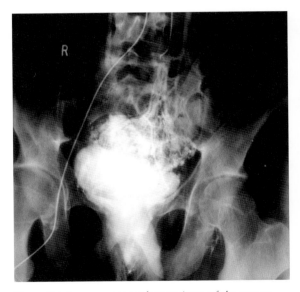

Figure 8.6 Large cavernous hemangioma of the rectum shown on selective mesenteric angiography.

schistosomiasis, sexually transmitted infections, infiltrative diseases such as lymphoma, rectal hemangioma, and solitary ulcers of the rectum. These may all present with recurrent rectal bleeding. A combination of flexible sigmoidoscopy and biopsy, endoanal ultrasonography, and rarely inferior mesenteric angiography may be necessary to achieve a diagnosis. Cavernous hemangioma of the rectum is a congenital condition manifesting as recurrent rectal bleeding – the flexible sigmoidoscopic appearance may be mistaken as inflammatory bowel disease. Rectal ulcers may be sometimes associated with cavernous hemangioma of the rectum.

References

1 Fijten GH, Blijham GH, Knottnerus JA. Occurrence and clinical significance of overt blood loss per rectum in the general population and in medical practice. *Br J Gen Pract* 1994;**44**:320–5.

2 Talley NJ, Jones M. Self-reported rectal bleeding in a United States Community: Prevalence, risk factors, and health care seeking. *Am J Gastroenterol* 1998;**92**:2179

3 Ford AC, Veldhuyzen van Zanten SJO, Rodgers CC, et al. Diagnostic utility of alarm features for colorectal cancer: systematic review and meta-analysis. *Gut* 2008; **57**:1545–53.

4 Nelson RL, Abcarian H, Davis FG, et al. Prevalence of benign anorectal disease in a randomly selected population. *Dis Colon Rectum* 1995;**38**:341–5.

5 Titi MA, Seow C, Molloy RG. Nicorandil-induced colonic ulceration: a new cause of colonic ulceration. Report of four cases. *Dis Colon Rectum* 2008;**51**: 1570–3.

6 Eisen GM, Dominitz JA, Faigel DO, et al. ASGE Standards of Practice Committee. Endoscopic therapy of anorectal disorders. *Gastrointest Endosc* 2001;**53**: 867–70.

7 Itzkowitz SH, Rochester J. Colonic polyps and polyposis syndromes. In: Feldman M, Friedman LS, Brandt LJ (eds), *Sleisenger and Fordtran's Gastrointestinal and Liver Disease*, 8th edn. Philadelphia, PA: Saunders, 2006: 2713–57.

8 Davila RE, Rajan E, Adler DG, et al. ASGE Guideline: the role of endoscopy in the patient with lower-GI bleeding. *Gastrointest Endosc* 2005;**62**:656–60.

9 Lieberman DA, Weiss DG, Bond JH, et al. Use of colonoscopy to screen asymptomatic adults for colorectal cancer. *N Engl J Med* 2000;**343**:169.

10 Davila RE, Rajan E, Baron TH. ASGE guideline: colorectal cancer screening and surveillance. *Gastrointest Endosc* 2006;**63**:546–57.

11 Winawer S, Zauber A, O'Brien M, et al. Randomized comparison of surveillance intervals after colonoscopic removal of newly diagnosed adenomatous polyps. *N Engl J Med* 1993;**328**:901–6.

12 Atkin WS, Saunders BP. Surveillance guidelines after removal of colorectal adenomatous polyps. *Gut* 2002;**51**(suppl V),v6–9.

13 Peura DA, Lanza FL, Gostout CJ, Fouch PG. The American College of Gastroenterology Bleeding Registry: preliminary findings. *Am J Gastroenterol* 1997;**92**: 924–8.

14 Jensen DM, Machicado GA. Diagnosis and treatment of severe hematochezia. The role of urgent colonoscopy after purge. *Gastroenterology* 1988;**95**:1569–74.

15 Eisen GM, Dominitz JA, Faigel DO, et al. ASGE Standards of Practice Committee. An annotated algorithmic approach to acute lower gastrointestinal bleeding. *Gastrointest Endosc* 2001;**53**:859–63.

16 Longstreth GF. Epidemiology and outcome of patients hospitalized with acute lower gastrointestinal hemorrhage: A population based study. *Am J Gastoenterol* 1997;**92**:419.

17 Parks TG. Natural history of diverticular disease of the colon. *Clin Gastroenterol* 1975;**4**:53–69.

18 Zuckerman GR, Prakash C. Acute lower intestinal bleeding. Part II: etiology, therapy and outcomes. *Gastrointest Endosc* 1999;**49**:228–38.

19 Green BT, Rockey DC, Portwood G, et al. Urgent colonoscopy for the evaluation and management of acute lower gastrointestinal hemorrhage: a randomized controlled trial. *Am J Gastroenterol* 2005;**100**:2395–402.

20 Jensen DM, Machicado GA, Jutabha R, Kovacs TOG. Urgent colonoscopy for the diagnosis and treatment of severe diverticular hemorrhage. *N Engl J Med* 2000;**342**: 78–82.

21 Fiorito JJ, Brandt LJ, Kozicky O, et al. The diagnostic yield of superior mesenteric angiography: correlation with the pattern of gastrointestinal bleeding. *Am J Gastroenterol* 1988;**84**:878–81.

22 Bandi R, Shetty PC, Sharma RP, et al. Superselective arterial embolization for the treatment of lower gastrointestinal hemorrhage. *J Vasc Interv Radiol* 2001;**12**: 1399–405.

23 Parkes BM, Obeid FN, Sorensen VJ, et al. The management of massive lower gastrointestinal bleeding. *Am Surg* 1993;**59**:676.

24 Adams JT. The barium enema as treatment for massive diverticular bleeding. *Dis Colon Rectum* 1974;**17**: 439–441.

25 Sylla P, Deutsch G, Luo J, et al. Cavernous arteriovenous and mixed hemangioma-lymphangioma of the rectosigmoid: rare causes of rectal bleeding – case series and review of the literature. *Int J Colorectal Dis* 2008;**23**: 653–8.

9 Multisystem Disorders and Gastrointestinal Disease

Lynne A. Meekison and John N. Plevris
The Royal Infirmary of Edinburgh, University of Edinburgh, Edinburgh, UK

Multisystem disorders often manifest with gastrointestinal (GI) symptoms as their first presentation. Sometimes the pattern of illness clearly indicates the underlying diagnosis; at other times the GI component of the illness may be thought to be an isolated problem initially, and it is only later that the systemic nature of the condition is recognized. Early diagnosis allows for earlier intervention, and vitally treatment of the systemic illness rather than the specific presenting symptoms, and may significantly alter prognosis. Illnesses such as diabetes and thyroid disorders are the most obvious endocrine examples, whereas underlying malignancy metastasizing to the GI tract or causing systemic effects with paraneoplastic syndrome causing intestinal pseudo-obstruction may present with the GI symptoms first. Inflammatory bowel disease and arthritis are common associations, whereas a number of GI pathologies leading to chronic blood loss can manifest as iron deficiency anemia. Hemolytic syndromes (e.g. Zieve's syndrome) can be directly associated to liver disease whereas gallstones are very common in patients with hemolytic syndromes such as sickle cell anemia. Skin manifestations are very common in GI and liver disease and often raise the suspicion of the underlying condition.

Case 1: dysphagia, regurgitation, and vomiting

Case presentation

The patient, KW – a woman aged 66 – presented over 10 years ago, aged 54, with longstanding troublesome symptoms of dysphagia, regurgitation, and vomiting. These symptoms persisted despite taking 40 mg of omeprazole daily. Regurgitation occurred after meals, drinks, and at night.

Her only comorbidity was obesity (BMI 32).

Past medical history included benign esophageal strictures with multiple previous dilations, and hypothyroidism for which she is on thyroxine replacement therapy.

On systemic inquiry, she reported dry mouth and eyes, and also had symptoms consistent with Raynaud's phenomenon. A routine complete blood count, and renal and liver function tests were (LFTs) normal except for γ-glutamyl transferase (GGT) which was 72 U/L (normal 10–55 U/L).

Clinical examination revealed sclerodactyly, a few dilated nailfold capillaries, telangiectasias on her left hand, but no evidence of calcinosis or scleroderma.

Upper GI endoscopy revealed a 3-cm hiatus hernia, and a 2-cm Barrett's esophagus (C2M2 by Prague

Problem-based Approach to Gastroenterology and Hepatology, First Edition. Edited by John N. Plevris, Colin W. Howden.
© 2012 Blackwell Publishing Ltd. Published 2012 by Blackwell Publishing Ltd.

C&M criteria) distally with no ulceration or stricture, but low-grade dysplasia on biopsies.

Questions

• What is the differential diagnosis?
• What other gastrointestinal investigations are appropriate?
• What further blood tests may be of value?
• Would you recommend any endoscopic surveillance?

Differential diagnosis

The differential diagnosis before investigations for the esophageal symptoms includes reflux esophagitis with stricture and the development of a stricturing adenocarcinoma. These have been excluded by endoscopy. The longstanding reflux may have caused a scarred immotile esophagus. Biopsies were taken to exclude eosinophilic esophagitis, although the history was of dysphagia not of the classic episodes of food bolus obstruction, and there were no endoscopic features such as diffuse narrowing, presence of concentric rings, or white spots or furrows along the esophagus. In addition, eosinophilic esophagitis affects more men than women, and it is more commonly found in younger patients.

The history is not classic for achalasia, but this diagnosis should be considered in patients who have dysphagia and an otherwise negative endoscopy.

The most likely cause of mild increase in GGT in this patient could be due to fatty liver secondary to obesity or due to an autoimmune condition such as primary biliary cirrhosis. Other common causes include gallstones in the common bile duct or liver metastases but this patient's symptoms together with negative endoscopy for malignancy make these unlikely.

Esophageal manometry and pH study

This revealed a lower esophageal sphincter resting pressure of just 6 mmHg, which is significantly reduced (normal values 14–34 mmHg). Relaxation of the sphincter was seen to be complete with wet swallows. Examination of the esophageal body motility demonstrated a total lack of esophageal peristalsis (Figure 9.1).

A pH study was then performed. This revealed significant excess acid exposure time at 26.8%

(normal value <6.95% of total recorded time). Detailed review of the traces demonstrated that there was pooling of acid, most pronounced in the supine position. Seven acid reflux episodes lasted more than 5 min. The longest episodes took 86 min to clear in the upright position, 74 min in the supine position.

Autoimmune screen, blood glucose level, and thyroid function tests

In view of the systemic symptoms and impaired peristalsis, an autoimmune screen was requested. This revealed a positive antinuclear antibody (ANA) with titer >1/640, and anti-centromere reactivity. She was also noted to have a positive anti-mitochondrial antibody at a titer of >1/160.

Thyroid function was rechecked and was normal. Thyrotoxicosis can present with abnormal liver function tests, namely raised serum alkaline phosphatase (ALP) and raised transaminases in a third of patients.

Diabetes was excluded in view of the history of thyroid disease. Uncontrolled diabetes may present with esophageal dysmotility.

This patient would merit endoscopic Barrett's surveillance. The endoscopy was repeated after 6 months and 1 year because of the detection of dysplasia, after maximizing acid suppression to eliminate acid-related inflammation, which can influence the interpretation of low-grade dysplasia. No new abnormalities were detected, and biopsies demonstrated no evidence of dysplasia. Thereafter, the patient was entered into the Barrett's surveillance program with 2-yearly endoscopies as per the recommendation of the British Society of Gastroenterology [1]. The patient remained on high-dose acid suppression with the addition of domperidone 10 mg tid as a prokinetic agent to improve gastric emptying.

She represented 3 years later with worsening dysphagia, and was also noted to have deterioration in the liver function tests with ALT 58 U/L, GGT 99 U/L, and ALP 209 U/L but normal bilirubin.

What investigations would be indicated?

• Repeat endoscopy and distal esophageal biopsies in case of an interval cancer. This demonstrated inflamed columnar-lined esophagus indefinite for dysplasia.
• Repeat esophageal manometry confirmed an undetectable pressure in the lower esophageal sphincter. All swallows were non-conducted in the esophageal

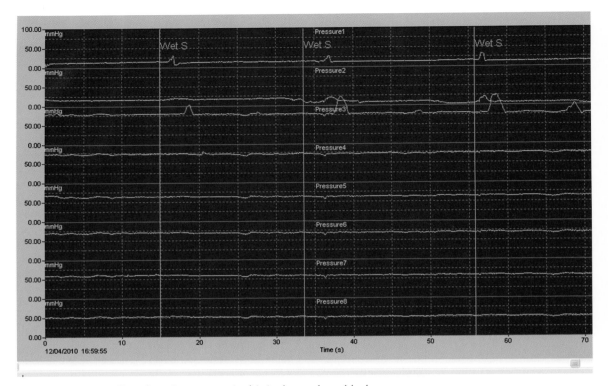

Figure 9.1 A wet swallow that triggers no peristalsis in the esophageal body.

body. These findings represented a further deterioration of the barrier function of the lower esophageal sphincter, and excluded achalasia (Figure 9.2).
• Repeat anti-mitochondrial antibodies; these remained positive, in keeping with primary biliary cirrhosis.
• Ultrasound scan excluded gallstones or any malignant process.

Diagnosis

Incomplete CREST syndrome associated with primary biliary cirrhosis (PBC).

Patient management

Esophageal dysmotility
This patient presented with symptoms suggestive of gastroesophageal reflux disease (GERD) and esophageal dysmotility, although a sinister pathology in the upper digestive system had to be excluded in view of her age. Dysmotility leading to dysphagia is common in CREST syndrome (calcinosis, Raynaud's, esophageal dysmotility, scleroderma, and telangiectasias). Unfortunately there is no intervention that will improve the esophageal dysmotility, which is part of CREST syndrome, as it does not respond to prokinetic agents such as domperidone. These drugs can, however, be of value in helping gastric emptying which may indirectly reduce the volume of reflux. Treatment with a high-dose proton pump inhibitor (PPI) is essential and often very high doses are required to heal persistent esophageal ulceration.

Barrett's esophagus
Such patients with longstanding acid reflux often develop Barrett's esophagus. This patient is entered into the authors' screening program for surveillance of Barrett's esophagus after discussing the implications of the condition and of surveillance itself.

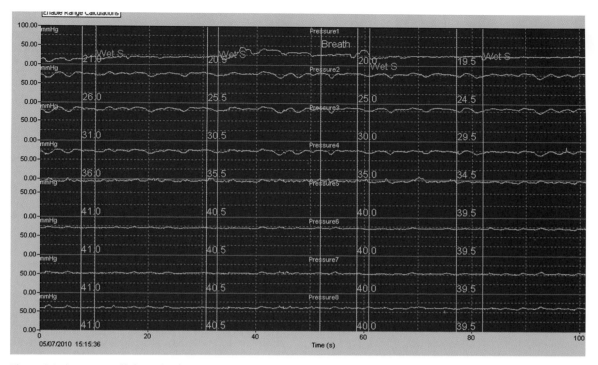

Figure 9.2 A station pull-through of the lower esophageal sphincter. The lower four channels are recording at the same level, and are unable to detect any resting pressure in the lower esophageal sphincter as the catheter is slowly pulled back.

Explanation was given about the underlying cancer risk of Barrett's esophagus, versus the morbidity and potential mortality of having screening endoscopies. A diagnosis of "indefinite for dysplasia" is most often made where there are changes suggestive of dysplasia but inflammatory changes make such a distinction impossible. The dose of PPI is maximized and repeat endoscopy performed at 6-monthly intervals. If two consecutive endoscopies fail to reveal definite evidence of dysplasia, i.e. apparent regression occurs, the patient can return to routine surveillance every 2 years according to the national and international guideline recommendations [1]. Patients with long-term GERD may be maintained on a PPI. There is a paucity of trials beyond 6 months to assess long-term symptom control. However, approximately 65–90% of patients are kept in clinical remission depending on the presence of esophagitis at baseline and the severity of the esophagitis. The presence of Barrett's esophagus would require the patient to be on long-term treatment with a PPI because such patients are more resistant to medical therapy; in addition PPIs may reduce the risk of progression of dysplasia although such risk is not eliminated [2].

An alternate treatment would be antireflux surgery. The REFLUX trial [3] compared otherwise healthy patients with GERD whose symptoms were controlled on a PPI, and who were randomly allocated either to laparoscopic Nissen fundoplication or continuation of PPI therapy. Antireflux surgery has given these patients superior results with regard to quality of life and patient satisfaction at 2 years, and the study is continuing to assess long-term results. In another study the risk of developing high-grade dysplasia or adenocarcinoma in patients with Barrett's esophagus was marginally lower in patients treated with surgery versus medical therapy but such a difference did not reach statistical significance [4].

Dysphagia may occur postoperatively in patients undergoing fundoplication [3,5]. Usually this is short-term dysphagia settling within 2–3 months. As many as 36% of patients may require further assessment postoperatively if dysphagia persists. Patients who have a total lack of peristalsis, similar to this patient, are at increased risk of postoperative dysphagia. In such circumstances some surgeons may consider offering antireflux surgery, but with a partial fundoplication instead (*Dor* [anterior] or *Toupet* [posterior]), but others may recommend maximizing medical management and avoiding surgery.

Primary biliary cirrhosis

Ursodeoxycholic acid is frequently prescribed in patients with PBC. In some studies it has been shown to improve biochemistry and perhaps delay disease progression, but in a recent Cochrane systematic review there was no reduction in mortality, improvement of itch, or delay in disease progression [6]. Furthermore, patients on ursodeoxycholic acid had weight gain as the main side effect.

Cholestyramine was recommended in the first instance for itch, and advice was also given about sodium bicarbonate baths to sooth itch.

Patients with PBC are at increased risk of osteoporosis, the cause of which is multifactorial. In addition, being on long term PPIs might contribute to the increased risk of osteoporosis although this is controversial. Such patients are advised to be on a high calcium intake diet (>1000 mg daily). They should take weight-bearing exercise, although this may be limited by fatigue. Screening for osteoporosis is performed with DXA (dual energy X-ray absorptiometry) scanning; this patient was found to have osteopenia of the spine, was prescribed calcium and vitamin D, and counseled about weight-bearing exercise. Monitoring of her bone density is arranged to assess for osteoporosis developing in the future, which may then require treatment. In such a case oral biphosphonates may be problematic in view of her esophageal pathology.

Screening for the complications of cirrhosis is required, with surveillance of varices by endoscopy and measurement of α-fetoprotein and 6-monthly liver ultrasonography for detection of hepatocellular carcinoma. The prevalence of hepatocellular carcinoma in PBC is approximately 3.3%, with an incidence of 0.35 per 100 patient-years, and it is more common in male PBC patients [7]. It should however

be noted that PBC is very uncommon in men (female to male ratio 9:1). The only effective treatment for advanced PBC is liver transplantation, but this patient is at an early stage of the disease with no evidence of cirrhosis.

Multisystem involvement

The association between systemic scleroderma and PBC is well recognized in women, but can rarely affect men [8]. Patients with CREST and PBC should be screened for other autoimmune manifestations such as celiac disease (anti-tissue transglutaminase or TTG antibodies), Hashimoto's thyroiditis (T_3/T_4 TSH, AND antibodies against thyroid peroxidase and/or thyroglobulins) well as the presence of rheumatoid arthritis.

Case 2: history of breast cancer in family

Case presentation

A 49-year-old woman with extensive family history of breast cancer was assessed by clinical genetics and found to carry the *BRCA*-1 gene.

At a preoperative assessment for prophylactic mastectomy, the patient was noted to have thrombocytosis with platelet count 578×10^9/L and mildly abnormal liver function tests (LFTs) with raised ALT 61 U/L and GGT 48 U/L.

There was no past history of thrombotic episodes. In her general health, she was obese and had hypertension. She was a non-smoker who consumed 34 units of alcohol per week.

Clinical examination revealed no breast lumps, lymphadenopathy, or hepatosplenomegaly.

Examination of the skin revealed excoriated papules and vesicles up to 1 cm in diameter on reddened skin, in particular on the elbows (Figure 9.3).

Investigations were as follows (normal values in brackets)
Hb 122 (115–165 g/l)
WBC 7.5 (4.0 – 11.0) $\times 10^9$/L
Platelets 578 (150–350) $\times 10^9$/L
Film: anisocytic normochromic
Vitamin B_{12} 247 (200–900) ng/L
Folate 2.2 (5–20) μg/L
Bilirubin 7 (3–16) μmol/L
ALT 74 (10–50) U/L

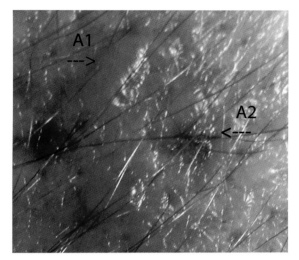

Figure 9.3 Dermatitis herpetiformis: blistering skin lesions (A1) in clusters are present causing intense itching which leads to scratching, breaking of the vesicles and crust formation (A2). Healing of the lesions is associated with some skin discoloration. (Image courtesy of Professor PC Hayes.)

ALP 84 (40–125) U/L
Albumin 40 (35–50) g/L
Ferritin 11 (14–50) µg/L

Questions

• What other tests would you consider?
• What is the differential diagnosis of thrombocytosis in this case?
• What are the skin lesions?

Other tests

Celiac antibodies
• Serum transglutaminase IgA was raised (>101 [5–30] U/mL)

Endoscopy and distal duodenal biopsy
• Endoscopy was normal but biopsies from distal duodenum showed increased intraepithelial lymphocytes and partial villous atrophy consistent with celiac disease

Bone marrow
• Reactive marrow was found not diagnostic of primary thrombocythemia, but with low iron stores.

Box 9.1 Causes of thrombocytosis

Primary: due to myeloproliferative disorders such as chronic myelogenous leukemia, polycythemia rubra vera, thrombocythemia, or myelofibrosis

Secondary or reactive due to inflammation or surgery

Hyposplenism

Persistent iron deficiency anemia or chronic blood loss

Active inflammatory bowel disease

Active rheumatoid arthritis

Bone or soft tissue sarcomatous tumors

Nephritis

Chronic bacterial infections

Drug-induced (e.g. Epinephrine, Tretinoin, Vincristine)

Differential diagnosis

The differential diagnosis for thrombocytosis is extensive (Box 9.1), but includes reactive iron deficiency. In this case underlying celiac disease has been the cause of the iron deficiency, thrombocythemia, and folate deficiency.

Patient markedly improved on gluten-free diet. The description of the skin rash is very suggestive of dermatitis herpetiformis. If there is uncertainty as to whether this patient has dermatitis herpetiformis or eczema/nodular prurigo, skin biopsy will be appropriate to clarify the diagnosis.

Her symptoms have worsened with stress and lack of compliance with diet. She proceeded to have a skin biopsy:

What are the characteristic findings of skin biopsy in dermatitis herpetiformis?
The microscopic appearance of dermatitis herpetiformis is characteristic.

The blister is subepidermal, the inflammatory cells (neutrophils and eosinophils) group in the dermal papillae, and direct immunofluorescence reveals IgA immunoglobulin in dermal papillae (Figure 9.4).

In dermatitis herpetiformis, blood tests are usually normal. However if gluten enteropathy is present, the following may be found:

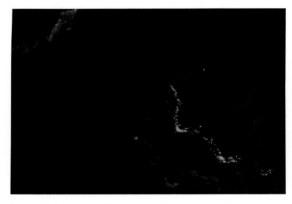

Figure 9.4 Immunofluorescence demonstrates IgA immunoglobulin in dermal papillae (Image courtesy of Dr Thomas Brenn.)

- Mild anemia
- Folic acid deficiency
- Iron deficiency.

How would you explain the abnormal LFTs?
LFTs remained mildly elevated with GGT 88 U/L and ALT 69 U/L. This is common in uncontrolled celiac disease (approximately 10–20% of patients with celiac disease may present with abnormal LFTs, with transaminases being the most common liver abnormality [9]. There is a recognized association between celiac disease and PBC.

A liver screen showed a normal autoantibody profile and in particular negative antimitochondrial antibodies and the hepatitis B and C screen was negative.

A liver ultrasound scan revealed a diffusely bright echotexture in keeping with fatty infiltration.

Patient management

- Patient was started on a gluten-free diet and confirmed to be compliant with the diet. Celiac antibodies anti-TTG IgA normalized to 4.9 U/mL, in keeping with good compliance with gluten-free diet.
- Skin review confirmed multiple excoriated lesions on the arms, leg, and upper back consistent with dermatitis herpetiformis. This was treated with a topic corticosteroid (clobetasol propionate) and has improved.
- Alternate treatment would be with dapsone

Clinical progress

This woman underwent an uncomplicated bilateral mastectomy, but, due to the stress of surgery, she complied poorly with her diet and developed further problems with her skin, with a worse rash on her arms and knees and hair loss, and itching, and had to be started on dapsone.

Discussion

Dermatitis herpetiformis (DH) is a chronic, blistering skin condition that affects 15–25% of people with celiac disease [10]. Most people with DH do not present with any other symptoms of celiac disease. The condition affects mainly adults and is more common in men in northern European countries.

The main pathophysiological event is an abnormal immune response to gluten in which IgA antibodies develop against the epidermal skin antigen transglutaminase. This triggers a more generalized immune skin reaction, resulting in recruitment of neutrophils and eosinophils, formation of microabscesses and development of blistering lesions, mainly at the elbows, knees, buttocks, back, or scalp which are extremely itchy.

The diagnosis is made by a positive transglutaminase blood screening test (IgA and IgG) and skin biopsy. A small bowel biopsy at endoscopy is often requested; this can be normal if the patient is not affected by celiac disease, but can also be falsely negative if the patient is already on a gluten-free diet, or the sample was taken from an unaffected site.

The main focus of treatment is a gluten-free diet, because it reduces the requirement for dapsone, it improves any associated gluten enteropathy, enhances nutrition and bone density and may reduce the risk of developing other autoimmune conditions as well as the risk of small bowel lymphoma.

Dapsone is the treatment of choice for DH; it is administered as an oral medication at a dose between 50 and 100 mg. It is a sulfone antibiotic medication that has been available for many years to treat leprosy. Dapsone is also used for treating various other skin conditions including vasculitis, pyoderma gangrenosum, Sweet's disease, aphthous ulceration, and granuloma anulare. Dapsone treatment requires careful laboratory monitoring because it is associated with a number of side effects such as hypersensitivity reactions, hemolysis particularly in patients with glucose-6-phosphate dehydrogenase (G6PD) deficiency, peripheral neuropathy, liver toxicity, and hematological problems such as agranulocytosis and aplastic anemia. It must be used with caution in patients who have cardiac and pulmonary disease, and avoided in porphyria.

Several other skin manifestations of gastrointestinal diseases are common or important to recognize. Typical skin lesions include erythema nodosum, pyoderma gangrenosum seen in about 15% of patients with inflammatory bowel disease, and more rarely necrotizing vasculitis, cutaneous polyarteritis nodosa and granulomatous perivasculitis.

Peutz–Jeghers syndrome (hamartomatous intestinal polyposis syndrome) is an autosomal dominant condition due to a mutation of the *STK11/LKB1* tumor-suppressor gene at chromosome 19. It is often the mucocutaneous lesions associated with hyperpigmentation in the mouth and on the hands and feet that raise the suspicion of this diagnosis.

Hereditary hemorrhagic telangiectasia (HHT) is another autosomal dominant condition characterized by mucocutaneous telangiectasias and iron deficiency anemia secondary to chronic blood loss. Epistaxis is the most common presentation followed by GI bleeding. More than 80% of all cases of HHT are due to mutations in either *ENG* or *ACVRL1* genes at chromosomes 9 and 12.

A very rare but important skin condition is the necrolytic migratory erythema which is classically associated with glucagon-secreting islet cell tumors of the pancreas, diabetes, and profound weight loss. The lesions are migratory, initially erythematous, progressing to raised bullous lesions and scaling. It is typically characterized by necrolysis of the upper epidermis with vacuolated keratinocytes on skin biopsy [11].

In conclusion there is a significant association between multisystem disorders and GI disease and early recognition of such associations can lead to earlier diagnosis and treatment, which in certain cases can alter prognosis.

References

1 Watson A, Heading RC, Shepherd NA. *Guidelines for the diagnosis and management of Barrett's columnar-lined oesophagus. A Report of the Working Party of the British Society of Gastroenterology.* 2005.

2 Wassenaar EB, Oelschlager BK. Effect of medical and surgical treatment of Barrett's metaplasia. *World J Gastroenterol* 2010;**16**:3773–9.

3 Grant AM, Wileman SM, Ramsay CR, et al., REFLUX Trial Group. Minimal access surgery compared with medical management for chronic gastro-oesophageal reflux disease: UK collaborative randomised trial. *BMJ* 2008;**337**:a2664.

4 Gatenby PA, Ramus JR, Caygill CP, Charlett A, Winslet MC, Watson A. Treatment modality and risk of development of dysplasia and adenocarcinoma in columnar-lined esophagus. *Dis Esoph* 2009;**22**:133–42.

5 Stark ME, Devault KR. Complications following fundoplication. *Tech Gastrointest Endosc* 2006;**8**: 40–53.

6 Gong Y, Huang ZB, Christensen E, Gluud C. Ursodeoxycholic acid for primary biliary cirrhosis. *Cochrane Database Syst Rev* 2008;(3):CD000551.

7 Cavazza A, Caballería L, Floreani A, et al. Incidence, risk factors, and survival of hepatocellular carcinoma in primary biliary cirrhosis: comparative analysis from two centers. *Hepatology* 2009;**50**:1162–8.

8 Douglas JG, Dewhurst NG, Finlayson NDC. Primary biliary cirrhosis and scleroderma in a man. *Br J Clin Pract* 1981;**35**:284–5.

9 Duggan JM, Duggan AE. Systematic review: the liver in coeliac disease. *Aliment Pharmacol Ther* 2005;**21**: 515–18.

10 Rodrigo L. Celiac disease. *World J Gastroenterol* 2006;**12**:6585–93.

11 van Beek AP, de Haas ERM, van Vloten WA, Lips CJM, Roijers JFM, Canninga-van Dijk MR. The glucagonoma syndrome and necrolytic migratory erythema: a clinical review. *Eur J Endocrinol* 2004;**151**:531–7.

PART TWO

Hepatology and Pancreatobiliary

10 Clinical Approach to Pancreatobiliary Disease

Erica J. Revie,[1] Lisa J. Massie,[1] Anne-Marie Lennon,[2] and O. James Garden[1]

[1]Clinical Surgery The Royal Infirmary, Edinburgh, UK
[2]Division of Gastroenterology and Hepatology, Johns Hopkins Hospital, Baltimore, MD, USA

Case 1: right upper quadrant pain and jaundice

Case presentation

A 27-year-old white man presented with a 6-week history of right upper quadrant (RUQ) pain radiating to his back, associated with dark urine and pale stools. For the previous 4 months, he had experienced passage of loose, pale bowel motions which were difficult to flush away and he had lost 14 lb over the preceding month. He was on no medications, was a non-smoker, and drank 25 units of alcohol per week. He was apyrexial, with blood pressure 112/63 mmHg, pulse rate 51 beats//min, respiratory rate 18/min with oxygen saturations of 99% on room air. Cardiovascular and respiratory examinations were unremarkable. The abdomen was soft, non-tender with active bowel sounds and no organomegaly. Rectal examination was normal and fecal occult blood testing was negative.

Initial investigations (normal values in brackets)
Hemoglobin 14.1 (12.5–16.5) g/dL
Normal mean corpuscular volume
WCC 6.2 (4–11) $\times 10^9$/L
Platelet count 200 (150–420) $\times 10^9$/L
Serum electrolytes normal
Albumin 40 (35–50) g/L
Alanine aminotransferase (ALT) 264 (10–50) IU/L
Alkaline phosphatase (ALP) 598 (40–125) IU/L
γ-Glutamyltransferase (GGT) 158 (10–55) IU/L

Bilirubin 9 (3–16) μmol/L
Prothrombin time normal
Fasting glucose 7.5 mmol/L
Calcium 2.33 (2.1–2.6) mmol/L
Triglycerides 1.3 (0.8–2.1) mmol/L
Amylase 56 (<100) IU/mL

Questions

• What further imaging investigations will you consider?
• What further investigations may be considered based on the above findings?
• What is the diagnosis based on the clinical presentation in this young patient and what are the main causes leading to this condition?

Further investigations

Imaging
Abdominal ultrasonography and abdominal computed tomography (CT) are the imaging investigations. Abdominal ultrasonography demonstrated multiple small calculi and sludge in the gallbladder. The common bile duct (CBD) was dilated (1.2 cm) with a possible calculus in the distal common bile duct. The pancreas was not visualized. There were no focal liver lesions or other abnormality. CT demonstrated an enlarged head of pancreas with heterogeneous low attenuation. A small rounded area of defined low attenuation (20 mm) was seen within the head of

---

Problem-based Approach to Gastroenterology and Hepatology, First Edition. Edited by John N. Plevris, Colin W. Howden.
© 2012 Blackwell Publishing Ltd. Published 2012 by Blackwell Publishing Ltd.

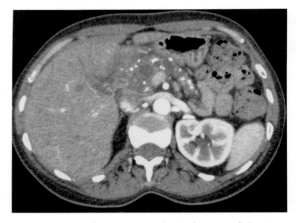

Figure 10.1 CT demonstrating classic features of chronic pancreatitis with slight enlargement of the pancreatic head, cystic changes in the head and neck of the gland, with diffuse calcification throughout the pancreatic parenchyma.

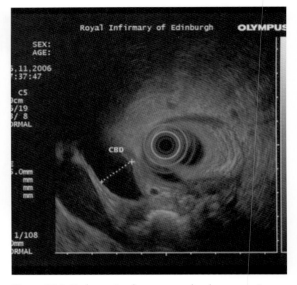

Figure 10.2 Endoscopic ultrasonography demonstrating 15 mm dilatation and smooth stricture within distal common bile duct (labeled).

the pancreas. There were multiple areas of calcification within a distended pancreatic duct as well as areas of calcification within the head of pancreas and the uncinate process (Figure 10.1).

The pancreatic tail was atrophic. The CBD was dilated (14 mm). The distal CBD tapered in the head of the pancreas with no obvious intraluminal calculus. Multiple lymph nodes measuring less than 1 cm were seen anterior to head of the pancreas.

Further imaging by magnetic resonance cholangio-pancreatography (MRCP) or endoscopic ultrasonography (EUS), depending on center availability, to characterize further the pancreatic lesion is favored by some. In the jaundiced patient, however, proceeding directly to endoscopic retrograde cholangiopancreatography (ERCP) is an alternate option because appropriate therapeutic intervention can be applied at the same time.

Serum IgG4 levels and genetic testing for hereditary pancreatitis should be carried out due to his age.

ERCP revealed a dilated pancreatic duct with a possible stricture at the lower end of the common bile duct. However, it was not possible to get adequate filling or a wire cannulation. MRCP confirmed a dilated CBD (18 mm) but no intraductal calculi were seen. The pancreatic features were similar to CT and it was concluded that the most likely diagnosis was chronic pancreatitis causing duct dilation but it

was impossible to rule out a malignant process. EUS revealed a diffusely enlarged head of pancreas with widespread calcification and stones within a dilated pancreatic duct. No focal mass was seen. No CBD stones or sludge were seen within a slightly dilated bile duct. There were multiple, small, reactive-looking lymph nodes and numerous collateral vessels around the stomach suggesting portal hypertension (Figure 10.2).

Diagnosis

The diagnosis is severe, calcific, chronic pancreatitis. The main causes are alcohol, hereditary pancreatitis, gallstone disease causing repeated episodes of pancreatitis, and autoimmune pancreatitis (unusual cause of calcification).

Differential diagnosis

The overall differential diagnoses in a patient with pain, obstructive jaundice, weight loss, and steatorrhea are given in Table 10.1. Likely causes include gallstones; primary sclerosing cholangitis and malignancy are possible given the weight loss. Chronic

Table 10.1 Causes of cholestasis

Obstructive	Gallstones
	Cancer of the pancreas or bile ducts
	Primary sclerosing cholangitis
	Biliary stricture
	Ischemic bile duct injury
	Acute or chronic rejection in a transplant patient
	Graft-vs-host disease
	Vanishing bile duct syndrome
Non-obstructive	
Infectious	Viral hepatitis, herpes and other viral infections
Toxic	Sepsis
Metabolic	Bacteremia
Infiltration and storage	Drugs, total parenteral nutrition
Canalicular transport	Wilson's disease
Miscellaneous	Amyloidosis
	Metastatic cancer
	Cholestasis of pregnancy
	Dubin–Johnson syndrome
	Benign recurrent intrahepatic cholestasis (BRIC)
	Rotor syndrome
	Shock/hypoperfusion
	Hypoxemia
	Hepatic sickle cell crisis
	Hodgkin's disease
	Paraneoplastic syndromes

Modified from Li MK, Crawford JM. The pathology of cholestasis. *Semin Liver Dis* 2004;**24**:1–39.

pancreatitis (CP) may cause a biliary stricture but classically presents with epigastric pain, radiating around to the back, associated with nausea and vomiting. Up to 20% of patients may present with signs of pancreatic insufficiency in the absence of pain [1]. When >90% of the pancreatic function is lost, patients can declare signs of pancreatic insufficiency. Failure to absorb fat causes loose, foul smelling, greasy stools which are difficult to wash away and absorption of the fat-soluble vitamins A, E, D and K may be impaired. Endocrine pancreatic insufficiency occurs late in the disease.

Risk factors for chronic pancreatitis

Alcohol excess accounts for up to 55–80% of cases (Table 10.2). Studies suggest that chronic pancreatitis occurs after ingestion of 140–400 g alcohol/day for 17–21 years [2,3]. However, only 10% of heavy alcohol drinkers develop pancreatic disease, suggesting that alcohol may be a cofactor and genetic susceptibility is important in its development. Tobacco smoking is an independent risk factor [4,5], although the mechanism for action is not known. Hyperlipidemia is associated with acute pancreatitis, and may account for a small number of chronic pancreatitis cases, although this is controversial [6]. This patient's ultrasound scan suggested a CBD stone but this was not confirmed by MRCP, ERCP, or EUS, all of which are more sensitive for detection. Pancreas divisum occurs when the dorsal and ventral pancreas fail to fuse and occurs in 7% of individuals. Some authors report that 60% of such patients benefit from surgical sphincteroplasty [7] whereas others report a similar incidence of pancreatitis in those with and without pancreas divisum [8]. Sphincter of Oddi dysfunction (SOD) has also been implicated.

In the absence of any obvious cause, autoimmune pancreatitis (AIP) must be considered. It was first described in 1961 by Sarles et al. [9], but it was not until 1995 that it was recognized as a disease in its own right [10]. It is twice as common in men, and mean age at diagnosis is 60 years with a range of 20–70. The most common presentation is painless jaundice, which is the presenting symptom in 86% of patients in one study due to either an inflammatory mass in the head of the pancreas or associated sclerosing cholangitis [11]. Abdominal pain and steatorrhea are unusual but weight loss is present in 35% of

Table 10.2 Risk factors for chronic pancreatitis

Ductal obstruction	Stone
	Tumor
	Trauma
	Pseudocyst
	Pancreas divisum[a]
	SOD[a]
	Periampullary duodenal wall cyst
	Postirradiation obstructive pancreatitis
Toxic/ Metabolic	Alcohol
	Tobacco
	Hypercalcaemia
	Hypertriglyceridemia[a]
	Hyperparathyroidism
	Chronic renal failure
Systemic diseases	SLE
	Cystic fibrosis
Tropical pancreatitis	
Autoimmune pancreatitis	Isolated autoimmune pancreatitis
	Associated with Sjögren's syndrome, IBD, PBC
Hereditary/ Genetic	Trypsinogen (codon 16, 22, 23, 29, 122) mutations
	CFTR mutations
	SPINK1 mutations
	α_1-Antitrypsin deficiency (possible)
Alcohol	
Medications/ Toxins	Phenacetin abuse
	Organotin compounds (e.g. DBTC or di-N-butyltin dichloride)

[a]Controversial.
IBD, inflammatory bowel disease; PBC, primary biliary cirrhosis; SLE, systemic lupus erythematosus; SOD, sphincter of Oddi dysfunction.

patients [12,13]. Up to 76% of patients have diabetes mellitus, which improves after the AIP is treated with steroids [14]. AIP is associated with sclerosing cholangitis, inflammatory bowel disease, bilateral swelling of the parotid or submandibular glands, disseminated lymphadenopathy, fever, retroperitoneal fibrosis with hydronephrosis, symptoms of IBD, pulmonary infiltration, and prostatitis [15]. Elevated levels of IgG4 can be found in serum in 15–76% [11,16,17]. Affected tissue can also be stained for IgG4. A variety of autoantibodies has been implicated but none is specific for AIP. The pancreas may present on imaging as diffusely enlarged and "sausage"-shaped or as a focal inflammatory mass with secondary ductal dilation of the CBD or pancreatic duct. Although calcification and pancreatic duct stones can occur, these are rare [11]. Enlarged peripancreatic lymph nodes up to 30 mm can be seen [18]. The Japanese Pancreatic Society has drawn up minimum consensus criteria for its diagnosis [19], while a Mayo Clinic group have developed the "HISORT" criteria which are based on histology, imaging, serology, other organ involvement, and response to steroid therapy [20]. Although this patient presented with painless obstructive jaundice and is male, he is young for a presentation of AIP. His imaging showed marked calcification of his pancreas which is an unusual finding in AIP, and his serum IgG4 was normal all of which make the diagnosis less likely.

Patients with mutations of the cystic fibrosis transmembrane conductance regulator (CFTR) gene can present with no other signs of cystic fibrosis except chronic pancreatitis. Most laboratories test routinely for 18–20 mutations in the CFTR gene; however, many more mutations exist. One study that examined 40 patients with chronic pancreatitis found that 18 (45%) had at least one abnormal allele when complete DNA analysis was performed [21]. Mutations in the trypsinogen gene, which are inherited in an autosomal dominant fashion, are found in patients with hereditary pancreatitis. The trypsinogen gene is found on the long arm of chromosome 7 and several genes have been implicated, with R122H substitution mutation, N29I, and 16V being the most common described [22–24]. A mutation in SPINK-1, which is a pancreatic trypsin inhibitor, has also been found in some patients with chronic pancreatitis [25]. Most patients with hereditary pancreatitis present with symptoms by the age of 20.

A genetic profile was requested in this patient; he was: *CFTR* gene negative, and *R122H*, *N29I*, and *A16V* mutations in cationic trypsinogen gene (*PRSS1*) negative. These results reduce the likelihood of, but do not exclude, hereditary pancreatitis.

Despite his age at presentation, this patient may well have a hereditary form of chronic pancreatitis despite the negative genetic tests. Some 100 genes have been described as involved in hereditary pancreatitis. Guidelines on genetic testing are available [26].

Differentiating pancreatic cancer from chronic pancreatitis can be very difficult and patients with chronic pancreatitis have a 16.5 increased relative risk of developing pancreatic cancer [27].

Clinical diagnosis

Idiopathic chronic pancreatitis with secondary CBD stenosis.

Patient management

The normal investigation of a patient with chronic pancreatitis consists of laboratory studies, pancreatic function tests, and imaging.

Laboratory tests

Routine blood tests include complete blood count, urea and electrolytes, lipid profile, calcium and glucose. Fecal elastase can be used to assess pancreatic exocrine function and genetic screening can be performed if indicated.

Imaging

Plain films Calcification can be seen on up to 30% of plain abdominal films in patients with CP and is seen commonly in tropical, alcohol and hereditary pancreatitis. It is rare in idiopathic cases.

Ultrasonography Transabdominal ultrasonography is non-invasive and readably available. It can assess the size, shape, contour, and echotexture of the gland, as well as identifying calcification and ductal dilation. It has a sensitivity of between 60% and 70% and a specificity of 80–90% for diagnosing chronic pancreatitis [28]. However, views of the pancreas are often obscured due to overlying bowel gas.

Computed tomography Findings on CT consistent with CP include calcification within the pancreatic ducts or parenchyma, and/or dilated main pancreatic ducts combined with parenchymal atrophy. CT has relatively good sensitivity for diagnosing moderate-to-severe chronic pancreatitis [29–32] as well as identifying the complications of chronic pancreatitis, including visualizing inflammatory or neoplastic masses larger than 1 cm [33].

Magnetic resonance imaging MRCP is non-invasive, avoids ionizing radiation and contrast administration, and does not routinely require sedation, making it the diagnostic procedure of choice. Early findings of chronic pancreatitis include low-signal-intensity pancreas on T1-weighted fat-suppressed images, decreased and delayed enhancement after intravenous contrast administration, and dilated side branches. Late findings include parenchymal atrophy or enlargement, pseudocysts, and dilation and beading of the pancreatic duct, often with intraductal calcifications [34]. The administration of secretin during the MRCP can improve the detection of subtle side-branch abnormalities and allows non-invasive assessment of exocrine pancreatic function. MRCP has an accuracy of 92% compared with ERCP for detecting either acute or chronic pancreatitis [35]. MRCP is also highly accurate for identifying pancreas divisum [36].

Endoscopic ultrasound EUS is minimally invasive and chronic pancreatitis is diagnosed based on the presence of a number of parenchymal and ductal criteria [37]. Chronic pancreatitis is unlikely in the absence of any criteria, and is highly likely in the presence of five or more criteria, whereas the clinical significance of one to four features is unclear. EUS appears to have very high sensitivity for disease and is thus valuable to "rule out" chronic pancreatitis in patients with non-specific abdominal pain; however, specificity is only moderate and likely requires other tests to confirm [38]. In non-calcific pancreatitis, EUS is very useful if a pancreatic mass is queried. It has a sensitivity of 96% (range 85–100%) [39–52] compared with 75% for ultrasonography, 77–80% for CT, and 89% for angiography [40,43,53,54] for detecting a pancreatic mass in a normal pancreas. EUS can identify pancreatic cancer in up to 8% of patients in whom CT has demonstrated a "full" or

121

enlarged pancreas but no mass [55]. EUS–fine needle aspiration (FNA) can be performed if a mass is found. However, EUS views are markedly limited by the presence of calcification.

Endoscopic retrograde cholangiopancreatogram
ERCP is the gold standard for diagnosing chronic pancreatitis in the absence of tissue, with a sensitivity and specificity of 90% and 100% respectively [56]. ERCP classification of chronic pancreatitis is based on the Cambridge classification [57]. In early or mild disease side branches and smaller ducts become dilated and irregular. As the disease progresses, these changes can be found in the main pancreatic duct. In severe disease, there is evidence of tortuosity, strictures, calcification, and cyst formation.

Pancreatic function testing
Pancreatic function testing can diagnose pancreatic insufficiency, aid in the evaluation of chronic pancreatitis, and provide a basis for rational treatment. Few centers perform direct testing of pancreatic exocrine secretion because this involves the administration of a meal or hormonal secretagogues followed by the collection and analysis of duodenal fluid to quantify normal pancreatic secretory content (i.e. enzymes and bicarbonate). These tests often use different stimulants and measure different parameters. Furthermore, the lack of appropriate control populations and technical variability make the test difficult to interpret [6].

Indirect measures of pancreatic function include staining a spot specimen with Sudan stain, but this is less reliable than a 72-hour quantitative measurement of fecal fat. Measurements of fecal chymotrypsin on a spot stool sample show a sensitivity of 85% for advanced chronic pancreatitis, but only 49% for mild or moderate pancreatic exocrine insufficiency [58]. Patients must stop their exogenous enzymes 2 days before the test and levels may not be reliable if the patient has concomitant diarrhea. Fecal pancreatic elastase-1 also measures fecal chymotrypsin and has the advantage of being independent of pancreatic enzyme replacement therapy. Studies have shown that it has a sensitivity of 100% for severe, 77–100% for moderate, and 0–63% for mild pancreatic exocrine insufficiency, with a specificity of approximately 93% [59–62]. The specificity of the test is reduced in patients with Crohn's disease, gluten-sensitive enteropathy, or short gut syndrome test [63]. The pancreo-

lauryl test measures the hydrolysis of fluorescein dilaurate by arylesterase. Although the sensitivity of this test is improved with administration of secretin, some authors feel that it may not be specific for pancreatic disease [6].

Complications
Splenic vein thrombosis can result in portal hypertension and gastric varices. Splenectomy is usually curative for patients who develop bleeding from varices. Pseudocyst occurs due to duct disruption in approximately 10% of patients with chronic pancreatitis. Pseudocysts can be differentiated from other cystic lesions of the pancreas due to the lack of an epithelial lining. Most pseudocysts are asymptomatic but they can cause pain, infection, pseudoaneurysm formation, and fistula formation into the chest or abdomen, resulting in pleural effusion or pancreatic ascites. Expansion of the pseudocyst can cause biliary, duodenal, or vascular obstruction. This patient had biliary stenosis but related to inflammation or fibrosis of the pancreatic head.

Follow-up
The patient subsequently underwent a duodenum-preserving Frey procedure with drainage of the pancreatic duct in an attempt to improve ongoing pain. Histology taken at surgery confirmed diffuse fibrosis with no evidence of vasculitis. The appearances were compatible with chronic pancreatitis but with non-specific appearances regarding etiology. The histology from the removed gallbladder was entirely normal with no evidence of stones. The patient is well and asymptomatic 36 months later, on pancreatic enzyme supplements.

Case 2: epigastric and RUQ pain

Case presentation

A 55-year-old woman presented as an emergency with a 2-day history of epigastric and right upper quadrant pain, radiating to her back. She attended her general practitioner on the first day of illness when the pain was initially mild, had blood investigations undertaken, was given analgesia, and asked to return for review the next day. However, the next morning she attended hospital as an emergency, having started to vomit and to feel hot and shivery overnight. She also reported new, loose, pale-colored stools and very dark urine. She admitted to similar episodes of pain previously, but these had always settled spontaneously, and had never been associated with vomiting or fever.

Other than mild asthma, she had no past medical history of note. She used a salbutamol inhaler and occasionally took an antacid. She worked as a receptionist, was a non-smoker, and drank approximately 18 units of alcohol per week. She lived with her husband and three children. There was no recent foreign travel.

Examination revealed a BMI of 30. She was jaundiced, perspiring, and had a temperature of 39.2°C. Pulse rate was 115 beats/min and BP 102/65 mmHg. Examination of cardiovascular and respiratory systems was otherwise normal. The abdomen was soft, but tender in the RUQ and epigastrium. Murphy's sign was negative. There was no organomegaly and bowel sounds were quiet. Rectal examination was normal with minimal soft pale stool (fecal occult blood [FOB] negative).

This patient is clinically jaundiced. The results of the investigations taken at the general practice (Table 10.3) to investigate this patient's jaundice suggest a hepatic parenchymal etiology, yet the pale stools and dark urine suggest post-hepatic or obstructive jaundice.

Questions

- How can these findings be reconciled?
- What is the most likely underlying pathology?
- What further investigations may be considered?
- How would you decide which imaging or therapeutic procedure should be performed next in this patient?
- What other key priorities are there in managing this patient?

Differential diagnosis

When differentiating hepatic from obstructive jaundice, it is worth noting that pale stools and dark urine are usually associated with obstructive jaundice, but *can* occur transiently in acute hepatic illnesses [64]. Furthermore, liver function tests may show a mixed picture of derangement and elevated aminotransferases (usually associated with parenchymal disease) may occur in biliary obstruction, occasion-

Table 10.3 Case 2: blood results

	Reference range	At GP	On admission
Hb (g/dl)	11.5–15	13.1	12.1
WCC (× 10⁹/L)	4–11	12.5	18.6
Platelets (× 10⁹/L)	150–400	367	465
MCV (fL)	76–98	95	94
INR	0.9–1.2		1.0
Urea (mmol/L)	2.5–6.5	6.2	11.2
Creatinine (μmol/L)	50–120	107	137
Na⁺ (mmol/L)	135–145	136	143
K⁺ (mmol/L)	3.5–5.0	4.1	3.8
ALT (IU/L)	5–30	153	324
GGT (IU/L)	5–30	34	1256
Bilirubin (μmol/L)	2–17	15	78
ALP (IU/L)	30–130	112	534
Albumin (g/L)	35–55	40	35
Amylase (IU/L)	0–50		121
Glucose (mmol/L)	3.5–5.5	4.7	7.1

ALP, alkaline phosphatase; ALT, alanine aminotransferase; GGT, γ-glutamyltransferase; INR, international normalized ratio; MCV, mean corpuscular volume; WCC, white cell count.

ally before significant elevation of alkaline phosphatase and γ-glutamyltransferase (GGT) [65]. Similarly, swollen, damaged hepatocytes seen in hepatitis often cause a degree of intrahepatic biliary obstruction. The blood tests taken by the GP should therefore be considered in the context of other features of the patient's presentation, and repeated to identify any trend.

There is clearly a concomitant infective process occurring in this patient. The fever associated with viral hepatitis is usually low grade, whereas high-grade fever is more in keeping with ascending biliary infection or hepatic abscess. Ultrasonography of the liver and biliary tree should be performed to clarify this, and other sources of infection should also be sought and ruled out.

The triad of RUQ pain, jaundice, and fever, is in keeping with a diagnosis of cholangitis. All three features of Charcot's triad are seen only in 50–70% of patients with cholangitis [66–69], and atypical presentation can lead to a delay in diagnosis. This is especially true of elderly people for whom a high index of suspicion must be maintained [70]. Rigors are very suggestive of biliary sepsis.

Cholangitis has a number of possible etiologies. Gallstones, benign strictures, malignancy, pancreatitis, and endoscopic manipulation of the biliary tree are all implicated in the development of biliary infection [71,72].

Gallstones are by far the most likely cause in this patient. Excluding those patients who have undergone biliary procedures, gallstones remain the most common cause of cholangitis. This patient not only demonstrates risk factors for the development of gallstones, but her history of recurrent pain over the years is consistent with episodes of biliary colic. Gallstones may impede bile flow not only by impaction in the distal CBD, but also by external compression of the common hepatic duct by a stone lodged in the cystic duct or Hartmann's pouch (Mirizzi's syndrome). Rarely, an inflamed and edematous gallbladder may compress the CBD.

During an episode of pancreatitis, significant swelling and inflammation of the pancreatic tissue surrounding the distal common bile duct can also impede biliary flow. It can often be difficult to determine whether pancreatitis is a *cause* or a *consequence* of CBD blockage, as a distal CBD stone may only transiently block the pancreatic duct, initiating pancreatitis, before passing spontaneously. Pancreatic enzymes should always be measured in patients presenting with obstructive jaundice, and where raised, prognostic scoring systems should be employed to predict severity (Table 10.4).

Cholangitis is seen much less frequently in malignant biliary obstruction such as that due to an ampullary tumor, than it is in choledocholithiasis, but should be borne in mind. Where it does occur, it is usually associated with biliary instrumentation. With no history of weight loss, and episodes of pain occurring over *years*, malignancy is unlikely in this patient.

Diagnostic findings

The results of blood tests taken on admission are shown in Table 10.3. Urine dipstick shows bilirubin strongly positive and ketones positive.

Chest and abdominal radiography were normal. Around 10% of gallstones are radio-opaque but occasionally a plain abdominal radiograph may reveal some of the complications of gallstone disease.

TABLE 10.4 Glasgow criteria for predicting severity of acute pancreatitis

On admission	
Age	>55 years
White cell count	$>15 \times 10^9$/L
Glucose	>10 mmol/L (no history of diabetes)
Serum urea	>16 mmol/L
Arterial oxygen saturation	<8 kPa
Within 48 h	
Serum calcium	<2 mmol/L
Serum albumin	<32 g/L
LDH	>600 U/L
AST/ALT	>200 U/L

ALT, alanine aminotransferase; AST, aspartate aminotransferase; LDH, lactate dehydrogenase.

Assuming no recent instrumentation, air in the biliary tree suggests the presence of a biliary–enteric fistula. This may be accompanied by small bowel obstruction, if a large gallstone has become lodged at the ileocecal junction (gallstone ileus). In cholecystitis, the presence of gas-forming organisms may be suspected if air is seen in the wall of the gallbladder and a porcelain gallbladder may also be seen on a plain radiograph.

Ultrasonography demonstrated a dilated CBD measuring 16 mm in diameter. It is the first-line investigation for imaging the liver and biliary tract. In experienced hands, this inexpensive, non-invasive test disease can detect biliary obstruction and stones in the gallbladder with high diagnostic accuracy [73]. However, the distal CBD is often poorly visualized, leaving uncertainty as to the cause of biliary obstruction. Given all the available information, the most likely diagnosis in this patient is a gallstone in the distal CBD. However, where uncertainty exists, the clinical picture then dictates how this is further investigated.

Options may include repeat ultrasound scan, further imaging by CT or MRCP, or more invasive investigation by ERCP or percutaneous transhepatic cholangiography (PTC). Abdominal CT is useful for imaging the pancreas, and often employed when pancreatic malignancy is suspected. MRCP allows more accurate imaging of the biliary tree and detection of stones in the bile ducts. ERCP and PTC have the advantage that a diagnostic procedure can be combined with a therapeutic one, in the form of biliary decompression, but both are invasive and not without risk. There is rarely a role for surgery in the immediate management of biliary obstruction.

Diagnosis

This is choledocholithiasis with cholangitis.

Patient management

Mortality rates in cholangitis range from 13% to 88%, and rise with increasing age. Prompt diagnosis and management are therefore vital, and treatment priorities include resuscitation, antibiotic therapy, and decompression of the biliary tree.

Acute renal failure is a marker of poor prognosis in cholangitis [71], and careful attention should be paid to fluid balance and renal function. Antibiotic therapy should be started empirically as soon as blood cultures have been taken. The causative organisms vary with underlying pathology and geographic location, and cover should generally be broad spectrum. When cholangitis is secondary to choledocholithiasis, Gram-negative organisms such as *Klebsiella* spp., *Pseudomonas aeruginosa*, and *Escherichia coli* are most frequently implicated [74]. In this situation, third-generation cephalosporins, ureidopenicillins, fluoroquinolones, and carbapenems provide good cover. The ureidopenicillins, piperacillin and mezlocillin, have the added advantage of being excreted at high concentrations in the bile.

In a proportion of patients, cholangitis may be treated adequately with antibiotics alone. Those who are reasonably well, or respond well to antibiotic therapy, may undergo further imaging of the biliary tree by MRCP. However, it appears that bile duct stones are much less likely to pass spontaneously in jaundiced or cholangitic patients, compared with those with cholecystitis [75]. Therefore, patients who fail to respond should proceed to biliary decompression without delay.

ERCP is the procedure of choice in the septic patient with an obstructed biliary system. PTC is reserved for those patients where ERCP fails, due to technical or anatomic reasons. With a very short history of obstructive jaundice, the synthetic function of the liver is unlikely to be significantly impaired, but coagulation defects should be identified and corrected before intervention is undertaken because "subclinical" biliary obstruction may deplete vitamin K levels.

At ERCP, the anatomy of the biliary tree and the level of obstruction can be clarified, brushings can be taking if any potentially malignant lesion is identified, and sphincterotomy and balloon trawl can be performed to relieve obstruction secondary to stones. For elderly people or those with extensive comorbidity, this may constitute definitive management. All other patients who are fit enough should proceed to early cholecystectomy to prevent recurrence of bile duct stones and avoid gallbladder symptoms in the future.

Case 3: epigastric pain radiating to the back

Case presentation

A 57-year-old man had presented to hospital 5 months previously with epigastric pain radiating to his back. Bloods taken on admission had revealed new-onset type 2 diabetes mellitus and an abdominal CT showed changes suggestive of chronic pancreatitis. Two months before review he developed symptoms of obstructive jaundice and underwent ERCP. This revealed a tapered stricture in the distal bile duct suspicious of malignancy and a stent was inserted to good effect. The patient was referred to the hepatobiliary clinic for further investigation.

At review, the patient admitted to feeling very tired and that he had lost 6 kg in weight over the past few months. He denied any symptoms of steatorrhea. Past medical history included longstanding hypertension and hypercholesterolemia. He lived with his wife, smoked 30 cigarettes a day, and denied any alcohol excess. His mother had died of gastric cancer.

Drug history: atenolol, simvastatin, aspirin, co-dydramol, dihydrocodeine.

There was no evidence of jaundice, anemia, finger clubbing, or lymphedema. The abdomen was soft and non-tender with no organomegaly or masses. Examination of the chest was unremarkable.

125

Bloods taken at the clinic reveal normal hematology and renal function; however, bilirubin levels were 36 (2–17) μmol/L.
ALT 146 (5–30) IU/L
ALP 247 (30–130) IU/L
Amylase 126 (0–50) IU/L.

A repeat CT scan showed a heterogeneous 4-cm diameter mass containing multiple small cysts in the head of the pancreas. There was dilation of the distal pancreatic duct. A few small lymph nodes (<1 cm) were seen in the peripancreatic fat.

Differential diagnosis

In this case, the patient's history of abdominal pain, weight loss, and obstructive jaundice, in addition to the CT findings of a mass in the head of the pancreas, make pancreatic malignancy an important diagnosis to exclude; however, there are other diagnoses that should be kept in mind.

Adenocarcinoma

The most common tumor originating in the pancreas is ductal adenocarcinoma; this accounts for over 90% of pancreatic tumors and presents frequently with obstructive jaundice, which may be painless. The jaundice may result from the primary tumor obstructing the biliary system in the head of the pancreas, or from hepatic metastases or nodal involvement at porta hepatis. Courvoisier's syndrome of a palpable gallbladder in a patient with painless jaundice is frequently seen in patients with pancreatic adenocarcinoma.

New-onset diabetes mellitus should raise suspicion of the possibility of an underlying pancreatic cancer. Up to 70% of patients with pancreatic cancer have diabetes or impaired glucose tolerance [76]. Type 2 diabetes mellitus may be a risk factor for pancreatic cancer but is also a symptom in itself. The patient in this case also demonstrates one of the most well-documented risk factors of pancreatic adenocarcinoma: cigarette smoking.

There are also hereditary syndromes that predispose to development of pancreatic adenocarcinoma including FAMMM (familial atypical mole-multiple melanoma), BRCA-2 expression, HNPCC (hereditary non-polyposis colorectal cancer syndrome), and Peutz–Jehgers syndrome [77]. It is therefore important to ask about a family history of pancreatic cancer because between 5 and 10% of pancreatic adenocarcinomas are thought to have a genetic component.

Cystic lesions

The presence of a cystic lesion in the pancreas raises further diagnostic issues. Such lesions can be divided into neoplastic and non-neoplastic lesions. The most common cystic lesions are non-neoplastic, namely pancreatic pseudocysts, localized collections of inflammatory fluid. The diagnosis can be suspected from a history of pancreatitis (or, more rarely, trauma), alcohol abuse, and radiological appearances [78]. If there is doubt as to the diagnosis, cyst fluid aspirate may be obtained. Pseudocyst fluid typically has raised amylase levels.

Cystic neoplasms, although rare, may present with similar symptoms to adenocarcinoma; however, they can be an incidental finding on cross-sectional imaging. Serous cystic neoplasms are the most common. They are typically benign, and either polycystic and oligocystic. Diagnosis can be made on CT or MRI. Cyst fluid analysis typically shows low levels of amylase, Carcinoembryonic antigen (CEA) and CA19-9. Patients with small, asymptomatic neoplasms may be observed with regular imaging; however, surgical resection should be performed if the neoplasm is large, symptomatic, or there is uncertainty about the diagnosis.

Mucinous cystic neoplasms (MCNs) and intraductal papillary mucinous neoplasms (IPNMs) are usually premalignant or malignant. IPMNs are more common in the head of the pancreas and may present with features of obstructive jaundice. MCNs are typically located in the body or tail of the pancreas and therefore rarely present with jaundice. MCNs tend to affect women aged 30–50, whereas IPMNs typically affect older patients, with males affected equally [78]. Surgical resection is the treatment of choice, given the difficulty in differentiating between invasive and non-invasive disease.

Diagnostic findings

Tumor markers

CA19-9 can be used as a tumor marker for pancreatic adenocarcinoma with a sensitivity of approximately 85%, but it is it may be elevated in other conditions such as hepatitis, pancreatitis, and extrapancreatic malignancies [79].

What modalities are useful in staging pancreatic cancer?
Abdominal CT, endoscopic ultrasonography, and laparoscopic ultrasonography are useful.

Staging of pancreatic tumors
CT is the first-line investigation in imaging pancreatic lesions, because it is non-invasive and able to provide accurate TNM staging if a tumor is present, and therefore determine resectability. Endoscopic ultrasonography, although more invasive than CT, is particularly useful in cases such as this one where the CT features are not diagnostic of neoplasia. Fine needle aspirates can be taken during the procedure to provide diagnosis. Endoscopic ultrasonography is very effective for detecting small masses (<35 mm) and peripancreatic lymph node involvement. It is not as effective, however, in the detection of liver metastases or tumor spread to blood vessels [80].

Diagnosis

In this patient, approximately five cysts were identified in the head of the pancreas with changes suggestive of chronic pancreatitis, but no discrete mass was seen. However, fine needle aspirate from the head of the pancreas revealed atypical cells highly suspicious of carcinoma.

Further management

The patient proceeded to laparotomy for resection of the tumor. At the time of surgery, the pancreas was found to be diffusely thickened with dilated common bile and pancreatic ducts, in keeping with a diagnosis of pancreatic adenocarcinoma. There was evidence of local infiltration of the peritoneum adjacent to the tumor and on intraoperative ultrasonography the tumor extended to involve the superior mesenteric/portal vein junction. It was felt that resection was unlikely to be curative and palliative hepaticojejunostomy and gastroenterostomy were performed. TruCut core biopsy obtained at surgery confirmed the diagnosis to be pancreatic adenocarcinoma.

Discussion

Surgical resection provides the only chance of cure for patients with pancreatic adenocarcinoma. The vast majority of patients present late in the disease process and less than 20% will be suitable for resection. In this case, conventional preoperative staging was not successful. There has been much debate as to whether laparoscopic staging in such patients is useful. Proponents of the technique point to the 20% nontherapeutic laparotomy rate in such patients, whereas others highlight the need to consider palliative bypass in patients whose disease is found to be unresectable at operation. In this patient, laparoscopy was not performed because of doubts about the underlying diagnosis, the suspicion of a cystic neoplasm, and the absence of a substantial mass.

The American Joint Commission on Cancer staging system is useful in management. Stage I (disease confined to pancreas) and stage II (disease extends beyond pancreas but does not involve celiac axis or superior mesenteric artery) tumors are both potentially resectable whereas stage III (disease extends beyond pancreas and involves celiac axis and superior mesenteric artery) and stage IV (metastatic disease) tumors are unresectable [81].

If a patient is deemed to have a resectable tumor in the head of the pancreas (normally stage I/II), the most common procedure undertaken is Whipple's procedure (pancreaticoduodenectomy). Pylorus-preserving pancreaticoduodenectomy can also be performed with the aim of reducing postoperative complications such as reflux and dumping syndrome. However, there is no difference in morbidity or mortality or of long-term survival rates between the two procedures [82].

Five-year survival rates in patients who undergo potentially curative surgery are 7–25%. Adjuvant chemotherapy with 5-fluorouracil or gemcitabine has been shown to improve disease-free and median survival; however, the role of chemoradiotherapy is less clear [83].

Patients with advanced disease at presentation have very poor prognosis with median survival of up to 6 months. Endoscopic stenting (plastic or metal) is the main treatment for the relief of biliary obstruction; however, plastic stents tend to occlude after a few months and may need to be replaced, whereas metal stents may remain patent for longer. Surgical bypass or percutaneous biliary drainage is an alternative if endoscopic stenting is unsuccessful.

For most patients with advanced pancreatic cancer the focus is on palliative management. Although chemotherapy has been shown to prolong survival in some this may be at the expense of quality of life. Pancreatic insufficiency should be addressed with the use of oral pancreatic enzyme supplements. Pain relief can be difficult to manage and the use of celiac plexus block may be considered for intractable pain.

Conclusion

These three cases have highlighted the various challenges of managing patients with pancreatobiliary disease. It is crucial to take a careful history and interpret clinical findings and results of investigations based on the initial presentation. Case 1 demonstrates the considerable diagnostic difficulties that may arise in the patient presenting with jaundice due to pancreatic pathology. An extensive array of blood and radiological investigations may still leave the clinician in doubt as to the cause of chronic pancreatic inflammation, even when tissue is available for histological analysis after surgery. Case 2 demonstrates how rapidly patients with an acutely obstructed biliary system can become unwell, and reminds us of the importance of adequate resuscitation and early biliary decompression. The case also serves to demonstrate the increasing reliance of the clinician on radiological and endoscopic diagnosis and intervention for patients with gallstone-related disease. Case 3 highlights the difficulties of establishing a diagnosis of pancreatic carcinoma and of staging the disease accurately. This case also illustrates well the dismal prognosis for patients with pancreatic cancer and the need for better therapeutic options.

References

1 Layer P, Yamamoto H, Kalthoff L et al. The different courses of early- and late-onset idiopathic and alcoholic chronic pancreatitis. *Gastroenterology* 1994;**107**: 1481–7.

2 Dani R, Penna FJ, Nogueira CE. Etiology of chronic calcifying pancreatitis in Brazil: a report of 329 consecutive cases. *Int J Pancreatol* 1986;**1**:399–406.

3 Durbec J, Sarles H. Multicenter survey of the etiology of pancreatic diseases. Relationship between the relative risk of developing chronic pancreatitis and alcohol, protein and lipid consumption. *Digestion* 1978;**18**: 337–50.

4 Talamini G, Bassi C, Falconi M et al. Cigarette smoking: an independent risk factor in alcoholic pancreatitis. *Pancreas* 1996;**12**:131–7.

5 Lin Y, Tamakoshi A, Hayakawa T, et al. Cigarette smoking as a risk factor for chronic pancreatitis: a case-control study in Japan. Research Committee on Intractable Pancreatic Diseases. *Pancreas* 2000;**21**: 109–14.

6 Etemad B, Whitcomb DC. Chronic pancreatitis: Diagnosis, classification, and new genetic developments. *Gastroenterology* 2001;**120**:682–707.

7 Lehman G, Sherman S. Pancreas divisum. Diagnosis, clinical significance, and management alternatives. *Gastrointest Endosc Clin North Am* 1995;**5**:145–70.

8 Delhaye MEL, Cremer M. Pancreas divisum: congenital anatomic variant or anomaly? Contribution of endoscopic retrograde dorsal pancreatography. *Gastroenterology* 1985;**89**:951–8.

9 Sarles H, Sarles JC, Muratore R, et al. Chronic inflammatory sclerosis of the pancreas an autonomous pancreatic disease? *Am J Dig Dis* 1961;**6**:688–9.

10 Yoshida K, Toki F, Takeuchi T, et al. Chronic pancreatitis caused by an autoimmune abnormality. Proposal of the concept of autoimmune pancreatitis. *Dig Dis Sci* 1995;**40**:1561–8.

11 Takayama M, Hamano H, Ochi Y, et al. Recurrent attacks of autoimmune pancreatitis result in pancreatic stone formation. *Am J Gastroenterol* 2004;**99**:932–7.

12 Okazaki K. Autoimmune pancreatitis: etiology, pathogenesis, clinical findings and treatment. The Japanese experience. *JOP* 2005;**6**(1 suppl):89–96.

13 Kloppel G, Lüttges J, Löhr M, et al. Autoimmune pancreatitis: pathological, clinical, and immunological features. *Pancreas* 2003;**27**:14–19.

14 Kim KP, Kim MH, Song MH, et al. Autoimmune chronic pancreatitis. *Am J Gastroenterol* 2004;**99**:1605–16.

15 Pickartz T, Mayerle J, Lerch MM. Autoimmune pancreatitis. *Nature Clinical Practice Gastroenterol Hepatol* 2007;**4**:314–23.

16 Uchida K, Okazaki K, Asada M et al. Case of chronic pancreatitis involving an autoimmune mechanism that extended to retroperitoneal fibrosis. *Pancreas* 2003;**26**: 92–4.

17 Kamisawa T, Egawa N, Nakajima H et al. Clinical difficulties in the differentiation of autoimmune pancreatitis and pancreatic carcinoma. *Am J Gastroenterol* 2003;**98**:2694–9.

18 Sahani DV, Kalva SP, Farrell J, et al. Autoimmune pancreatitis: imaging features. *Radiology* 2004;**233**: 345–52.

19 Kim KP, Kim MH, Kim JC, et al Diagnostic criteria for autoimmune chronic pancreatitis revisited. *World J Gastroenterol* 2006;**12**:2487–96.

20 Chari ST, Smyrk TC, Levy MJ, et al. Diagnosis of autoimmune pancreatitis: the Mayo Clinic experience. *Clin Gastroenterol Hepatol* 2006;**4**:1010–16.

21 Bishop M, Freedman SD, Zielenski J, et al. The cystic fibrosis transmembrane conductance regulator gene and ion channel function in patients with idiopathic pancreatitis. *Hum Genet* 2005;**118**:372–81.

22 Whitcomb DC, Gorry MC, Preston RA, et al. Hereditary pancreatitis is caused by a mutation in the cationic trypsinogen gene. *Nat Genet* 1996;**14**:141–51.

23 Gorry M, Gabbaizedeh D, Furey W, et al. Mutations in the cationic trypsinogen gene are associated with recurrent acute and chronic pancreatitis. *Gastroenterology* 1997;**113**:1063–8.

24 Witt H, Luck W, Becker M. A signal peptide cleavage site mutation in the cationic trypsinogen gene is strongly associated with chronic pancreatitis. *Gastroenterology* 1999;**117**:7–10.

25 Witt H, Luck W, Hennies HC, et al. Mutations in the gene encoding the serine protease inhibitor, Kazal type 1 are associated with chronic pancreatitis. *Nat Genet* 2000;**25**:213–16.

26 Ellis I, Lerch MM, Whitcomb DC. Genetic testing for hereditary pancreatitis: guidelines for indications, counselling, consent and privacy issues. *Pancreatology* 2001;**1**:405–15.

27 Lowenfels AB, Maisonneuve P, Cavallini G, et al. Pancreatitis and the risk of pancreatic cancer. *N Engl J Med* 1993;**328**:1433–7.

28 Bolondi L, Li Bassi S, Gaiani S, et al. Sonography of chronic pancreatitis. *Radiol Clin North Am* 1989;**27**:815–33.

29 Malfertheiner P, Buchler M. Correlation of imaging and function in chronic pancreatitis. *Radiol Clin North Am* 1989;**27**:51–64.

30 Buscail L, Escourrou J, Moreau J, et al. Endoscopic ultrasonography in chronic pancreatitis: a comparative prospective study with conventional ultrasonography, computed tomography and ERCP. *Pancreas* 1995;**10**:251–7.

31 Malfertheiner P, Buchler M, Stanescu A, et al. Exocrine pancreatic function in correlation to ductal and parenchymal morphology in chronic pancreatitis. *Hepatogastroenterology* 1986;**33**:110–14.

32 Kusano S, Kaji T, Sugiura Y, et al. CT demonstration of fibrous stroma in chronic pancreatitis: pathologic correlation. *J Comput Assist Tomogr* 1999;**23**:297–300.

33 Freeny P, Marks WM, Ryan JA, et al. Pancreatic ductal adenocarcinoma: diagnosis and staging with dynamic CT. *Radiology* 1988;**166**:125–33.

34 Miller FH, Keppke AL, Wadhwa A, et al. MRI of pancreatitis and its complications: Part 2, chronic pancreatitis. *AJR* 2004;**183**:1645–52.

35 Sica G, Braver J, Cooney MJ, et al. Comparison of endoscopic retrograde cholangiopancreatography with MR cholangiopancreatography in patients with pancreatitis. *Radiology* 1999;**210**:605–10.

36 Bret PM, Reinhold C, Taourel P, et al. Pancreas divisum: evaluation with MR cholangiopancreatography. *Radiology* 1996;**199**:99–103.

37 Raimondo M, Wallace MB. Diagnosis of early chronic pancreatitis by endoscopic ultrasound (Are we there yet?) *J Pancreas* 2004;**5**:1–7.

38 Wallace M. Imaging the pancreas: into the deep. *Gastroenterology* 2007;**132**:484–7.

39 Yasuada K, Mukai H, Fujimoto S, et al. The diagnosis of pancreatic cancer by endoscopic ultrasonography. *Gastrointest Endosc* 1988;**34**:1–8.

40 Rosch MT, Lorenz R, Braig C, et al. Endoscopic ultrasound in pancreatic tumor diagnosis. *Gastrointest Endosc* 1991;**37**:347–52.

41 Rosch T, Braig C, Gain T, et al. Staging of pancreatic and ampullary carcinoma by endoscopic ultrasonography. Comparison with conventional sonography, computed tomography, and angiography. *Gastroenterology* 1992;**102**:188–99.

42 Snady H, Cooperman A, Siegel J. Endoscopic ultrasonography compared with computed tomography with ERCP in patients with obstructive jaundice or small peri-pancreatic mass. *Gastrointest Endosc* 1992;**38**:27–34.

43 Palazzo L, Roseau G, Gayet B, et al. Endoscopic ultrasonography in the diagnosis and staging of pancreatic adenocarcinoma. Results of a prospective study with comparison to ultrasonoraphy and CT scan. *Endoscopy* 1993;**25**:143–50.

44 Muller MF, Meyenberger C, Bertschinger P, et al. Pancreatic tumors: evaluation with endoscopic US, CT, and MR imaging. *Radiology* 1994;**190**:745–51.

45 Marty O, Aubertin JM, Bouillot JL, et al. Prospective comparison of ultrasound endoscopy and computed tomography in the assessment of locoregional invasiveness of malignant ampullary and pancreatic tumors verified surgically. *Gastroenterol Clin Biol* 1995;**19**:197–203.

46 Gress F, Hawes RH, Savides TJ, et al. Role of EUS in the preoperative staging of pancreatic cancer; a large single-center experience. *Gastrointest Endosc* 1999;**50**:786–91.

47 Midwinter M, Beveridge CJ, Wilsdon J, et al. Correlation between spiral computed tomography, endoscopic ultrasonography and findings at operation in pancreatic and ampullary tumours. *Br J Surg* 1999;**86**:189–93.

48 Mertz H, Seschopoulos P, Delbeke D, et al. EUS, PET, and CT scanning for evaluation of pancreatic adenocarcinoma. *Gastrointest Endosc* 2000;**52**:367–71.

49 Rivadeneira D, Pochapin M, Frobmyer SR, et al. Comparison of linear array endoscopic ultrasound and helical computed tomography for the staging of periampullary malignancies. *Ann Surg Oncol* 2003;**10**:890–7.

50 Ainsworth A, Rafaelsen SR, Wamberg PA, et al. Is there a difference in diagnostic accuracy and clinical impact between endoscopic ultrasonography and magnetic resonance cholangiopancreatography? *Endoscopy* 2003;**35**:1029–32.

51 Agarwal B, Abu-Hamda E, Molke KL, et al. Endoscopic ultrasound-guided fine needle aspiration and multidetector spiral CT in the diagnosis of pancreatic cancer. *Am J Gastroenterol* 2004;**99**:844–50.

52 DeWitt J, Deveraux B, Chriswell M, et al. Comparison of endoscopic ultrasound and multidetector computed tomography for the detection and staging of pancreatic cancer. *Ann Intern Med* 2004;**141**:753–63.

53 Yasuda K, Mukai H, Nakajaima M. Endoscopic ultrasonography diagnosis of pancreatic cancer. *Gastrointest Endosc*, 1995;**5**:699–712.

54 DeWitt J. EUS in pancreatic neoplasms. In: Hawes RH, Fockens P (eds), *Endosonography*. Philadelphia, PA: Saunders Elsevier, 2006:177–204.

55 Ho S, Bonasera RJ, Pollack BJ, et al. A single-center experience of endoscopic ultrasonography for enlarged pancreas on computed tomography. *Clin Gastroenterol Hepatol* 2006;**4**:98–103.

56 Caletti G, Brocchi E, Agostini D, et al. Sensitivity of endoscopic retrograde pancreatography in chronic pancreatitis. *Br J Surg* 1982;**69**:507–9.

57 Axon A, Classen M, Cotton PB, et al. Pancreatography in chronic pancreatitis: international definitions. *Gut* 1984;**25**:1107–12.

58 Niederau C, Grendell JH. Diagnosis of chronic pancreatitis. *Gastroenterology* 1985;**88**:1973–95.

59 Dominguez-Munoz JE, Hieronymus C, Sauerbruch T, et al. Fecal elastase test: evaluation of a new noninvasive pancreatic function test. *Am J Gastroenterol* 1995;**90**:1834–7.

60 Gullo L, Ventrucci M, Tomassetti P, et al. Fecal elastase 1 determination in chronic pancreatitis. *Dig Dis Sci* 1999;**44**:210–13.

61 Beharry S, Ellis L, Corey M, et al. How useful is fecal pancreatic elastase 1 as a marker of exocrine pancreatic disease? *J Pediatr* 2002;**141**:84–90.

62 Loser C, Mollgaard A, Folsch UR. Faecal elastase 1: a novel, highly sensitive, and specific tubeless pancreatic function test. *Gut* 1996;**39**:580–6.

63 Carroccio A, Verghi F, Santini B, et al. Diagnostic accuracy of fecal elastase 1 assay in patients with pancreatic maldigestion or intestinal malabsorption: a collaborative study of the Italian Society of Pediatric Gastroenterology and Hepatology. *Dig Dis Sci* 2001;**46**:1335–42.

64 Beckingham IJ, Ryder SD. Investigation of liver and biliary disease – ABC of diseases of liver, pancreas and biliary system. *BMJ* 2001;**322**:33–6.

65 Johnston DE. Special considerations in interpreting liver function tests. *Am Family Physician* 1999;**59**:2223–32.

66 Boey JH, Way LW. Acute cholangitis. *Ann Surg* 1980;**191**:264–70.

67 Csendes A, Diaz JC, Burdiles P, et al. Risk factors and classification of acute suppurative cholangitis. *Br J Surg* 1992;**79**:655–8.

68 Welch JP, Donaldson GA. The urgency of diagnosis and surgical treatment of acute suppurative cholangitis. *Am J Surg* 1976;**131**:527–32.

69 O'Connor MJ, Schwartz ML, McQuarrie DG, Sumer HW. Acute bacterial cholangitis: an analysis of clinical manifestation. *Arch Surg* 1982;**117**:437–41.

70 Rahman SH, Larvin M, McMahon MJ, Thompson D. Clinical presentation and delayed treatment of cholangitis in older people. *Dig Dis Sci* 2005;**50**:2207–10.

71 Gigot JF, Leese T, Dereme T, et al. Acute cholangitis: multivariate analysis of risk factors. *Ann Surg* 1989;**209**:435–8.

72 Kimura Y, Takada T, Kawarada Y, et al. Definitions, pathophysiology, and epidemiology of acute cholangitis and cholecystitis: Tokyo guidelines. *J Hepatobiliary Pancreat Surg* 2007;**14**:15–26.

73 Lindsell DM. Ultrasound imaging of the pancreas and biliary tract. *Lancet* 1990;**335**:390–3.

74 Bornman PC, van Beljon JI, Krige JEJ. Management of cholangitis. *J Hepatobiliary Pancreat Surg* 2003;**10**:406–14.

75 Tranter SE, Thompson MH. Spontaneous passage of bile duct stones: frequency of occurrence and relation to clinical presentation. *Ann R Coll Surg Engl* 2003;**85**,174–7.

76 Yalniz M, Pour PM. Diabetes mellitus: a risk factor for pancreatic cancer? *Langenbecks Arch Surg* 2005;**390**:66–72.

77 Cowgill SM, Muscarell P. The genetics of pancreatic cancer. *Am J Surg* 2003;**186**:279–86.

78 Katz MHG, Mortenson MM, Wang H, et al. Diagnosis and management of cystic neoplasms of the pancreas: an evidence-based approach. *J Am Coll Surg* 2007;**207**:106–20.

79 Safi F, Schlosser W, Kolb G, Berger HG. Diagnostic value of CA 19-9 in patients with pancreatic cancer and non-specific gastrointestinal symptoms. *J Gastrointest Surg* 1997;**1**:106–12.

80 Legmann P, Vignaux O, Dousset B, et al. Pancreatic tumours: comparison of dual phase helical CT and endoscopic sonography. *Am J Roentgenol* 1998;**170**:1315–22.

81 Katz MHG, Hwang R, Fleming JB, Evans DB. Tumor-node-metastasis staging of pancreatic adenocarcinoma. *CA Cancer J Clin* 2008;**58**:111–25.

82 Diener MK, Heukaufer C, Schwarzer G, et al. Pancreatoduodenectomy (classic Whipple versus pylorus-preserving pancreaticoduodenectomy (Whipple for surgical treatment of periampullary and pancreatic car-cinoma). *Cochrane Database Syst Rev* 2008;**16**: CD006053.

83 Boeck S, Ankerst DP, Heinemann V. The role for adjuvant chemotherapy for patients with resected pancreatic cancer: systematic review of randomized control trials and meta-analysis. *Oncology* 2007;**72**: 314–21.

11 The Problem of Right Upper Quadrant Pain

Malcolm B. Barnes[1] and Simon Glance[2]

[1]Monash Medical Centre, Clayton, Victoria, Australia
[2]The Northern Hospital, Melbourne Australia.

Right upper quadrant (RUQ) pain is a common reason to present for medical assessment. Often both gastroenterologists and gastrointestinal surgeons are consulted to determine the underlying etiology and its subsequent management. In western societies, the most common cause of RUQ pain is gallstones. This may manifest as cholecystitis or choledocholithiasis, with possible complications of empyema, cholangitis, or acute biliary pancreatitis. The removal of stones for acute resolution of symptoms and prevention of future attacks may require a cholecystectomy or less often an endoscopic retrograde cholangiopancreatography (ERCP).

However, the assessment of RUQ pain is not always clear-cut – particularly if no calculi are identified with first-line imaging. The advent of newer, more powerful diagnostic imaging modalities has improved our ability to assess the hepatopancreatobiliary system for microlithiasis. Magnetic resonance cholangiopancreatography (MRCP), in particular, has dramatically reduced the need for unwarranted operations and diagnostic ERCP, and avoids the potential complications of such interventions. In the absence of demonstrated calculi, biliary motility disorders such as sphincter of Oddi dysfunction (SOD) must also be considered, particularly in middle-aged women.

Case 1: right upper quadrant pain and jaundice

Case presentation

A 62-year old-white man is admitted to the emergency department on Thursday evening after he reports feeling unwell for the past 24 hours with fever, sweats, and RUQ pain. He describes rigors and has noted the presence of dark urine for 3 days. He has no past history of similar events and his gallbladder remains *in situ*. He denies headache, cough, chest pain, or dysuria. He has no pruritus or weight loss.

Of significance is a past history of mitral valve replacement (MVR) 5 years ago for severe mitral regurgitation from childhood rheumatic fever. He takes 5 mg warfarin daily to maintain an international normalized ratio (INR) of between 2.5 and 3.5. His last recorded INR was 2.8. His cardiologist has told him that he has a mild impairment in overall cardiac function although he manages a round of golf once a week with minimal breathlessness. His other medications are amiodarone 200 mg daily and ramipril 5 mg. He has had no other operations and has no allergies.

On examination, his temperature is 38.8°C, he has an irregular pulse of 115 beats/min, with a blood pressure of 90/55 mmHg lying and 85/50 mmHg sitting.

Problem-based Approach to Gastroenterology and Hepatology, First Edition. Edited by John N. Plevris, Colin W. Howden.
© 2012 Blackwell Publishing Ltd. Published 2012 by Blackwell Publishing Ltd.

Table 11.1 Case 1: investigation results

Investigation (normal values)	On admission	+ 12 hours	Post-ERCP
WCC (×10⁹/L) (4–11)	17.7	18.2	11.5
Platelets (×10⁹/L) (150–420)	107	91	145
Urea (mmol/L) (2.5–7.8)	15	22	10
Creatinine (μmol/L) (50–120)	161	239	130
Albumin (g/L) (35–50)	36	30	28
ALP (IU/L) (30–120)	111	240	71
GGT (IU/L) (5–35)	408	622	224
ALT (IU/L) (9–40)	310	315	63
Bilirubin (μmol/L) (<17)	98	136	41
INR (1–1.2)	5.4	5.1	2.5
CRP (mg/L) (<5)	160	204	81

ALP, alkaline phosphatase; ALT, alanine transaminase; CRP, C-reactive protein; GGT, γ-glutamyltransferase; WCC, white cell count.

He has mild scleral icterus with no stigmata of chronic liver disease. His prosthetic valve is audible and his abdominal examination reveals a mildly tender RUQ with no guarding or rebound tenderness. He has no peripheral edema.

His initial blood investigations are shown in Table 11.1.

He has already been given 1 L of crystalloid stat before you are called for your opinion and assessment.

Questions

• What is the most likely diagnosis?
• How urgent and aggressive should his initial management be?
• What would you consider as the first-line image of choice?
• What further therapeutic intervention may be necessary?
• Given the clinical deterioration what further therapeutic intervention would you recommend?

Diagnosis

Our patient's presentation is typical for acute cholangitis; however, additional cholecystitis or acute biliary pancreatitis has not been excluded. Fevers, jaundice,

and RUQ pain make up Charcot's triad. It should be noted, however, that not every patient with cholangitis presents in such classic fashion. Elderly patients, for example, may not mount an obvious febrile response and the jaundice may be subtle, whereas others may present solely with confusion. Hypotension and confusion/coma in addition to Charcot's triad are termed Reynold's pentad. It signifies a severe attack of cholangitis and septicemia and is still associated with significant mortality.

Initial management

The patient needs aggressive resuscitation to counter the vasodilatory effects of sepsis or the systemic inflammatory response syndrome (SIRS). Although initially this can be with fluid, close attention must be paid to his central venous pressure because of his cardiac condition. Inotropic support may be required. Antibiotics are mandatory and should be broad spectrum to cover the likely causative bacteria. Commonly *Escherichia coli*, *Klebsiella* spp., and other Gram-negative organisms are found. Triple antibiotics (ampicillin, gentamicin, and metronidazole) are usual first-line therapy, but, given this man's raised creatinine, aminoglycosides should be avoided. In this instance, a third-generation cephalosporin (such as ceftriaxone) can be combined with metronidazole. More powerful antibiotics such as timentin, tazocin, and meropenem are efficacious but should be reserved as second-line therapy.

Investigations

Abdominal ultrasonography is the first-line imaging modality required. This provides a quick, inexpensive, non-invasive assessment of the gallbladder for calculi and wall thickness, biliary ducts for dilation, and the liver parenchyma to exclude abscess formation.

Although 80–90% of patients with cholangitis will respond to conservative therapy, the remainder require urgent decompression of the biliary ducts [1]. Endoscopic drainage is the most effective drainage technique in acute cholangitis [2–6] (Figure 11.1). It has been demonstrated to effectively lower bile and serum endotoxin levels and aborts the process of SIRS [7]. The decision about the timing of an "urgent" ERCP is always difficult. The literature on urgent

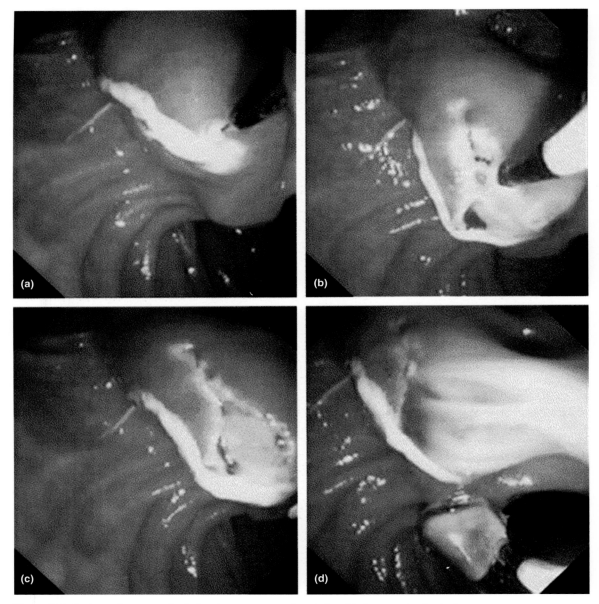

Figure 11.1 Endoscopic retrograde cholangiopancreatography: cholangitis from retained calculus.

ERCP reports an average or median time to performing an ERCP of less than 24 h [4,8,9]. Logistic considerations (such as distance from a center able to perform ERCP, weekend staffing levels, etc.) will always impact on this.

The markers of severity for cholangitis (and thus indicators of who will benefit from urgent decompression) were detailed in a study by Hui et al. [10]; 142 consecutive patients with cholangitis were commenced on broad-spectrum antibiotics and their progress monitored in the ensuing 24 h. The four factors that were statistically significant in predicting the need for an urgent ERCP were: a tachycardia (>100), albumin <30, bilirubin >50, and a prothrombin time >14 s. The authors concluded that the presence of at least one of these factors should lead to an ERCP being performed within 48 h.

Diagnosis and initial management in this case

Following intravenous antibiotics and fluid resuscitation, an abdominal ultrasound scan is ordered and demonstrates a 14-mm common bile duct (CBD) with no obvious filling defects but poor views of the distal duct due to overlying gas. The gallbladder has normal wall thickness and multiple small, mobile stones are seen. He is Murphy's sign negative. The liver, pancreas, and spleen are unremarkable. His serum amylase is 73 (<100) IU/L and his lipase 22 (<60) IU/L. His warfarin is withheld and he has received vitamin K 1 mg i.v.

After 12 hours it is now Friday morning and he has received a total of 5 L fluid and produced 45 mL/h urine. His temperature remains 38°C, his BP is 95/55 mmHg lying with no significant postural drop, but his pulse remains at 110 beats//min. His liver enzymes have deteriorated (see Table 11.1).

Further therapeutic options

The authors have already detailed their concerns about delaying biliary decompression in this patient due to his comorbidities and the number of positive predictors for failure of conservative management. His worsening liver enzymes in conjunction with the ultrasound findings of a dilated CBD are suspicious for an obstructing distal calculus. Furthermore, the thin-walled, non-tender gallbladder on ultrasonography, and the normal lipase, exclude the presence of additional cholecystitis and pancreatitis respectively.

The diagnosis is therefore one of acute, severe cholangitis that has failed to respond to conservative therapy. As the realities of medical care dictate that the appropriate expert staff are often less likely to be available on a Saturday, he requires an ERCP and biliary decompression today.

The biliary infection and consequent endotoxemia and SIRS can all be resolved by allowing the infected bile to drain into the duodenum. The placement of a plastic stent (or indeed a nasobiliary catheter), or performing an endoscopic sphincterotomy and definitive stone extraction, is of equal effect in the short term for cholangitis. In principle, the larger 10 Fr stents provide better drainage than the smaller 7 Fr stents for thick, viscous bile.

In this patient, two factors favor the first option. First, a stent alone is quicker and technically easier, which reduces the overall procedure time and inherent risks of anesthesia, which are not inconsiderable. Second, his INR remains high and at such a level precludes a sphincterotomy being safely performed. The INR remains high due to a combination of his anticoagulant therapy and his inability to adequately absorb the fat-soluble vitamin K. Although it is possible to quickly and completely reverse his coagulopathy with clotting factors, we also need to be mindful of the thromboembolic potential of his prosthetic mitral valve. This risk can be reduced by limiting the time off full anticoagulation therapy in the form of warfarin, heparin, or low-molecular-weight heparin.

Patient management

An ERCP is successfully performed using minimal contrast to avoid a septic shower. The cholangiogram demonstrates a 15-mm CBD with a 15-mm stone impacted at the ampulla. A 10 Fr plastic stent is inserted, pushing the stone proximally with excellent flow of inspissated bile, and streaks of pus following.

The patient's hemodynamics and liver enzymes rapidly improve (see Table 7.1) and he remains afebrile over the weekend. He is commenced on heparin when his INR <2.5. Five days later he undergoes a second ERCP off anticoagulation therapy. The previously placed stent is removed before a large sphincterotomy is performed. The stone is broken into fragments with a mechanical lithotripsy basket and completely removed using a combination of the basket and a balloon. The final cholangiogram is clear.

Questions

Your patient wants to know if he will need to have his gallbladder removed to prevent future episodes. What would you recommend?

It is strongly suggested that in this case laparoscopic cholecystectomy is warranted and should be done while the patient is an inpatient and off his anticoagulation therapy. The patient has been extremely unwell and must be protected from suffering further attacks. It is known that, in western populations, 95% of patients with a CBD stone have coexisting gallbladder stones [10,11]. Furthermore, recurrent bile duct stones after endoscopic sphincterotomy occur in 4–24% of patients [12,13]. Therefore, although endoscopic sphincterotomy alone *may* be successful in preventing complications of choledocholithiasis, it is really appropriate only for elderly people or those with significant medical impediments to surgery. The risk factors for stone recurrence include age >80 years, an intact gallbladder, persistent CBD dilation >13 mm, and anatomic considerations such as the presence of a periampullary diverticulum and distal duct angulations [12–14].

Preoperative assessment by a cardiologist and anesthetist will be required and, once the decision has been taken, it would be most appropriate to perform the operation while he is still an inpatient and his coagulation state is controlled, thus minimizing both bleeding and thromboembolic complications.

The laparoscopic approach to cholecystectomy is undertaken in approximately 90% of cholecystectomies. Complications from this approach (such as bile duct injury) were initially blamed on the operator "learning curve" for the technique. A recent 10-year review confirmed that, although the frequency of complications has certainly stabilized, they do still occur despite the ever-increasing experience of operators [15]. Similarly, there is still a need for open cholecystectomy in 10% of operations if surgical difficulties are encountered. These usually relate to intra-abdominal adhesions, unusual anatomy, intraoperative complications, or large ductal stones.

Commentary

This case highlights one of the common complications caused by gallstones. Cholangitis is a significant and serious infection with an appreciable mortality rate. It must be recognized early and treated aggressively with antibiotics and biliary decompression. The timing of endoscopic drainage should be determined based on the degree of hemodynamic compromise, presence of persisting fevers, coagulopathy,

and the levels of albumin and bilirubin. Once the acute situation has stabilized, if the gallbladder remains *in situ*, a cholecystectomy should then be performed to prevent complications of recurrent choledocholithiasis.

Case 2: right upper quadrant pain

Case presentation

A 42-year-old woman is referred by her GP with RUQ pain after presenting to her with multiple similar episodes during the past 18 months. A typical episode would last for between 2 and 3 hours, with waves of disabling pain that require opiate analgesia. In between episodes she denies any symptoms. She describes the sensation as similar to the pain that she experienced from gallstones, for which she underwent a laparoscopic cholecystectomy 4 years ago. She denies jaundice, pruritus, fever, weight loss, or a change in the color of her stool or urine. She describes herself as "lactose intolerant" and she has been told that she has irritable bowel syndrome (IBS). She denies taking any regular medication, although she was on an antidepressant 3 years ago after she and her husband divorced. She drinks 4 units alcohol/day and smokes five cigarettes. Examination reveals a slim woman with a soft, non-tender abdomen and no organomegaly. Her pain has eased following an opiate injection.

Her liver enzymes are performed and demonstrate (normal range): alanine transaminase (ALT) 158 (9–40) IU/L, alkaline phosphatase (ALP) 221 (30–120) IU/L, bilirubin 6 (<17) μmol/L, serum amylase 36 (<100) IU/L, and lipase 22 (<60) IU/L. An abdominal ultrasound scan is undertaken and reported as normal with an absent gallbladder and a 7-mm CBD with no filling defects. The liver and pancreas are normal.

Questions

- What is the differential diagnosis?
- What further investigations would you consider?
- What management option(s) would you choose?

Differential diagnosis

At this early stage further information is needed about the integrity of the biliary system before subjecting the patient to an ERCP and sphincterotomy.

Patients with known or suspected SOD are five times more likely to develop pancreatitis after biliary sphincterotomy than patients with other indications such as removal of stones [16]. Similarly, it would be premature and unfair to dismiss this woman as being narcotic dependent. There is no evidence of chronic pain, malabsorptive diarrhea, or diabetes to suspect chronic pancreatitis, although documented normal lipase levels during previous attacks of RUQ pain would assist in excluding this differential. The CBD diameter is mildly dilated for her age but is consistent with her having had a cholecystectomy. At this juncture, the most likely diagnosis is one of a small retained stone that episodically and briefly obstructs the narrowest portion of the CBD near the ampulla. In the absence of calculi, the differential must always include SOD. This is particularly so given her age, sex, and associated IBS.

Further investigations

An abdominal computed tomography (CT) scan would provide an additional assessment of the pancreatic parenchyma. An MRCP would provide important information about whether a small retained stone at the lower end of the common bile duct is present.

In this case . . .
A contrast CT scan of the abdomen is performed to assess the liver, pancreas, and surrounds in detail. It is reported as normal, specifically commenting that there is no evidence of either acute or chronic pancreatitis or mass lesions within the pancreas. The CBD is confirmed at 7 mm with no filling defects.

Her pain has now resolved and she is keen to return home. She is, however, anxious for a diagnosis to be made. Given the ongoing suspicion for a retained stone, an outpatient MRCP is arranged.

The MRCP is also reported as normal, with a 7-mm CBD, with normal distal taper and normal pancreatic duct. There are no filling defects or strictures. Furthermore, she has remained pain free and her latest liver enzymes have returned to normal.

Patient management

You are now faced with a number of management options for this patient:

- She should undergo an ERCP + endoscopic sphincterotomy (ES) and balloon trawl because there are still suspicions of a stone.
- She should be considered as having SOD and may require an ERCP + manometry and ES.
- If available, endoscopic ultrasonography (EUS) would complement the MRCP and (if normal) provide further evidence against biliary pathology such as small calculi.
- She should be managed conservatively and her progress assessed over the next 12 months. With each attack, liver enzymes and lipase levels should be recorded.

Further differential diagnoses

In the absence of causative pathology, it is necessary now consider the possible differential diagnosis of SOD. The fluctuating liver enzymes together with pain are consistent with both a mobile calculus and SOD. However, the absence of either a significantly dilated duct or any filling defects on MRCP counts strongly against a calculus. MRCP has a sensitivity of 85% and a specificity of 93% for choledocholithiasis, with a negative predictive value of 92% [17].

EUS does provide an adjuvant modality to assess the biliary system and should be utilized if available. When choledocholithiasis is suspected, EUS has a sensitivity of >90% for detection of stones [18] and is comparable to ERCP.

In centers where neither EUS nor manometry is available, given her current stable state and the lack of positive data thus far, one could follow her progress over the next year. However, if the episodes of pain persist, with associated documented rises in liver enzymes, she should be referred to a tertiary centre where the diagnosis of SOD can be fully assessed.

The Rome II diagnostic criteria for SOD [19] were established in 1999 to assist in what has always been a difficult area. They include episodes of severe epigastric or RUQ abdominal pain in addition to all of the following:
- Symptom episodes lasting 30 min or more with pain-free intervals.
- Symptoms have occurred on one or more occasions in the previous 12 months.
- The pain is steady and interrupts daily activities or requires consultation with a physician.

Table 11.2 Modified Hogan–Geenen biliary sphincter of Oddi classification system [20]

Biliary type 1	Patients with biliary-type pain, ALT/AST/ALP 1.1 × normal documented on any occasion, and bile duct >10 mm diameter
Biliary type 2	Patients with biliary-type pain but only one of the above criteria
Biliary type 3	Patients with only biliary-type pain and no other abnormalities

ALP, alkaline phosphatase; ALT, alanine transaminase; AST, aspartate transaminase.

- There is no evidence of structural abnormalities to explain the symptoms.

There may be transient elevation of liver enzymes but these are present in less than 50% of patients [20].

Once the diagnosis of SOD is suspected, the patient can be classified according to the Hogan-Geenen SOD classification system (Table 11.2) in its modified form [21]. Importantly, this gives a guide to which patients should undergo biliary manometry. It is not recommended in all suspected cases due to the risk of post-ERCP pancreatitis, which has been reported to be as high as 31% [22].

In this case . . .
An EUS is performed and excellent views are obtained of normal biliary and pancreatic ducts. Under the same sedation, duodenoscopy is utilized to exclude an ampullary lesion.

At this juncture, the working diagnosis is of suspected SOD, biliary type II. Manometry via ERCP is recommended, and if SOD is confirmed a sphincterotomy will be performed. Informed consent is obtained for the potential risks of pancreatitis.

An ERCP is undertaken with an anesthetist providing i.v. propofol sedation to ensure no movement artifact. A baseline duodenal manometry tracing is first recorded before selective deep cannulation of both the bile and the pancreatic ducts. Contrast is first injected into both ducts and excludes other pathology. Manometry is then performed with the tracings confirming a raised pressure of 65 mmHg (<35 mmHg) for the biliary sphincter, with a normal tracing of 10 mmHg for the pancreatic sphincter. With a firm diagnosis of SOD, a biliary sphincterotomy is performed without complication. A small (3F) stent is then inserted into the pancreatic duct to lower the risk of pancreatitis.

Our patient remains well following the procedure with no evidence of pancreatitis. A plain abdominal radiograph 2 weeks post-procedure confirms the spontaneous passage of the pancreatic stent. At 6-month follow-up she had had no further episodes of pain.

SOD; principles of management

Functional gastrointestinal disorders are complex in that diagnosis relies on a constellation of symptoms rather than the positive results of an investigation. Fortunately, the diagnosis and management of SOD have benefited from the number of trials and publications that have enabled more concise categorization. This has given clear guidelines as to when to perform manometry and (importantly) when to perform an endoscopic sphincterotomy.

SOD is most common in middle-aged women [20]. It can involve abnormalities in either the biliary or the pancreatic sphincter or both. Diagnosis is based on the Rome II criteria and the absence of alternate pathology on investigation. As a result of the associated risks, invasive testing with ERCP and manometry should be reserved for patients with a high index of suspicion (as per the Hogan–Geenen classification) and those in whom definitive therapy in the form of an endoscopic sphincterotomy is planned. A number of non-invasive investigations of SOD have been reported. They include hepatobiliary scintigraphy to assess bile flow, secretin-stimulated EUS or MRCP, and a morphine provocation test. All have proven disappointing and are not currently recommended for screening [20].

Endoscopic sphincterotomy is the most effective treatment. Clinical improvement ranging from 55% for biliary type III to 95% for biliary type I has been reported [23]. A randomized controlled trial of type II patients post-cholecystectomy demonstrated that 17 of 18 patients with proven SOD on manometry benefited from sphincterotomy, whereas, in patients with normal sphincter pressures, sphincterotomy was no more beneficial than placebo therapy [24]. Recent studies have assessed the effectiveness of botulinum toxin (Botox), a smooth muscle relaxant, in lowering the sphincter pressure. Although its effects are temporary (3–6 months), it may help identify patients most likely to benefit from an endoscopic sphincterotomy without the inherent risks [25,26].

Concerns about the rate of pancreatitis after ERCP and/or sphincterotomy have led to numerous trials on medical therapy to attempt to lower the rate. None has proven efficacious. Suspected SOD is an independent risk factor by multivariate analysis of post-ERCP pancreatitis [27]. Initially this was thought to be due to procedure-related factors such as repeated duct instrumentation and contrast injection. More recently, pancreatic sphincter hypertension (PSH) has been implicated. In a randomized trial of pancreatic duct stenting after biliary sphincterotomy in SOD patients, the risk of post-ERCP pancreatitis decreased from 26% to 7% with the use of a pancreatic stent [28]. The barbs are removed to enable most of the stents to pass spontaneously 24–96 h post-insertion.

Discussion

RUQ pain is a very common reason for presentation to GPs or emergency departments. As both are so busy, a quick and easy distinction must be made about the underlying pathology. Essentially, we must separate biliary causes of pain from non-biliary causes.

Biliary versus non-biliary pain

Although history, examination, and clinical acumen were traditionally used to make this distinction, increasingly in modern medicine it is the quick access to blood and ultrasound results that has supplanted it. In most instances, the results of such tests are available before the involvement of the gastroenterology registrar or consultant. In this way, non-biliary causes of RUQ pain, such as the capsular stretch pain of acute hepatitis or the subacute distension from multiple metastatic deposits, can quickly be identified through an ALT >1000 or ultrasound findings of multiple space-occupying lesions respectively.

Once such pathology has been excluded, it is possible to further separate biliary pain as arising from the gallbladder (and/or fossa) or the bile ducts (including both intra- and extrahepatic ducts). Such distinc-

tion may be important in centers to determine to which unit (medical or surgical) a patient is admitted.

The most common cause of RUQ pain in the western world is from gallstones. Parasites such as *Ascaris lumbricoides* are common worldwide and can obstruct the ducts, causing cholangitis or pancreatitis [29]. Malignancies such as cholangiocarcinoma or pancreatic cancer most often present with a painless obstruction; however, ampullary lesions may mimic the symptoms of stone disease.

Biliary colic occurs when a small, mobile calculus is temporarily caught in the cystic duct and the usual peristaltic contractions bring strong, episodic waves of quite disabling pain. Opiate or opioid analgesia may be required for relief. Presentation to a doctor for analgesia may precipitate the initial investigation into the cause. Such typical pain, in association with abdominal ultrasonography demonstrating calculi in the gallbladder, is diagnostic for *cholelithiasis*. The presence of a thickened gallbladder wall, often in association with abnormal liver enzymes and fever, is consistent with *cholecystitis*. Management of both conditions requires a cholecystectomy, the timing of which depends on the severity and frequency of attacks, the presence of complications, and waiting lists! A cholecystectomy removes the reservoir of stones and in so doing serves to prevent future attacks of pain, as well as the potential complications of an obstructing calculus such as cholangitis or acute biliary pancreatitis. It has been reported that 10% of patients who undergo a cholecystectomy have CBD stones [10,11]. The situation is somewhat different in Asian populations where primary CBD stones are more common [30,31].

Determining the underlying etiology (and thus the appropriate management) often depends upon the combination of radiological and endoscopic imaging modalities.

Ultrasonography

This quick, non-invasive scan is the first choice investigation for the hepatopancreatobiliary system. The liver and pancreas parenchyma are assessed for lesions, the bile ducts for dilatation and the presence of any filling defects and the gallbladder can be assessed for wall thickness and the presence of stones.

The presence of a dilated CBD raises the suspicion of calculi within the ducts. A useful rule of thumb for the expected diameter of the CBD is 1mm for every decade of life: therefore the expected normal duct diameter in a 60 year old man would be 6mm. Further mild (1–2 mm) dilatation is acceptable if the patient has previously had a cholecystectomy.

Whilst the U/S can occasionally demonstrate a filling defect within the duct, it's usually the combination of a dilated CBD with obstructive liver enzymes (raised ALP, GGT and bilirubin) which alerts us to the likelihood of a distal stone being present.

CT

Despite the evidence for ultrasonography as the first step for suspected calculi, often if the abdominal pain is non-specific (and particularly if there are features of peritonitis) a CT of the abdomen may be performed. This is becoming increasingly common in emergency departments where busy doctors are anxious not to miss pathology. Although the sensitivity for calculi is only 65% [32], it does enable excellent views of the solid organs and can exclude the presence of free gas or fluid. Further detail is possible with triple-phase CT scans which perform additional views in the arterial and portal phases. This is particularly useful in further elucidating mass lesions, assessing their vascularity and association with surrounding anatomy. The sensitivity and specificity of CT for the diagnosis of malignancy in biliary strictures are 77% and 63% respectively [33].

A CT cholangiogram is used to isolate the bile ducts and determine if any filling defects or strictures are present. However, due to an inability to adequately concentrate the contrast in an obstructed system, this scan can be used only if the bilirubin is <40 μmol/L. Furthermore, an adequately functioning renal system is required to process such large volumes of contrast.

MRCP

The advent of MR technology has had a huge impact in the hepatopancreatobiliary field. It uses T2-weighted sequences to highlight the fluid-containing biliary and pancreatic ducts (Figure 11.2). MRCP has an overall sensitivity of 85% and specificity of 93% for choledocholithiasis [17] and, with the advantage

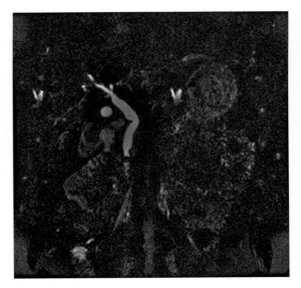

Figure 11.2 Magnetic resonance cholangiopancreatography: distal common bile duct calculus.

of no complications such as pancreatitis, has virtually replaced the need for diagnostic ERCP. It is also able to assess strictures for malignancy with a sensitivity of 85% [33] and highlight anatomic anomalies such as pancreatic divisum, which may be seen in up to 7% of individuals [34]. Furthermore, it can provide useful information on the location of strictures (particularly hilar lesions) before a therapeutic ERCP [35].

This technique is not suitable for patients with significant claustrophobia and most importantly those with implanted metal (clips, pacemakers, bullets!). Its other limitations include access and availability, cost, and sensitivity to movement artifact.

Endoscopic ultrasonography

As EUS has become more widely available, its use as an additional endoscopic imaging modality for patients with previously identified lesions of the gastrointestinal tract, mediastinum, and surrounding organs has increased. However, access to equipment and availability of appropriately trained staff does continue to limit its use outside tertiary centers.

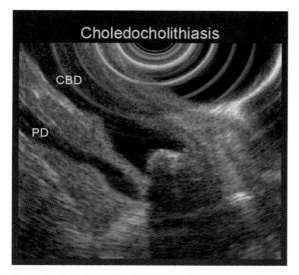

Figure 11.3 Endoscopic ultrasonography: common bile duct stone with distal shadowing.

Initially the benefits of EUS were for identifying and staging esophageal and pancreatic lesions, and enabling fine-needle aspiration and firm tissue diagnosis of pancreatic lesions in particular. Now its varied uses include: mediastinal lymph node biopsies, access for pancreatic cyst drainage, and assessment of various lesions identified on CT. It is also very useful for determining the presence or absence of calculi as a cause for RUQ pain and fluctuating liver enzymes (Figure 11.3). When choledocholithiasis is suspected, EUS has a sensitivity of 93% for the detection of CBD stones, and is comparable to MRCP and ERCP [17]. Although EUS does not have the therapeutic advantage of ERCP, it has been shown to be a cost-effective initial screening study for patients with low-to-intermediate risk of bile duct stones before ERCP [36]. Ideally, if there is some doubt about the pathology, an EUS would be performed before an ERCP, and if a stone or lesion is detected the operator can progress to an ERCP under the same anesthetic. It is likely that such an approach will become more widespread as more interventional endoscopists become skilled in both techniques.

ERCP

The role of ERCP has changed in the past decade with the widespread use of more sensitive and specific imaging modalities such as MRCP and EUS, rendering the diagnostic cholangiogram obsolete. As a result of the risk of pancreatitis, only rarely is there an acceptable reason to perform a diagnostic rather than therapeutic ERCP. Despite multiple trials with various substances, no medication has yet been able to reduce the incidence of post-ERCP pancreatitis which occurs in approximately 5% of cases overall [37,38]. Imaging is therefore utilized to confirm the presence of a stone, stricture, or pancreatic lesion before the procedure.

As the number of overall procedures lessens, the number of specialists in this area has also diminished. Furthermore, recent evidence has suggested that inpatients who undergo ERCP at high-volume (>200 cases/year) hospitals have a shorter length of stay and lower procedural failure rates than those undergoing ERCP at low-volume centers [39].

Despite the reduced number of procedures, the therapeutic utility of ERCP remains strong. It enables:
• direct assessment of the ampulla and biopsy of potential lesions
• removal of calculi with either balloon or basket
• assessment and sampling of strictures with biliary brushings and biopsy
• performance of an endoscopic sphincterotomy for the above and for treatment of SOD
• insertion of a plastic stent for the relief of obstruction or multiple stents to dilate strictures
• the insertion of metal stents for the palliation of malignant (and some benign) strictures
• pancreatic duct access for stone removal, stenting of persisting ductal injury, and therapy for SOD.

Conclusion

The two cases have served as a template for discussing some of the important issues with RUQ pain. There is no doubt that improving technology has assisted with determining the causative etiology. Practitioners must have an appreciation of the risks and benefits of both endoscopic and surgical interventions so that their patients can be fully informed about their options.

References

1 Ng Enders KW, Chung S. Common bile duct stones and cholangitis. In: Cotton PB, Leung J (eds), *Advanced*

Digestive Endoscopy: ERCP. Oxford:. Blackwell Publishing, 2006: 88–119.

2 Leung JWC, Chung SCS, Sung JJY, et al. Urgent endoscopic drainage for acute suppurative cholangitis. *Lancet* 1989;**10**:1307–9.

3 Ikeda S, Tanaka M, Yoshimoto H, et al. Endoscopic biliary drainage for acute obstructive cholangitis: an analysis of 100 consecutive patients. *Dig Endosc* 1990;**2**:214–17.

4 Lai EC, Mok FP, Tan ES, et al. Endoscopic biliary drainage for severe acute cholangitis. *N Engl J Med* 1992;**326**:1582–6.

5 Lee DWH, Chan ACW, Lam YH, et al. Biliary decompression by nasobiliary catheter or biliary stent in acute suppurative cholangitis: a prospective randomized trial. *Gastrointest Endosc* 2002;**56**:361–5.

6 Sharm BC, Kumar R, Agarwal N, et al. Endoscopic biliary drainage by nasobiliary drain or by stent placement in patients with acute cholangitis. *Endoscopy* 2005;**37**:439–43.

7 Lau JY, Chung SC, Leung JW, Ling TK, Yung MY, Li AK. Endoscopic drainage aborts endotoxaemia in acute cholangitis. *Br J Surg* 1996;**83**:181–4.

8 Hui CK, Liu CL, Lai KC, et al. Outcome of emergency ERCP for acute cholangitis in patients 90 years and older. *Aliment Pharmacol Ther* 2004;**19**:1158–68.

9 Kumar R, Sharma BC, Singh J, Sarin SK. Endoscopic biliary drainage for severe acute cholangitis in biliary obstruction as a result of malignant and benign diseases. *J Gastroenterol Hepatol* 2004;**19**:994–7.

10 Moreaux J. Prospective study of open cholecystectomy for calculus biliary disease. *Br J Surg* 1994;**81**:116–19.

11 Morgenstern L, Wong L, Berci G. Twelve hundred open cholecystectomies before the laparoscopic era. A standard for comparison. *Arch Surg* 1992;**127**:400–3.

12 Keizman D, Shalom MI, Konikoff FM. Recurrent symptomatic common bile duct stones after endoscopic stone extraction in elderly patients. *Gastrointest Endosc* 2006;**64**:60–5.

13 Kim DI, Kim M, Lee SK, et al. Risk factors for recurrence of primary bile duct stones after endoscopic biliary sphincterotomy. *Gastrointest Endosc* 2001;**54**:42–8.

14 Pereira-Lima JC, Jakobs R, Winter UH, et al. Long-term results (7 to 10 years) of endoscopic papillotomy for choledocholithiasis. Multivariate analysis of prognostic factors for the recurrence of biliary symptoms. *Gastrointest Endosc* 1998;**48**:457–65.

15 Khan MH, Howard TJ, Fogel EL, et al. Frequency of biliary complications after laparoscopic cholecystectomy detected by ERCP: experience at a large tertiary referral center. *Gastrointest Endosc* 2007;**65**:247–57.

16 Freeman ML, Nelson DB, Sherman S, et al. Complications of endoscopic biliary sphincterotomy. *N Engl J Med* 1996;**335**:909–18.

17 Verma D, Kapadia A, Eisen GM, Adler DG. EUS vs MRCP for detection of choledocholithiasis. *Gastrointest Endosc* 2006;**64**:248–54.

18 Buscarini E, Tansini P, Vallisa D, et al. EUS for suspected choledocholithiasis: do benefits outweigh costs? A prospective, controlled study. *Gastrointest Endosc* 2003;**57**,510–18.

19 Corazziari E, Shaffer EA, Hogan W, Sherman S, Toouli J. Functional disorders of the biliary tract and pancreas. *Gut* 1999;**45**(suppl 2):48–54.

20 Fogel EL, Sherman S. Sphincter of Oddi dysfunction. In: Cotton PB, Leung J (eds), *Advanced Digestive Endoscopy: ERCP*. Oxford: Blackwell Publishing, 2006:165–98.

21 Eversman D, Fogel EL, Rusche M, Sherman S, Lehman GA. Frequency of abnormal pancreatic and biliary sphincter manometry compared with clinical suspicion of sphincter of Oddi dysfunction. *Gastrointest Endosc* 1999;**50**:637–41.

22 Sherman S, Troiano FP, Hawes RH, Lehman GA. Sphincter of Oddi manometry: decreased risk of clinical pancreatitis with the use of a modified aspirating catheter. *Gastrointest Endosc* 1990;**36**:462–6.

23 Hogan W, Sherman S, Pasricha P, Carr-Locke DL. Sphincter of Oddi manometry. *Gastrointest Endosc* 1997;**45**:342–8.

24 Geenen JE, Hogan WJ, Dodds WJ, Toouli J, Venu RP. The efficacy of endoscopic sphincterotomy after cholecystectomy in patients with sphincter-of-Oddi dysfunction. *N Engl J Med* 1989;**320**:82–7.

25 Pasricha PJ, Miskovsky EP, Kalloo AN. Intrasphincteric injection of botulinum toxin for suspected sphincter of Oddi dysfunction. *Gut* 1994;**35**:1319–21.

26 Wehrmann T, Seifert H, Seipp M, et al. Endoscopic injection of botulinum toxin for biliary sphincter of Oddi dysfunction. *Endoscopy* 1998;**30**:702–7.

27 Freeman ML, DiSario JA, Nelson DB, et al. Risk factors for post-ERCP pancreatitis: a prospective, multicenter study. *Gastrointest Endosc* 2001;**54**:425–34.

28 Tarnasky PR, Palesch YY, Cunningham JT, Mauldin PD, Cotton PB, Hawes RH. Pancreatic stenting prevents pancreatitis after biliary sphincterotomy in patients with sphincter of Oddi dysfunction. *Gastroenterology* 1998;**115**:1518–24.

29 Cho YD, Kim YS, Cheon K, Shim CS, Hong SS. Ascaris-induced acute pancreatitis treated endoscopically. *Gastrointest Endosc* 2007;**66**:1226–7.

30 Lau JY, Leow CK, Fung TM, et al. Cholecystectomy or gallbladder in situ after endoscopic sphincterotomy and bile duct stone removal in Chinese patients. *Gastroenterology* 2006;**130**:96–103.

31 Ko CW, Lee SP. Epidemiology and natural history of common bile duct stones and prediction of disease. *Gastrointest Endosc* 2002;**56**:S165–9.

32 Neitlich JD, Topazian M, Smith RC, et al. Detection of choledocholithiasis: comparison of unenhanced helical CT and endoscopic retrograde cholangiopancreatography. *Radiology* 1997;**203**:753–7.

33 Rosch T, Meining A, Fruhmorgen S, et al. A prospective comparison of the diagnostic accuracy of ERCP, MRCP, CT and EUS in biliary strictures. *Gastrointest Endosc* 2002;**55**:870–6.

34 Cano DA, Herbrok M, Zenker M. Pancreatic development and disease. *Gastroenterology* 2007;**132**: L745–762.

35 Yeh TS, Jan YY, Tseng JH, et al. Malignant perihilar biliary obstruction: magnetic resonance cholangiopancreatographic findings. *Am J Gastroenterol* 2000;**95**: 432–40.

36 Canto MF, Chak A, Stellato T, et al. Endoscopic ultrasonography versus cholangiography for the diagnosis of choledocholithiasis. *Gastrointest Endosc* 1998;**47**: 439–48.

37 Cotton PB, Lehman G, Vennes J, et al. Endoscopic sphincterotomy complications and their management: an attempt at consensus. *Gastrointest Endosc* 1991;**37**:383–93.

38 Sherman S, Lehman GA. ERCP-and endoscopic sphincterotomy-induced pancreatitis. *Pancreas* 1991;**6**: 350–67.

39 Varadarajulu S, Kilgore ML, Wilcox CM, Eloubeidi MA. Relationship among hospital ERCP volume, length of stay, and technical outcomes. *Gastrointest Endosc* 2006;**64**:338–47.

12 Abnormal Liver Function Tests: Diagnostic Approach

Timothy T. Gordon-Walker and John P. Iredale

Centre for Liver & Digestive Disorders, The Royal Infirmary and Centre for Inflammation Research, Queen's Medical Research Institute, University of Edinburgh, Edinburgh, UK

The interpretation of liver function tests (LFTs) is essential to the diagnosis and management of liver disease. The term "liver function tests" is in itself a misnomer. It is commonly applied to a group of laboratory tests that measure the levels of serum liver enzymes, and therefore more precisely reflect cholestasis and hepatocyte integrity rather than liver function. Furthermore, changes in serum albumin and prothrombin time, although they may be associated with reduced hepatic synthetic function, are not specific to liver disease, e.g. hypoalbuminemia may occur in malnutrition, sepsis, and protein-losing states.

Standard liver panels include bilirubin (total/conjugated), aspartate aminotransferase (AST), alanine aminotransferase (ALT), alkaline phosphatase (ALP), γ-glutamyl transferase (GGT), albumin and prothrombin time (Table 12.1) [1,2]. Dynamic tests of liver function, such as galactose and aminopyridine clearance, are not widely available.

In this chapter the authors consider the interpretation of LFT abnormalities in relation to a series of common clinical cases. Defined patterns of LFT abnormalities may arise in association with signs and symptoms of overt liver disease, or may occur unexpectedly in an asymptomatic patient. The latter is an increasingly common occurrence due to the widespread inclusion of LFTs in "routine blood tests." It is therefore important to develop a clear diagnostic strategy, to identify those patients in whom LFT abnormalities indicate clinically significant liver disease, while avoiding investigations that may be unnecessarily costly or potentially injurious.

There are significant limitations to both the sensitivity and the specificity of LFTs. By definition, the "normal" range for any test represents the mean value ± two standard deviations, as observed in a reference population, with as many as 2.5% of "normal" patients demonstrating abnormally elevated LFTs [2]. Conversely, 15–50% of patients with chronic hepatitis C infection will have a persistently normal aminotransferase level [3–6], whereas as many as 78% of patients with non-alcoholic fatty liver disease (NAFLD) will have normal LFTs at any one time [7,8].

Systematic approach to the interpretation of liver function tests

Clinical assessment

Liver function tests should be interpreted not in isolation, but rather interpreted in the context of the individual patient. This includes recognition of how factors such as age, gender, race, and geographic location will affect the likely differential diagnosis [1].

The importance of thorough clinical history and examination cannot be overstressed. Apparently vague symptoms of lethargy, anorexia, nausea, and fever may be suggestive of underlying liver disease. Meanwhile jaundice, itch, pale stools, and discoloration of urine are indicative of biliary obstruction. The

Problem-based Approach to Gastroenterology and Hepatology, First Edition. Edited by John N. Plevris, Colin W. Howden.
© 2012 Blackwell Publishing Ltd. Published 2012 by Blackwell Publishing Ltd.

Table 12.1 The origin and significance of standard liver function tests [1,2]

	Marker	Origin	Relationship to liver disease
Synthetic function	Albumin	Hepatocytes	Serum albumin is reduced in progressive liver disease due to decreased synthetic function. Levels are also affected by nutrition, sepsis, gastrointestinal, and urinary losses
	Prothrombin time (PT)	Hepatocytes	Liver-produced clotting factors contribute to coagulation cascade. This includes the vitamin K-dependent clotting factors (II, VII, IX and X). PT reflects the rate of conversion of prothrombin to thrombin, requiring factors II, V, VII and X. PT prolongation occurs in liver disease, vitamin K malabsorption, warfarin therapy, and disseminated intravascular coagulation
Cholestasis	Bilirubin	Heme degradation product that is excreted in bile after conjugation in hepatocytes.	Elevated bilirubin occurs in a range of prehepatic, hepatic, and extrahepatic disorders
	Alkaline phosphatase (ALP)	Membrane-bound enzyme found in both hepatocytes and biliary epithelium. ALP also present in various other tissues, notably bone and placenta	Elevated in cholestatic disease due to release of membrane-bound enzyme into the bloodstream
	γ-Glutamyltransferase (GGT)	Membrane-bound enzyme found in found in both hepatocytes and biliary epithelial cells. GGT also present in a various non-hepatic tissues	Elevated GGT in association with increased ALP occurs in hepatobiliary injury. GGT also elevated in response to chronic alcohol misuse
Hepatocyte Integrity	Alanine aminotransferase (ALT):aspartate aminotransferase (AST)	Hepatocytes. ALT/AST also present in various non-hepatic tissues, notably heart, skeletal muscle, brain, and erythrocytes	Cytosolic (ALT/AST) and mitochondrial (AST) enzymes involved in gluconeogenesis. Elevated in hepatocellular injury

occurrence of abdominal pain in the context of jaundice is classically associated with extrahepatic biliary obstruction due to gallstones. Conversely, painless jaundice often heralds a diagnosis of malignant biliary obstruction or intrahepatic cholestasis. However, clinical symptoms themselves are rarely sufficient for diagnosis.

In respect of clinical assessment, particular attention should be paid to alcohol consumption and risk factors for transmission of viral hepatitis, including: intravenous drug use, blood transfusions, tattoos, and body piercings. Past medical history can provide important clues to etiology through recognized disease associations, e.g. ulcerative colitis (primary sclerosing cholangitis) and hyperlipidemia/type 2 diabetes mellitus (non-alcoholic fatty liver disease). A complete drug history is vital and should include recent antibiotic exposure, herbal/over-the-counter medicines, and the use of vitamin supplements (e.g. vitamin A). However, although certain drugs are commonly associated with hepatotoxicity, most drugs can cause liver injury infrequently [9]. Therefore,

145

Table 12.2 The relationship between magnitude of alanine aminotransferase (ALT):aspartate aminotransferase (AST) elevation and differential diagnosis [8,12]

Liver disease	Peak aminotransferase level (×ULN)	Peak bilirubin (×ULN)	Pattern of resolution
Acute viral hepatitis	10–40 (sustained)	5–10	Typically associated with gradual reduction in ALT and AST
Acute ischemic injury	>40 (early)	<5	Rapid reduction in ALT and AST following initial peak
Toxic injury	>10 (early)	<5	Similar pattern to ischemic injury
Acute biliary obstruction	5–10 (early)	5–10 to >10	Rapid elevation and fall in ALT and AST typically precedes rise in Bilirubin and ALP
Alcoholic hepatitis	5–10 (sustained)	5–10 to >10	Associated with prolonged elevation of ALT and AST. AST:ALT ratio typically >2

particular attention should be paid to how changes in medication relate temporally to LFT disturbance. Finally, family history can point towards the presence of inherited (e.g. hemochromatosis, Wilson's disease, α_1-anti-trypsin deficiency) or autoimmune disease.

Clinical examination may reveal evidence of chronic liver disease, including: palmar erythema, spider nevi, body hair loss, caput medusae, and hepatosplenomegaly. In addition, features of hepatic decompensation may be present, including: fetor hepaticus/asterixis (hepatic encephalopathy), ascites/pleural effusion/caput medusae (portal hypertension/hypoalbuminemia), and peripheral edema (hypoalbuminemia). Finally, specific examination features may be suggestive of the etiology of liver disease, e.g. bronze complexion/cardiomegaly (hemochromatosis), obesity (non-alcoholic fatty liver disease), or xanthelasma/prominent scratch marks (primary biliary cirrhosis).

The pattern of LFT disturbance

When presented with a set of abnormal LFTs an attempt should be made to systematically characterize the pattern of liver enzyme alteration. A number of parameters should be considered [2].

First, effort should be made to identify the predominant pattern of LFT disturbance. Most common liver enzyme alterations can be broadly categorized into either hepatocellular or cholestatic-predominant subgroups.

Second, the magnitude of enzyme alteration should be considered. With respect to elevated aminotransferase levels, the magnitude of enzyme elevation can help discriminate between competing diagnoses (Table 12.2).

Third, we should consider the rate of change and course of enzyme alteration, which will typically follow a stereotyped and well-defined pattern in specific liver diseases.

Hepatocellular-predominant liver function disturbance

The aminotransferase enzymes ALT (alanine aminotransferase) and AST (aspartate aminotransferase) play a critical role in hepatic gluconeogenesis. They are responsible for catalyzing the transfer of amino groups from alanine and aspartate to form oxaloacetic acid and pyruvic acid, respectively. Although both are sensitive indicators of hepatocyte integrity and thus hepatocellular injury, neither enzyme is specific to the liver. AST, with both cytosolic and mitochondrial isoenzymes, is found in the liver, cardiac muscle, skeletal muscle, lungs, kidneys, pancreas, erythrocytes, and leukocytes. Elevated AST may therefore occur in myocardial ischemia or skeletal muscle injury. By contrast, ALT, a cytosolic enzyme, although widely expressed, is more specific for liver disease.

The AST:ALT ratio can help discriminate between different forms of hepatic injury. In alcoholic hepatitis, the AST:ALT ratio is typically elevated to >2.0. This can be explained by a number of factors. First, mitochondrial AST is more sensitive to the effects of alcohol-related mitochondrial injury. Second, AST is found in its maximal concentration in the perivenular region (zone 3) of the hepatic acinus that is most adversely affected in alcoholic liver disease (ALD). Third, both AST and ALT require pyridoxal-5-phosphate (vitamin B_6) for their enzymatic activity. Pyridoxal-5-phosphate deficiency is common in ALD and ALT is more sensitive to the effects of its deficiency. In acute viral hepatitis, it is more usual for ALT to exceed AST. However, an AST:ALT ratio >2 can occur in acute viral hepatitis, where it is associated with poor prognosis [10]. Furthermore, in both chronic viral hepatitis [11] and NAFLD [12], there is evidence to suggest that a rising AST:ALT ratio (>1.0) parallels progression of hepatic fibrosis.

Case 1: high aminotransferase levels in an unconscious patient

Case presentation

A 64-year-old man is admitted to the emergency department of his local hospital. The patient is known to have a history of alcohol dependency and schizophrenia. He was found unconscious by his neighbors on the floor of his apartment, having not been seen for several days. Numerous empty bottles of spirits and medication containers were strewn about the room. Examination revealed the following findings:
- The patient was hypothermic (temperature 34.2°C) and markedly hypoxic (oxygen saturations 81% on air). He had a reduced level of consciousness (Glasgow Coma Scale or GCS 8/15). No stigmata of chronic liver disease were present.
- He was hypotensive (BP 76/46 mmHg) with a sinus tachycardia (rate 120 beats/min). Clinical examination revealed reduced air entry and bronchial breathing at the right lung base. The abdomen was soft and non-tender. A smooth liver edge was palpable 2 cm below the costal margin. No splenomegaly was present.

The patient was immediately intubated and ventilated before transfer to intensive care. CT of the head showed no evidence of intracranial bleeding. Chest radiograph confirmed findings consistent with right basal consolidation. He received intravenous fluid resuscitation and commenced on third generation cephalosporin and metronidazole for treatment of presumed aspiration pneumonia.

Investigations were as follows (normal values in brackets):
Hb 13.8 (13.5–17.5) g/dL
MCV 92 (76–98) fL
WCC 18 (4–11) × 10^9/L
Platelets 146 (150–400) × 10^9/L
Bilirubin 34 (2–17) μmol/L
AST 3650 (10–40) IU/L
ALT 2960 (5–30) IU/L
GGT 180 (5–30) IU/L
Albumin 31 (35–55) g/L
Urea 16.2 (2.5–6.5) mmol/L
Creatinine 178 (50–120) μmol/L
ALP 140 (30–130) IU/L
PT 16 s (control 9 s)
APTT 33 s (32 s)
Na^+ 138 (135–145) mmol/L
K^+ 5.6 (3.5–5.0) mmol/L

Questions

- What is the likely cause for this patient's presentation?
- What blood tests could be undertaken to confirm the hepatic origin of the aminotransferase elevation?
- What are the possible causes of this patient's renal impairment?

Differential diagnosis

This example illustrates a case of acute liver injury. Indeed aminotransferase levels seldom exceed 10 times the upper limit of normal (ULN) except after an acute hepatic insult [13]. Furthermore, ALP is elevated in excess of three times the ULN in less than 10% of cases of acute liver injury [14]. In the context of this case the differential diagnosis would include acute viral hepatitis, acute ischemic hepatitis, and acute toxic injury. *Alcoholic hepatitis* would normally present with a more modest elevation in aminotransferase levels, rarely exceeding 10 × ULN. Other less common causes of this pattern of acute liver injury include autoimmune hepatitis and Budd–Chiari syndrome. Acute bile duct obstruction may be associated with a rapid and transient elevation in amino-transferase levels, although enzyme activity would rarely exceed >2000 IU/L [15]. In this context, aminotransferase levels would typically return to normal within 10 days, even in the presence of ongoing obstruction.

Acute viral hepatitis is typically characterized by a self-limiting illness. However, fulminant liver failure may occur, culminating in either death or liver transplantation. After a suitable incubation period, a steady increase in aminotransferase levels will be observed, usually peaking at 7–14 days and typically resolving over 4–6 weeks. Bilirubin levels lag behind aminotransferase elevation with peak levels delayed by up to 1 week, followed by gradual decline thereafter. The incidence of jaundice in acute viral hepatitis varies from 70% in cases of acute hepatitis A virus (HAV) infection, to 33–50% and 20–33% in acute HBV and HCV infection, respectively [11]. Chronic infection may occur in a minority of patients with HBV infection and a significantly greater proportion of patients with HCV infection. A full discussion of viral hepatitis is outwith the scope of this chapter and is considered elsewhere.

Acute toxic liver injury may occur as an idiosyncratic reaction to prescribed medication or following accidental or deliberate drug overdose. Paracetamol (acetaminophen) poisoning is currently the most common cause for acute liver failure in the USA [16]. The diagnosis may be apparent from clinical history alone. However, measurement of paracetamol levels should be undertaken, both to support diagnosis and to determine whether specific treatment with N-acetylcysteine is required. It is important to recognize that paracetamol levels will be unreliable after late presentation or staggered drug overdose. Peak ALT and AST levels are often greater than those seen in acute viral hepatitis, often exceeding 100 times ULN [17,18].

Ischemic hepatitis, also referred to as "shocked liver," results from sudden reduction in systemic blood flow or increased hepatic venous congestion, as may occur in sepsis or cardiogenic shock. As such, it is more prevalent in patients with underlying cardiovascular disease. The pattern of LFT disturbance is similar to that seen in acute toxic liver injury with markedly elevated aminotransferase levels. Indeed ischemic or toxic liver injury is the cause of >90% of cases of acute liver injury with AST >3000 U [19].

Transaminase levels will typically peak within the first 24–48 h and fall rapidly over the subsequent days. Prothrombin time prolongation is a common early finding after both ischemic and toxic liver injury, whereas significantly elevated bilirubin levels are uncommon in these circumstances.

Diagnosis

The diagnosis in this case was that of ischemic hepatitis. The patient has presented with septic shock in the context of aspiration pneumonia. The precise circumstances surrounding his collapse are unclear, but there would be clinical suspicion of drug or alcohol ingestion that should be thoroughly pursued. Wherever possible a collateral history should be obtained. The pattern of LFT disturbance, with markedly elevated aminotransferase levels, is most in keeping with an ischemic or toxic liver injury. Cardiac enzymes (creatine kinase [CK] and cardiac troponin) should be measured to confirm hepatic origin of the raised aminotransferase levels. Renal failure was present in this case due to acute tubular necrosis in the context of prolonged hypotension, although it would also be important to exclude rhabdomyolysis.

A standard set of investigations should be undertaken in any case of acute liver injury. Paracetamol level and toxicology screen should be sent, even where there is a low clinical suspicion of drug overdose. It is also important to exclude acute viral hepatitis. Standard work-up of patients suspected of being at risk of acute viral hepatitis includes IgM antibody tests for HAV and HBV core antibody, HBV surface antigen, and HCV antibodies. Less common causes of acute viral hepatitis would include hepatitis D (HDV), hepatitis E (HEV), herpes simplex (HSV), varicella-zoster (VZV), cytomegalovirus (CMV), Epstein–Barr virus (EBV), enterovirus, cornavirus, adenovirus, and reovirus infections.

Autoimmune hepatitis may rarely present with fulminant hepatic failure and blood should be sent for serum immunoglobulins and autoantibodies (including antinuclear antibodies [ANAs] and smooth muscle antibodies [SMAs]).

Radiological imaging of the abdomen should be undertaken with either abdominal ultrasonography or computed tomography (CT). This is to enable identification of any focal lesions (e.g. abscess, metastases) or evidence of biliary obstruction or cirrhosis. Assessment of intact blood supply and venous drainage should also be performed in order to exclude Budd–Chiari syndrome.

Patient management

The patient's initial management is essentially supportive. Ischemic hepatitis typically occurs in the context of severe hemodynamic instability and multiorgan failure, usually necessitating management in a high-dependency or intensive care environment. In this case, liver screening investigations were unrevealing. The patient's aminotransferase levels and coagulopathy improved markedly over the following days. Both the clinical history and the pattern of LFT disorder were consistent with a diagnosis of ischemic hepatitis. The patient remained in intensive care for 2 weeks until he could be successfully weaned from the ventilator. He sustained no long-lasting liver impairment.

Case 2: abnormal LFTs in an asymptomatic patient

Case presentation

A 47-year-old accountant presented to his family doctor for a routine medical examination. Routine blood tests were undertaken and revealed liver function test abnormalities.

On further questioning, the patient reported mild lethargy. Past medical history included osteoarthritis. The patient was on no regular prescribed medication but used ibuprofen intermittently for joint pain. The patient was a non-smoker and drank 16 units of alcohol each week.

On clinical examination the patient appeared tanned and mildly obese (BMI 32 kg/m^2). Palmar erythema was present. On cardiovascular examination heart sounds I and II were present and there was a soft (2/6) pansystolic murmur, loudest at the apex. The abdomen was soft and non-tender. The liver edge was palpable 3 cm beneath the costal margin.

Laboratory investigations (normal values in brackets)
Hb 18.1 (13.5–17.5) g/dL
MCV 92 (76–98) fL
WCC 5.0 (4–11) × 10^9/L
Platelets 205 (150–400) × 109/L

Bilirubin 12 (2–17) µmol/L
AST 120 (10–40) IU/L
ALT 133 (5–30) IU/L
GGT 35 (5–30) IU/L
Albumin 35 (35–55) g/L
Urea 5.4 (2.5–6.5) mmol/L
Creatinine 98 (50–120) µmol/L
ALP 120 (30–130) IU/L
PT 9S (control 9 s)
Sodium 137 (135–145) mmol/L
Potassium 4.2 (3.5–5.0) mmol/L
Fasting Glucose 8.2 (3.5–5.0) mmol/L
Ferritin 2340 (20–250) µg/L
Transferrin saturation 78 (22–40)%
Ceruloplasmin 42 (>35)
Antinuclear antibody negative
Anti-smooth muscle antibody negative
Anti mitochondrial antibody negative

Questions

• What is the differential diagnosis in this patient?
• What features on clinical examination may be suggestive of the underlying cause of this man's liver dysfunction?
• What specific diagnostic tests should be undertaken to confirm this patient's diagnosis?
• How should this patient be managed?

Differential diagnosis

This case is intended to demonstrate a common clinical scenario, that of an asymptomatic patient presenting with a mildly elevated ALT. When confronted with this situation, the first step should be to confirm the abnormality with repeat blood tests. If the abnormality persists, appropriate and timely investigation is required to avoid the sequelae of ongoing liver injury. It is therefore entirely appropriate that any patient presenting with evidence of chronic liver injury should undergo a battery of standard baseline tests chosen to exclude common and clinically relevant liver diseases (Table 12.3) [13].

Drug-induced liver injury may present as acute hepatitic, cholestatic, or mixed hepatitic/cholestatic patterns. Hepatocellular drug-induced injury will typically present with elevated ALT and AST. The degree of ALT elevation does not reflect severity. However, in the context of hepatocellular drug-induced injury

Table 12.3 Routine screening tests employed in patients with liver function test (LFT) disturbance [13]

Classification	Cause	Screening investigation	Notes
Viral hepatitis	Hepatitis A	HAV IgM	
	Hepatitis B	HBsAg, Anti-HB core IgM	
	Hepatitis C	Anti-HCV IgM	
Autoimmune disease	Autoimmune hepatitis (AIH)	Antinuclear (ANA), anti-smooth-muscle (ASMA) and anti-liver–kidney–microsomal (LKM) antibodies	Type I AIH is associated with positive ANA and ASMA
			Type II AIH is associated with presence of LKM
		Hypergammaglobulinemia typically present	Type III is uncommon and associated with soluble liver antigen/liver pancreas antibodies (SLA/LP)
	Primary biliary cirrhosis (PBC)	Anti-mitochondrial antibody (AMA) Associated with elevated total IgM	
	Primary sclerosing cholangitis (PSC)	Anti-neutrophil cytoplasmic antibody (p-ANCA).	ANA and ASMA may also be positive
Metabolic disease	Hemochromatosis	Markedly elevated ferritin Transferrin saturation >45%	Genetic testing for common HFE mutations (C282Y/H63D) is available
	Wilson's disease	Low ceruloplasmin	Reduced in 85% of patients with Wilson's Disease. May also be reduced in advanced liver disease
	α_1-Anti-trypsin deficiency	α_1-Anti-trypsin activity and phenotype analysis	
Miscellaneous	Celiac disease	Anti-endomysial and anti-tissue transglutaminase (TTG) antibodies	Recognized cause of otherwise unexplained elevated transaminase levels

and in the absence of biliary obstruction or Gilbert's syndrome, hyperbilirubinemia (more than three times the ULN) is associated with increased mortality. Although almost any drug may cause hepatotoxicity infrequently, certain drugs are more commonly implicated and represent the major clinical load (Table 12.4).

Chronic viral hepatitis is a common cause of persistent LFT abnormalities. Between 300 and 500 million people worldwide are estimated to have chronic HBV infection. The global prevalence of chronic HCV infection is estimated to be 3% [20], with the prevalence in the USA reaching 1.8% [21]. Chronic viral hepatitis will typically present with mild persistent elevation in aminotransferase levels. However, aminotransferase levels may fluctuate and 15–50% of patients with chronic HCV infection will have normal LFTs.

Alcoholic liver disease (ALD) refers to a spectrum of disease, ranging from asymptomatic LFT abnormalities to severe alcoholic hepatitis and decompensated cirrhosis. How chronic alcohol intake affects the liver depends on a complex interplay of genetic and environmental factors. Reliable alcohol history can be notoriously difficult to obtain. Biochemical abnormalities include isolated elevation of GGT or persistently raised aminotransferase levels. AST:ALT ratio >2.0 is highly suggestive of ALD. Surrogate

Table 12.4 List of drugs commonly associated with liver function test (LFT) disturbance

Pattern of liver injury	Drugs associations
Dose-dependent hepatotoxicity	Acetaminophen (paracetamol), nicotinic acid
Hepatitis/ Hepatocellular Injury	Amiodarone, dantrolene, disulfiram, halothane, labetolol, statins, isoniazid, ketoconazole, phenytoin, terbinafine, sulfonamides, diclofenac, etidronate, flucloxacillin, methotrexate, methyldopa, minocycline, nitrofurantoin, propylthiouracil, rifampacin, and valproate
Granulomatous hepatitis	Allopurinol, carbamazepine, hydralazine, quinine, quinidine
Cholestasis	ACE inhibitors, amoxicillin/clavulanic acid, erythromycin, flucloxacillin, trimethoprim/sulfamethoxazole, chlorpromazine, dextropropoxyphene, tricyclic antidepressants, oral contraceptive pill, estrogens, and androgens

markers of alcohol excess, including GGT and elevated mean corpuscular volume (MCV), are non-specific.

Autoimmune hepatitis (AH) is characterized by persistent inflammation of the liver of unknown cause. It will classically present in middle-aged woman (female:male ratio 4:1 [22]). The patient may have a personal or family history of associated autoimmune disease. The characteristic finding is of persistent elevation of transaminase levels, in the absence of any other identifiable cause. Polyclonal γ-globulins are elevated in 80% of patients [23]. Autoantibody tests include ANA, ASMA, liver–kidney–microsomal antibody (LKM), and antibodies to soluble liver antibodies. Types 1, 2, and 3 AH are defined by the pattern of autoantibody expression (see Table 12.3). Criteria for the diagnosis of AH have been defined [24]. Liver biopsy may be required for firm diagnosis.

Non-alcoholic fatty liver disease (NAFLD) is now the most common cause of mild LFT abnormalities in the western world with an estimated prevalence of 23% among American adults [25]. NAFLD is commonly associated with type 2 diabetes and obesity. It is now recognized as the hepatic component of metabolic syndrome. Insulin resistance leads to metabolic changes, which promotes the accumulation of fatty acids and triglycerides within the liver. Subsequent to this, increased oxidative stress, bacterial endotoxin, and the generation of inflammatory cytokines, such as tumor necrosis factor α (TNFα), are thought to promote inflammation and ultimately fibrosis. Mildly elevated aminotransferase levels may be the only abnormality on routine LFTs, although aminotransferase levels are frequently normal. Indeed, there is convincing evidence that the current ULN for ALT fails to identify a significant proportion of patients with underlying liver disease, and indeed it has been suggested that the ULN for ALT should be decreased to 30 U/L in men and 19 U/L in women [26], in order to increase the sensitivity of this test for the detection of liver injury.

Similarly, factors including age, gender, race, and BMI are known to be independently associated with ALT levels and should be taken into account when interpreting laboratory results of patients with suspected liver disease [1]. Aminotransferase elevation (if present) is usually less than four times ULN. AST:ALT ratio is typically <1.0, although it is recognized that the AST:ALT ratio may increase with progressive liver fibrosis. Liver ultrasonography or CT may demonstrate fatty infiltration of the liver. Serological tests are essential to exclude viral and autoimmune liver disease. Detectable ANA and ASMA tests at low titer may be present, but are not likely to be of clinical significance. Findings at liver biopsy are indistinguishable from ALD. Indeed, the cut-off limit for alcohol consumption to distinguish between NAFLD and ALD is not known. An arbitrary limit of 14 units/ week for woman and 21 units/weeks for men is usually employed. Histology demonstrates steatosis, with a variable degree of non-alcoholic steatohepatitis (NASH) and liver fibrosis. NAFLD is considered in more detail elsewhere.

Wilson's disease is a rare inherited (autosomal recessive) disorder of biliary copper excretion that may present with raised aminotransferase levels. Excessive copper is deposited in the liver and brain resulting in progressive liver damage and neuropsychiatric symptoms, including behavioral abnormalities and movement disorders. Clinical onset of symptoms is typically between the ages of 5 and 25, but the diagnosis should be considered in patients up to the age of 40 years. Serum ceruloplasmin will be reduced in 85% of patients with Wilson's disease [22]. Kayser–Fleischer rings may be present but may require slit-lamp examination for their identification. A 24-hour urinary copper excretion of >100 µg is suggestive of Wilson's disease. The gold standard diagnostic test, liver biopsy, will confirm the diagnosis if hepatic copper levels exceed 250 µg/g dry weight. Wilson's disease is caused by mutations in the *ATP7B* gene on chromosome 13. However, reliable genetic testing is not yet available due to the number of different mutations seen.

α_1-*Antitrypsin deficiency* is an uncommon cause of chronic liver disease. Mutations in the α_1-antitrypsin (α_1AT) gene may cause accumulation of this protein in the liver and progressive liver injury. An associated reduction in serum levels of α_1AT is responsible for the association with emphysema in some forms of α_1AT deficiency. Reduced levels of α_1AT may be measured directly or by the lack of a peak in the α-globulin band on serum electrophoresis. Diagnosis is best established by phenotypic analysis. Homozygosity for the Z variant of α_1-antitrypsin, termed Pi (protease inhibitor) ZZ, results in the most severe form of α_1AT deficiency.

Occult *celiac disease* is a recognized cause of otherwise unexplained modestly raised aminotransferase levels. In a study of 140 asymptomatic patients referred to liver clinic for investigation of chronically elevated aminotransferase levels, 13 patients were found to have celiac disease [27]. Patients with unexplained aminotransferase levels should therefore be screened with tissue transglutaminase and anti-endomysial antibody tests. Celiac disease is also associated independently with other autoimmune liver diseases, notably primary biliary cirrhosis (PBC).

Diagnosis

The diagnosis in this patient was *hereditary hemochromatosis* (HH). HH is a common autosomal recessive disorder affecting 1 in 200 people of northern European ancestry. It is characterized by increased intestinal absorption of iron and its subsequent deposition in the liver, heart, joints, pancreas, and other endocrine organs. Clinical manifestations include cutaneous pigmentation, dilated cardiomyopathy, arthropathy, diabetes mellitus, chronic liver disease, hypogonadism, and pituitary and adrenal insufficiency. Liver disease is characterized by LFT disturbance with raised aminotransferase levels, progressing to cirrhosis and hepatocellular carcinoma. Blood tests will reveal evidence of iron overload with elevated ferritin and transferrin saturation (serum iron divided by iron-binding capacity). A transferrin saturation exceeding 45% is suggestive of hemochromatosis [28]. Liver biopsy remains the gold standard diagnostic test, allowing assessment of hepatic iron index and liver fibrosis.

The results of this patient's liver biopsy showed significant iron overload (Figure 12.1). Hepatic iron index (hepatic iron level in micromoles per gram dry weight divided by patient's age) >1.9 is consistent with a diagnosis of hemochromatosis [28]. Genetic testing is now available to identify common defects in the hemochromatosis (*HFE*) gene. Two point mutations in the *HFE* gene, *C282Y* and *H63D*, have been identified that account for most *HFE* defects. The risk of iron overload is greatest in patients homozygous for the *C282Y* mutation. Iron overload may also occur in conjunction with defects in a number of other genes involved in iron transport, including hemojuvelin, transferrin receptor-2 and ferroportin.

Patient management

Treatment requires regular venesection to reduce iron overload. The removal of 1 unit of blood (450–

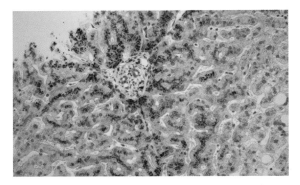

Figure 12.1 Liver biopsy (Perl's Prussian blue stain) from a patient with hereditary hemochromatosis, showing excessive deposition of iron in hepatocytes and cholangiocytes. (Image courtesy of Dr Timothy Kendall.)

500 mL) results in the loss of 200–250 mg iron. Initial phlebotomy should be performed weekly with the aim of reducing serum ferritin to below 50 ng/mL, without inducing anemia. A secondary aim is to reduce transferrin saturation to below 50% [29]. In cases where phlebotomy is not tolerated or refractory anemia is present, iron chelation therapy (e.g. desferrioxamine) may be considered. Treatment with venesection should result in a dramatic improvement in LFTs, although hepatic cirrhosis, if present, is irreversible. Patients may report improvement in symptoms such as tiredness, abdominal discomfort, and skin pigmentation. However, arthropathy and hypogonadism do not improve with phlebotomy.

Screening should be undertaken to detect other complications of HH, including secondary diabetes mellitus and cardiomyopathy. In this case, the patient underwent an echocardiogram which showed reduced right and left ventricular ejection fraction, suggestive of dilated cardiomyopathy. Fasting glucose measurement was 8.2 mmol/L (normal range 3.5–5.0 mmol/L) consistent with a diagnosis of type 2 diabetes mellitus. Patients with HH are at increased risk of developing hepatocellular carcinoma (HCC) and cirrhotic patients should be screened every 6 months with ultrasound and α-fetoprotein (a serum marker for HCC). The risk of HCC is reduced by venesection. Finally, it is important that genetic counseling and testing of family members should be offered in cases of confirmed cases of HH.

Cholestatic-predominant liver function test disturbance

Cholestasis is characterized biochemically by elevated levels of serum bilirubin, alkaline phosphatase ALP, and GGT. Bilirubin is produced as the end-product of heme breakdown in the reticuloendothelial system. Water-insoluble unconjugated bilirubin cannot be excreted directly in urine and is transported to the liver bound to albumin. In the liver it is conjugated to form water-soluble bilirubin glucuronide, which is subsequently excreted in the bile. A proportion of the conjugated bilirubin that is excreted into the gut is reabsorbed as urobilinogen, and is subsequently excreted in the urine. Total bilirubin is normally 80% unconjugated. Any cause of increased heme breakdown (Table 12.5) [2,30] will lead to increased levels of unconjugated bilirubin (>80% total). In contrast, hepatocellular disease will lead to increased conju-

Table 12.5 Causes of unconjugated/conjugated hyperbilirubinemia [2,30]

Unconjugated bilirubin	Conjugated bilirubin
Increased bilirubin production	Hepatocellular disease
Hemolytic anemia	
Blood transfusion	Dubin–Johnson syndrome
Ineffective hemopoiesis	Rotor syndrome
Resorption of large hematoma	
Reduced hepatic uptake/ conjugation	Intra- and extrahepatic biliary obstruction
Neonatal jaundice	
Gilbert's syndrome	Total parenteral nutrition
Types 1 and 2 Crigler–Najjar syndrome	
Drugs, e.g. rifampicin	

gated bilirubin (20–60% total), whereas intrahepatic and extrahepatic biliary obstruction may cause greater increases in conjugated bilirubin (>70% total) [31]. The caveat is that conjugated bilirubin may occasionally be increased to >70% in some cases of severe hepatocellular injury causing intrahepatic obstruction.

Obstructive jaundice is characterized clinically by progressive jaundice accompanied by dark urine and pale stool. This reflects obstruction to bile flow into the gut and resulting excretion of conjugated bilirubin in the urine. The presence of abdominal pain may be suggestive of gallstones, whereas painless jaundice is usually a more ominous occurrence, often heralding a diagnosis of malignant biliary obstruction (e.g. pancreatic carcinoma, cholangiocarcinoma, HCC). In acute biliary obstruction a rapid and transient elevation of ALT and AST may precede rising ALP and GGT.

Although differential bilirubin levels may help discriminate between different types of jaundice, this may not be readily available. Prompt imaging with ultrasonography or CT is required to confirm or refute the presence of obstruction. The precise cause of obstruction may not be immediately obvious, in which case further imaging with magnetic resonance cholangiopancreatography (MRCP) or endoscopic retrograde cholangiopancreatography (ERCP) may be required. ERCP has the advantage that it may be possible to perform a therapeutic procedure (e.g. ductal gallstone removal or biliary stent insertion) but does carry with it the risk of iatrogenic injury (e.g. pancreatitis, bleeding).

Gilbert's syndrome is a common cause of unconjugated hyperbilirubinemia, due to an inherited (autosomal dominant) defect in UDP-glucuronyltransferase. Serum bilirubin levels may be exacerbated by fasting and intercurrent illness, but do not usually exceed 68 μmol/L and occur in the absence of any additional LFT abnormalities [32]. Gilbert's syndrome is an entirely benign disorder and no specific treatment is required. Genetic testing is available.

ALP refers to a family of membrane-bound enzymes that catalyze the hydrolysis of phosphate esters at alkaline pH. Alkaline phosphatase is present (in deceasing abundance) in placenta, ileal mucosa, kidney, bone, and liver [1]. Elevated ALP may therefore be found in a number of conditions (Box 12.1) [2,22,30]. In addition, there is significant gender- and age-specific variation in ALP levels and separate reference intervals are required for children and pregnant

women. Specificity for liver disease may be increased by measurement of tissue-specific isoenzymes. The hepatic origin of an elevated ALP measurement may also be corroborated by the measurement of GGT. The membrane-bound enzyme GGT is found in a wide variety of tissues and is a highly sensitive, but non-specific, indicator of liver injury. Precisely because of its limited specificity, the measurement of GGT should arguably be reserved for this purpose.

Case 3: cholestatic LFTs in a young male patient

Case presentation

A 36-year-old man is referred to the liver clinic for investigation of persistently abnormal LFTs. The patient had initially presented to his family doctor with increasing lethargy, accompanied by widespread itch, which prevented him from sleeping. Past medical history included longstanding irritable bowel syndrome. He was on no regular medication but remembered receiving a course of antibiotics 6 months earlier for treatment of a sore throat. He was an ex-smoker and consumed 10 units of alcohol each week.

On clinical examination the patient was of slim build. The presence of numerous scratch marks was noted. There were no stigmata of chronic liver disease. The abdomen was soft and non-tender. The liver and spleen were not palpable.

Laboratory investigations (normal values in brackets)
Hb 14.1 (13.5–17.5) g/dL
MCV 97 (76–98) fL
WCC 6.2 (4–11) $\times 10^9$/L
Platelets 325 (150–400) $\times 10^9$/L
Albumin 38 (35–55) g/L
Bilirubin 23 (2–17) μmol/L
AST 28 (10–40) IU/L
ALT 25 (5–30) IU/L
GGT 150 (5–30) IU/L
Urea 4.0 (2.5–6.5) mmol/L
Creatinine 104 (50–120) μmol/L
ALP 340 (30–130) IU/L
PT 10s (control 9s)
Na$^+$ 138 (135–145) mmol/L
K$^+$ 3.7 (3.5–5.0) mmol/L
HBsAg/HBcAb/HCVAb negative

Box 12.1 Common causes of elevated alkaline phosphatase (ALP) [2,22,30]

Physiological

Adolescence (related to increased ALP from bone during growth spurt)

Pregnancy (increased placental ALP in third trimester)

Benign/Familial (increased intestinal ALP)

Pathological

Intra-/extrahepatic bile duct obstruction

Primary biliary cirrhosis

Primary sclerosing cholangitis

Hepatocellular disease, e.g. alcoholic liver disease, viral hepatitis, cirrhosis

Drug-induced cholestasis

Vanishing bile duct syndrome

Metastatic liver disease/Hepatocellular carcinoma

Infiltrative disease, e.g. sarcoidosis, tuberculosis

Bone disease, e.g. fracture, hyperparathyroidism, Paget's disease, bony metastases

---

Ferritin 123 (20–250) μg/L
Transferrin saturation 25 (22–40)%
Ceruloplasmin 50 (>35)
Antinuclear antibody negative
Anti-smooth muscle antibody negative
Anti-mitochondrial antibody negative
p-ANCA strongly positive
Abdominal ultrasonography was reported as showing
  no abnormalities

Questions

• What is the differential diagnosis?
• How might the patients past medical history relate
to his final diagnosis?
• How might you proceed with the further investigation of this patient?

Differential diagnosis

The case represents that of a patient presenting with
tests suggestive of chronic cholestasis. ALP is present
on the surface of bile duct epithelia and any cause
of cholestasis will enhance its release into the
bloodstream.

Drug reactions are a common cause of cholestatic
LFT disturbance, characterized by elevation in ALP
and bilirubin. Commonly implicated drugs include
antibiotics, angiotensin-converting enzyme inhibitors,
antidepressants, and the oral contraceptive pill. The
overwhelming majority of drug reactions are self-
limiting following discontinuation of the offending
drug. However, progression to fulminant hepatic
failure is not uncommon. LFT abnormalities will typically resolve over the course of several months, more
slowly than would be the case following hepatocellular injury.

Primary biliary cirrhosis (PBC) is a chronic autoimmune liver disease that is characterized by autoimmune destruction of intrahepatic bile ducts, leading
to progressive liver fibrosis and ultimately cirrhosis
[33]. It typically presents in middle-aged women
(female:male ratio 9:1) and in association with other
autoimmune diseases, particularly Sjögren's syndrome
and rheumatoid arthritis. It may present initially in
asymptomatic patients with elevated ALP and GGT
on routine biochemical tests. AST and ALT may be
elevated in up to 50% of cases, but would not usually
exceed twice the ULN [34]. The pre-symptomatic
phase may extend for two or more decades. As the
disease progresses, symptoms of lethargy and pruritis
become prominent. Clinical signs include hyperpigmentation, hepatosplenomegaly, and xanthelasma.
Jaundice develops late in disease. PT prolongation
may reflect vitamin K malabsorption or advanced
fibrotic liver disease. The autoimmune marker, AMA,
will be present in most patients with PBC, but may
be found in association with other diseases. The M2
variant of AMA, directed against the pyruvate dehydrogenase complex, is more specific for PBC. Levels
of serum IgM immunoglobulins are also elevated in
PBC. Liver biopsy will show inflammatory destruction of intrahepatic bile ducts and granuloma
formation.

Elevated ALP may also be found in association
with HCC, hepatic metastases, lymphoma, and infiltrative disorders such as sarcoidosis. In addition, ALP
may be elevated in certain malignancies without
hepatic/bony involvement, due to the production of
an ALP isoenzyme ("Regan isoenzyme").

Diagnosis

The diagnosis in this patient is primary sclerosing
cholangitis (PSC). PSC is a chronic cholestatic liver
disease of unknown etiology, characterized by progressive inflammatory destruction and fibrosis of both
the intra- and extrahepatic bile ducts. PSC is more
common in males and in association with inflammatory bowel disease (IBD). IBD is present in 75% of
patients with PSC. Of these patients, 87% have ulcerative colitis and 13% have Crohn's disease [35]. PSC
may precede the diagnosis of IBD and patients presenting with PSC may describe symptoms suggestive
of hitherto undiagnosed IBD.

PSC is characterized clinically by an insidious onset
and fluctuating course. Elevated ALP (3–10 × ULN)
is the characteristic biochemical finding. ALT and
AST levels may be elevated (2–3 × ULN). Scarring
and stricture formation in the extrahepatic bile ducts
may be associated with rapid deterioration in liver
function and secondary biliary cirrhosis. In addition,
these patients are at risk of recurrent episodes of
ascending cholangitis. There is also an increased risk
of cholangiocarcinoma, which occurs in 10–30% of
patients with PSC [36].

The diagnosis of PSC is established by demonstrating the classical "beaded" cholangiographic findings
in the context of cholestatic liver dysfunction (Figure

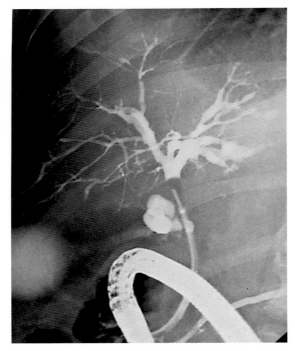

Figure 12.2 Endoscopic retrograde cholangiopancreatogram (ERCP) showing characteristic "beaded" appearance of the biliary tree in primary sclerosing cholangitis, due to the presence of multifocal intra- and extrahepatic biliary strictures. (Image courtesy of Dr Doris Redhead.)

12.2). This appearance results from the presence of multifocal intra- and extrahepatic biliary strictures. Non-invasive MRCP has increasingly replaced ERCP as the investigation of choice in the diagnosis of PSC. Perinuclear anti-neutrophil cytoplasmic antibodies (p-ANCAs) are present in around two-thirds of patients with PSC but are non-specific [37,38]. Liver biopsy may be required to support the diagnosis of PSC. PSC is characterized histologically by inflammation and concentric fibrosis ("onion-skinning") around bile ducts with eventual obliteration of their lumina. These changes ultimately lead to cirrhosis.

Patient management

At present there is no effective medical therapy for the treatment of PSC. The most extensively studied drug is the synthetic hydrophobic bile acid, ursode-oxycholic acid (UDCA). The evidence for the efficacy of ursodeoxycholic acid in the treatment of PSC is limited [39]. A number of trials have demonstrated that the use of ursodeoxycholic acid is associated with an improvement in LFTs. However, comparatively few studies have been able to demonstrate any improvement in liver histology. It has been suggested that high-dose ursodeoxycholic acid (22–25 mg/kg) may be more effective than standard doses of this drug (13–15 mg/kg). Biliary enrichment with ursode-oxycholic acid increases with escalating dose, reaching a plateau at 22–25 mg/kg [40]. Furthermore, in a small trial, the use of high-dose ursodeoxycholic acid (22–25 mg/kg) was associated with improvements in both liver fibrosis and cholangiographic appearance.

A number of agents, including corticosteroids, ciclosporin, tacrolimus, methotrexate, and D-penicillamine, have been proposed for use in PSC. However, at the time of writing, there is no conclusive evidence for the routine use of these agents.

Patients who develop dominant strictures may be treated endoscopically with balloon dilation or biliary stent insertion. Furthermore, in selected patients, hepatojejunostomy may be considered. Benign dominant strictures may be difficult to differentiate from cholangiocarcinoma, for which there are no effective screening strategies for diagnosis. Diagnosis relies on critical interpretation of imaging, brush cytology, and non-specific tumor markers (e.g. CA19-9 and CEA). Liver transplantation remains the only definitive treatment for PSC, although disease recurrence is reported to occur in 20–40% [41]. Finally, patients with PSC and IBD have a markedly increased risk of developing colorectal neoplasia, compared with those with IBD alone. In view of this, current guidelines recommend that these patients receive annual screening colonoscopies, with random biopsies taken every 10 cm to detect developing dysplasia [42].

LFTs in pregnancy

The interpretation of liver function abnormalities in pregnancy poses particular problems for the clinician. It is estimated that liver disorders complicate 3% of all pregnancies [43]. Hepatic disease occurring in pregnancy can be divided into three categories: hepatic diseases peculiar to pregnancy, pre-existing liver disease exacerbated by pregnancy, and coincidental acute liver or gallstone disease [44]. In addition, the normal physiological adaptation that occurs in pregnancy is associated with predictable changes in liver function, which can itself cause diagnostic uncertainty. Plasma volume increases, leading to a decrease in serum albumin and reaching its nadir toward the end of pregnancy. Reduction in albumin-bound bilirubin and hemodilution is responsible for a reduction in total bilirubin. Placental and fetal production of ALP leads to a progressive rise in enzyme levels towards the end of pregnancy and renders it a poor marker for cholestasis. By contrast, levels of GGT, ALT, and AST are broadly unchanged in pregnancy and elevation in these enzymes should prompt further investigation to exclude underlying liver disease.

Case 4: pregnancy and abnormal LFTs

Case presentation

A 32-year-old pregnant woman presents to her local obstetric unit, at 36-weeks gestation, with a 1-week history of persistent nausea, vomiting, and dull right upper quadrant (RUQ) pain. She had also noticed mild yellow discoloration of her skin and eyes.

On examination, the patient was jaundiced. The patient displayed slow mentation and asterixis could be demonstrated. On cardiovascular examination pulse was 110 regular and blood pressure was 110/70. The abdomen was gravid with mild RUQ tenderness, but no guarding or rebound tenderness. The liver and spleen were not palpable.

Initial investigations (normal values in brackets)
Hb 10.1 (11.5–15.5) g/dL
MCV 77 (76–98) fL
WCC 13 (4–11) $\times 10^9$/L
Platelets 100 (150–400) $\times 10^9$/L
GGT 120 (5–30) IU/L
ALT 234 (5–30) IU/L
AST 216 (10–40) IU/L
Bilirubin 78 (2–17) μmol/L
Albumin 30 (35–55) g/L
Urea 6.5 (2.5–6.5) mmol/L
Creatinine 120 (50–120) μmol/L
Sodium 138 (135–145) mmol/L
Potassium 4.7 (3.5–5.0) mmol/L
ALP 120 (30–130) IU/L
PT 14 s (control 9 s)
APTT 40 s (control 32 s)

Fibrinogen 1.8 (1.5–4.0) g/L
Urinalysis showed mild proteinuria (+)

Questions

• What is the differential diagnosis in this patient and what initial investigations should be performed?
• What recommendations would you make about this patient's management?
• What factors may be contributing to the patient's coagulopathy?

Differential diagnosis

The differential diagnosis of hepatic dysfunction in pregnancy is influenced by the trimester in which biochemical changes occur. The precise diagnostic strategy employed should not differ from that employed in non-pregnant patients, except that a number of conditions specific to pregnancy should be considered (Table 12.6) [44–46]. Clinical signs of chronic liver disease may be difficult to interpret in pregnancy. The development of palmer erythema and spider nevi is promoted by elevated estrogen levels in pregnancy. In addition, it may be difficult to assess for the presence of hepatosplenomegaly and ascites in the presence of a gravid uterus.

The case described here is that of hepatocellular-predominant liver injury and acute liver failure. As in any case of hepatic dysfunction, a thorough history and examination is essential. This should be complemented by a set of routine blood tests and radiological investigations to exclude "common" causes of acute liver dysfunction (see Table 12.3). It should be recognized that pregnant patients remain susceptible to the same causes of liver dysfunction and acute liver injury as the general population. In particular, prompt diagnosis of hepatitis B is vital in order that passive and active immunization may be given at birth to reduce the risk of vertical transmission. Of those conditions specific to pregnancy, eclampsia, HELLP syndrome (hemolysis elevated liver enzymes and low platelets) and acute fatty liver of pregnancy (AFLP) are the most important causes of severe liver dysfunction. A further condition worthy of note is acute HEV. This virus is endemic in some developing countries and has a similar pattern of transmission as HAV infection. However, in pregnancy HEV infection may present with fulminant hepatic failure and

Table 12.6 Causes of LFT dysfunction in pregnancy [43–46]

Disease	Onset in pregnancy	Clinical features
Hyperemesis gravidarum (HG)	First trimester	HG characterized by severe nausea and vomiting that may require hospital admission. LFT disturbance occurs in up to 25% of patients with ↑ aminotransferase (<200 U), ↑ ALP (<2 × ULN) and mild unconjugated hyperbilirubinemia. Treated with supportive management
Preeclampsia/ Eclampsia	Second/third trimester	See below. LFT disturbance occurs in 20–30% of patients with preeclampsia with modestly elevated ALP and transaminase levels. Treatment by delivery/supportive management
HELLP syndrome	From mid-second trimester 30% occurs postpartum	See below. Defined as syndrome of hemolysis, elevated liver enzymes and low platelets. May occur as a complication of preeclampsia/eclampsia. Typical laboratory findings include: LDH >600 IU/L, bilirubin >20 μmol/L, ALT:AST (>70 IU/L), thrombocytopenia (<100 000/μL), and evidence of microangiopathic hemolytic anemia on blood film
Acute fatty liver of pregnancy (AFLP)	Third trimester	See below. Rare complication of pregnancy characterized by progressive fatty infiltration of the maternal liver. May present with vague abdominal pain, nausea and vomiting. May progress rapidly with increasing jaundice and acute hepatic failure
Intrahepatic cholestasis of pregnancy (ICP)	Third trimester	Rare disorder with incidence of 1 in 1000–10 000 of all pregnancies. May present with pruritis alone (80%) or in combination with jaundice (20%). Laboratory features: ↑ bilirubin (<100 μmol/L) and ↑ ALP (<4 × ULN). Elevated serum bile acids are the most sensitive test (10–25 × ULN). Treatment requires delivery at fetal maturity and ursodeoxycholic acid for itch
Liver hematoma/ Rupture	Late third trimester/ Postpartum	May occur as a complication of preeclampsia/eclampsia and HELLP syndrome. Diagnosis requires ultrasonography or contrast CT. Contained hematomas may be treated conservatively. Rupture requires emergency surgery
Liver adenoma	May increase in size during pregnancy	Uncommon benign neoplasm typically occurring in young women on taking the oral contraceptive pill. May also be associated with pregnancy, type 2 diabetes mellitus, and glycogen storage disease. Characteristically increase in size during pregnancy and may be complicated by liver hematoma and rupture. Small hematomas (<5 cm) should be monitored. Large (>5 cm) or symptomatic hematomas may require resection. Surgical resection in second trimester is considered safe

ALT, alanine aminotransferase; ALP, alkaline phosphatase; AST, aspartate aminotransferase; LDH, lactate dehydrogenase; LFT, liver function test; ULN, upper limit of normal.

maternal mortality of 16% [46]. Other conditions that may present more commonly in pregnancy include liver hematoma and rupture, often in association with preeclampsia and HELLP. There is also an increased incidence of Budd–Chiari syndrome, presumably due to hypercoagulability associated with pregnancy.

Preeclampsia is characterized by the triad of hypertension, proteinuria, and peripheral edema, and complicates 5–7% of pregnancies [46]. *Eclampsia* is characterized by seizures and coma in the presence of the clinical features of preeclampsia. Preeclampsia typically occurs in the second and third trimester. Risk factors include primiparity, extremes of maternal age, and multiple gestation. The pathophysiology of these conditions is believed to result from failure of placental implantation. The resulting placental ischemia causes endothelial activation with coagulation cascade initiation, increased platelet adhesiveness, and thrombogenicity. The resulting end-organ damage is responsible for associated morbidity and mortality. LFT abnormalities are present in 20–30% of patients, typically elevated ALP and ALT/AST [46]. Liver biopsy may show sinusoidal fibrin deposition, periportal hemorrhage, and liver cell necrosis. Maternal mortality rate is less than 1%. Some 80% of maternal deaths are due to central nervous system complications with hepatic complications (e.g. fulminant hepatic failure, subcapsular hematoma and rupture) accounting for most of the remaining mortality.

The *HELLP syndrome* is traditionally considered to be a complication of preeclampsia, although these two conditions differ in several respects. The condition affects 0.1–0.6% of all pregnancies and 4–12% of patients with preeclampsia. Approximately one-third of cases occur postpartum. The characteristic laboratory findings that define the HELLP syndrome result from endothelial and coagulation cascade activation. Laboratory tests show a microangiopathic hemolytic anemia with raised lactate dehydrogenase, elevated aminotransferase levels (2–10 × ULN), and thrombocytopenia. Patients will typically present in the third trimester of pregnancy with lethargy, nausea, vomiting, weight gain, and RUQ pain. Complications include disseminated intravascular coagulation, acute renal failure, placental abruption, pulmonary edema, subcapsular hematoma, and rupture. Overall maternal mortality rate is 1–3% and the risk of recurrence in further pregnancies is 3–27%.

Definitive treatment of both the HELLP syndrome and severe preeclampsia requires delivery of the fetus, although ongoing supportive management may be required for several days after delivery. Expectant management with delayed delivery may be considered for patients with mild preeclampsia presenting early in the third trimester. Expectant management of HELLP syndrome is somewhat more controversial. In patients presenting before 34 weeks, delivery may be delayed, with close monitoring of the patients, to allow administration of corticosteroids to promote fetal lung maturation. There is also some evidence that steroids may have beneficial effects for platelet counts and aminotransferase levels.

Diagnosis

The case described here is that of *acute fatty liver of pregnancy*. This is rare complication of pregnancy, affecting 1 in 13 000 pregnancies with significant maternal (18%) and fetal (23%) mortality. The disease will typically present late in the third trimester of pregnancy and it can be difficult to differentiate this condition from preeclampsia/HELLP syndrome (half of patients with AFLP have preeclampsia). Initial symptoms are non-specific and may include lethargy, anorexia, nausea, vomiting, and RUQ pain. Slowly progressive jaundice will occur as the disease progresses. The presence of encephalopathy and jaundice in the absence of the features of preeclampsia is suggestive of AFLP. Laboratory tests typically reveal elevated ALT and AST (<1000 IU/L), PT time prolongation, hypoglycemia, hyperbilirubinemia, and raised ammonia levels. AFLP is commonly complicated by disseminated intravascular coagulation (DIC). Ultrasonography or CT will typically demonstrate fatty infiltration of the liver. Liver biopsy will show pronounced microvesicular steatosis in the absence of significant inflammation or necrosis. It is now recognized that AFLP occurs in association with fetal deficiency in the enzyme long-chain 3-hydroxyacyl-CoA dehydrogenase (LCHAD). In normal circumstances, women heterozygous for this enzyme defect will have normal fatty acid oxidation. AFLP occurs when a heterozygous mother has a fetus that is homozygous for this enzyme defect. The fetus is unable to oxidize long-chain fatty acids, which accumulate in the maternal liver having been transferred across the placenta. Fatty acid accumulation leads to microvesicular steatosis, impairing hepatocyte function and resulting in hepatic failure.

Patient management

The only effective treatment is prompt delivery of the fetus, which removes the source of excess fatty acids and allows the maternal liver to recover, with no long-term sequelae. If left untreated, fulminant hepatic failure will develop. Patients may require admission to a high-dependency or intensive care unit for supportive management of acute hepatic failure. Associated complications of AFLP include pancreatitis, DIC, acute renal failure, seizures, coma, encephalopathy, gastrointestinal and uterine bleeding.

Conclusion

In this chapter a systematic approach to the interpretation of abnormal LFTs was discussed. Specific liver diseases produce distinct pattern of LFT disturbance. These can be described on the basis of the predominant pattern of LFT disturbance, the magnitude of enzyme alteration, and the rate of change/course of these changes. In categorizing LFT abnormalities in this manner, a differential diagnosis is produced and can be further refined through a standard set of laboratory and radiological investigations. It is the intention of this approach to tailor the path of investigation to the pattern of LFT disturbance, and thus lead to prompt and accurate diagnosis, while minimizing unnecessary and costly investigations. At the same time, it is important to recognize the limitations of any diagnostic algorithm. LFT abnormalities may not be easily categorized and specific pathological processes may coexist or produce unexpected patterns of disturbance. Indeed in some cases the diagnosis may not be apparent even after extensive investigation, including liver biopsy. However, in these difficult cases, thoughtful use and interpretation of laboratory and radiological investigations, in the context of thorough clinical assessment, is most likely to lead to a correct diagnosis.

References

1 Dufour DR, Lott JA, Nolte FS, et al. Diagnosis and monitoring of hepatic injury. I. Performance and characteristics of laboratory tests. *Clin Chem* 2000;**46**: 2027–49.

2 Giannini EG, Testa R and Savarino V. Liver enzyme alteration: a guide for clinicians. *Can Med Assoc J* 2005;**172**:367–79.

3 Inglesby TV, Raj R, Astemborski J, et al. A prospective community-based evaluation of liver enzymes in individuals with hepatitis C after drug use. *Hepatology* 1999;**29**:590–6.

4 Alter HJ, Conry-Cantilena C, Melpolder J, et al. Hepatitis C in asymptomatic blood donors. *Hepatology* 1997;**26**(suppl 1):29–33.

5 Mathurin P, Moussalli J, Cadranel JF, et al. Slow progression rate of fibrosis in hepatitis C patients with persistently normal alanine aminotransferase activity. *Hepatology* 1998;**27**:568–72.

6 Kenny-Walsh E. Clinical outcomes after hepatitis C infection from contaminated anti-D immune globulin. *N Engl J Med* 1999;**340**:1228–33.

7 Ipecki SH, Basaranoglu M, Sonsuz A. The fluctuation of serum levels of aminotransferase in patients with non-alcoholic steatohepatitis. *J Clin Gastroenterol* 2003; **36**:371.

8 Yano E, Tagawa K, Yamaoka K, et al. Test validity of periodic liver function tests in a population of Japanese male bank employees. *J Clin Epidemiol* 2001;**54**: 945–51.

9 Lee WM. Drug induced hepatotoxicity. *N Engl J Med* 2003;**349**:474–85.

10 Girlin N. The serum glutamic oxaloacetic transaminase/ serum glutamic pyruvic transaminase ratio as a prognostic index in severe acute viral hepatitis. *Am J Gastroenterol* 1982;**77**:2–4.

11 Sheth SG, Glamm SL, Gordon FD, et al. AST/ALT ratio predicts cirrhosis in patients with chronic hepatitis C virus infection. *Am J Gastroenterol* 1998;**93**: 44–8.

12 Sorbi D, Boynton J, Lindor KD. The ratio of aspartate aminotransferase to alanine aminotransferase: potential value in differentiating non-alcoholic steatohepatitis from alcoholic liver disease. *Am J Gastroenterol* 1999;**94**:1018–22.

13 Dufour DR, Lott JA, Nolte FS, et al. Diagnosis and monitoring of hepatic injury. II. Recommendations for use of laboratory tests in screening, diagnosis and monitoring. *Clin Chem* 2000;**46**:2050–68.

14 Ellis G, Goldberg DM, Spooner RJ. Serum enzyme tests in diseases of the liver and biliary tree. *Am J Clin Pathol* 1978;**70**:248–58.

15 Fortson WC Tedesco FJ, Starnes EC, et al. Marked elevation of serum transaminase activity associated with extrahepatic biliary tract obstruction. *J Clin Gastroenterol* 1995;**17**:502–5.

16 Larson AM, Polson J, Fontana RJ, et al. Acute Liver Failure Study Group. Acetaminophen-induced acute liver failure: results of a United States multicenter, prospective study. *Hepatology* 2005;**42**: 1364–72.

17 Singer AJ, Carracio TR, Mofenson HC. The temporal profile of increased transaminase levels in patients with acetaminophen-induced liver dysfunction. *Ann Emerg Med* 1995;**26**:49–53.

18 Zimmerman HJ, Maddrey WC. Acetaminophen (paracetamol) hepatotoxicity with regular intake of alcohol: analysis of instance of therapeutic misadventure. *Hepatology* 1995;**22**:767–73.

19 Johnson RD, O'Connor ML, Kerr RM. Extreme elevations of aspartate aminotransferase. *Am J Gastroenterol* 1995;**90**:1244–5.

20 Wasley A, Alter MJ. 2000;Epidemiology of hepatitis C: geo-graphic differences and temporal trends. *Semin Liver Dis* **20**:1–16.

21 Alter MJ, Kruszon-Moran D, Nainan OV, et al. The prevalence of hepatitis C virus infection in the United States, 1988 through 1995. *N Engl J Med* 1999;**341**:556–65.

22 Pratt DS, Kaplan MM. Evaluation of abnormal liver enzyme results in asymptomatic patients. *N Engl J Med* 2000;**342**:1266–71.

23 Krawitt EL. Autoimmune hepatitis. *N Engl J Med* 1996;**334**:897–903.

24 Czaja A, Freese DK. Diagnosis and treatment of autoimmune hepatitis. *Hepatology* 2002;**36**:470–97.

25 Harrison SA, Kadakia S, Lang KA, et al. Non-alcoholic steatohepatitis: what we know in the new millennium. *Am J Gastroenterol* 2002;**97**:2714–24.

26 Prati D, Taioli E, Zanella A, et al. Updated definitions of healthy ranges for serum alanine aminotransferase levels. *Ann Intern Med* 2002;**137**:1–9.

27 Bardella MT, Vecchi M, Conte D, et al. Chronic unexplained transaminasemia may be caused by occult celiac disease. *Hepatology* 1999;**29**:654–7.

28 Powell LW, George DK, McDonnell SM, et al. Diagnosis of hemochromatosis. *Ann Intern Med* 1998;**129**:925–31.

29 Tavil AS. Diagnosis and management of hemochromatosis. *Hepatology* 2001;**33**:1321–8.

30 Limdi JK, Hyde GM. Evaluation of abnormal liver function tests. *Postgrad Med J* 2003;**79**:313–19.

31 Knight JA. Liver function tests: their role in the diagnosis of hepatobiliary diseases. *J Infus Nursing* 2005;**28**:108–17.

32 Thomsen HF, Hardt F, Juhl E. The diagnosis of Gilbert's syndrome. *Scand J Gastroenterol* 1981;**16**:699–703.

33 Talwalkar JA, Lindor KD. Primary biliary cirrhosis. *Lancet* 2003;**362**:53–61.

34 Lohse AW, Meyer Zum Buschenfelde KH, Franz B, et al. Characterisation of the overlap syndrome of primary biliary cirrhosis (PBC) and autoimmune hepatitis: evidence for it being a hepatitis form of PBC in genetically susceptible individuals. *Hepatology* 1999;**29**:1078–84.

35 Kaplan MM. Toward better treatment of primary sclerosing cholangitis. *N Engl J Med* 1997;**336**:719–21.

36 Lazaridis KN, Gores GJ. Primary sclerosing cholangitis and cholangiocarcinoma. *Semin Liver Dis* 2006;**26**:42–51.

37 Mulder AH, Horst G, Haagsma EB, et al. Prevalence and characterisation of neutrophil cytoplasmic antibodies in autoimmune disease. *Hepatology* 1993;**17**:411–17.

38 Morena LLE, Gores GL. Advances in the diagnosis of cholangiocarcinoma in patients with primary sclerosing cholangitis. *Liver Transplant* 2006;**12**:S15–19.

39 Cullen SN, Chapman RW. Review Article: current management of primary sclerosing cholangitis. *Aliment Pharmacol Ther* 2005;**21**:933–48.

40 Rost D, Rudolf G, Kloeters-Plachky P, Stiehl A. Effect of high dose ursodeoxycholic acid on its biliary enrichment in primary sclerosing cholangitis. *Hepatology* 2004;**40**:693–8.

41 Gordon F. Recurrent primary sclerosing cholangitis: clinical diagnosis and longterm management issues. *Liver Transplant* 2006;**12**:S73–5.

42 Eaden JA, Mayberry JF. Guidelines for surveillance of asymptomatic colorectal cancer in patients with IBD. *Gut* 2002;**51**:V10–12.

43 Ch'ng CL, Morgan M, Hainsworth I, et al. Prospective study of liver dysfunction in pregnancy in southwest Wales. *Gut* 2002;**51**:876–80.

44 Guntupalli SR, Steingrub J. Hepatic disease and pregnancy: an overview of diagnosis and management. *Crit Care Med* 2005;**33**(10 suppl):S332–9.

45 Knox TA, Olans LB. Current concepts: liver disease in pregnancy. *N Engl J Med* 1996;**335**:569–75.

46 Benjaminov FS, Heathcote J. Liver disease in pregnancy. *Am J Gastroenterol* 2004;**99**:2479–88.

13 The Acute Liver Failure Patient

Neil C. Henderson and Kenneth J. Simpson

Centre for Liver & Digestive Diseases, Academic Hepatology and Scottish Liver Transplantation Unit,
Clinical and Surgical Sciences, The Royal Infirmary, University of Edinburgh, Edinburgh, UK

Acute liver failure is a rare but often devastating condition. Massive liver injury results in sudden loss of liver function, which may progress to multiorgan failure and death in a patient without pre-existing liver disease [1–3]. The development of clinical hepatic encephalopathy defines the syndrome, which characteristically is associated with coagulopathy, jaundice, and very abnormal liver function tests. Effective organ support can allow regeneration of the surviving liver; however, some patients require emergency liver transplantation and subsequent lifelong immunosuppression. It is one of the most challenging medical emergencies, because of multiorgan failure, the rapid evolution of the clinical condition, the need for multidisciplinary care, and the requirement for the clinician to prognosticate accurately to make best use of orthotopic liver transplantation (OLT) as a life-saving treatment [4].

After the initial definition of acute hepatic failure by Trey and Davidson in 1970 as a "potentially reversible condition, the consequence of severe liver injury with an onset of encephalopathy within 8 weeks of the appearance of the first symptoms and in the absence of pre-existing liver disease," the condition was later reclassified based on the time taken to develop hepatic encephalopathy (HE) after the first appearance of jaundice, as "hyperacute," "acute," and "subacute" liver failure referring to a jaundice-to-encephalopathy interval of 0–7, 8–28, and 29–84 days respectively. Paradoxically, the more acute the liver failure, the better the prognosis. However, potentially fatal complications such as cerebral edema are more common in this group of patients.

Case 1: paracetamol (acetaminophen) overdose

Case presentation

A 19-year-old student was admitted with jaundice, abdominal pain, nausea, and vomiting. Three days previously she had taken 90 paracetamol tablets (equivalent to 45 g paracetamol [acetaminophen]) and drank a bottle of wine after an argument with her boyfriend, in a deliberate attempt at suicide. She had no previous history of overdose, or drug or alcohol misuse. There was a past history of asthma for which she was using a salbutamol inhaler as required. There was no past history of gynecological problems.

Examination revealed jaundice but no other stigmata of chronic liver disease. She had a mild flapping tremor and hepatic fetor. She was slow on answering questions and had a Glasgow Coma Scale (GCS) score of 13, pulse 100 beats/min, BP 120/60 mmHg, respiratory rate 18/min. Examination of both the cardiovascular and respiratory systems was normal. Abdominal examination revealed right upper quadrant tenderness, with no organomegaly or ascites. There were no focal neurological abnormalities.

Investigations (normal values in brackets)
Hb 14.9 (115–165) g/dL
WCC 15.3 (4.0–11.0) × 10^9/L
Platelet count 40 (150–350) × 10^9/L
MCV 96 (78–98) fL
PT 120 (control 9) s
Urea 33.9 (2.5–6.6) mmol/L
Creatinine 512 (60–120) μmol/L
Na^+ 120 (135–145) mmol/L
K^+ 5.4 (3.6–5.0) mmol/L
Bicarbonate 11 (22–30) mmol/L
Bilirubin 180 (3–16) μmol/L
ALT 16 500 (10–50) U/L
ALP 110 (40–125) U/L
GGTP 128 (5–35) U/L
Albumin 30 (35–50) g/L
Total protein 49 (60–80) g/L
Ceruloplasmin 0.23 (0.20–0.60) g/L
Iron 16 (10–28) μmol/L
Transferrin saturation 23%
Ferritin 30 125 (14–150) μg/L
Paracetamol and salicylates undetectable
HAV IgM negative
HCV negative
HBsAg negative
HB IgM anticore negative
Pregnancy test negative
Ultrasonography: normal liver, spleen, and gallbladder; no biliary dilation; no ascites; patent hepatic and portal veins; empty uterus

Questions

- What initial management is required?
- What are the indications for transferring this patient to a specialist liver transplant unit?
- What is the patient's prognosis?

Differential diagnosis

This case describes the presentation of a young woman who had taken a paracetamol overdose 3 days before her admission. Clinical examination showed HE but no features characteristic of chronic liver disease. These are crucial clinical findings.

The presence of HE defines the syndrome of acute or fulminant liver failure (ALF). ALF was originally described as a reversible condition leading to the sudden onset of liver failure, characterized by the

---

Box 13.1 Etiology of acute liver failure

Drugs (70–80%):

Major cause is paracetamol

Idiosyncratic drug reactions, ecstasy, antituberculous drugs, antiepileptics

Infection (10–15%):

Hepatitis A, B, D, E, and non-A–E hepatitis (seronegative hepatitis or cryptogenic hepatitis)

Other viruses, e.g. Epstein–Barr virus or cytomegalovirus

Leptospirosis

Pregnancy-associated: acute fatty liver of pregnancy, HELLP

Miscellaneous (<5%):

Wilson's disease, shock, cardiac failure, Budd–Chiari syndrome

Poisons (<5%):

Carbon tetrachloride, Amanita phalloides (death cap mushroom)

---

presence of HE within 8 weeks of the onset of symptoms and in the absence of pre-existing liver disease; is therefore distinct from decompensated chronic liver disease or acute-on-chronic liver failure. This simple definition has been much debated, but for the purposes of discussion of most cases this definition is perfectly adequate. ALF has many causes (Box 13.1). However, in this case investigations show marked prolongation of the prothrombin time (PT), renal failure, and marked liver dysfunction with gross elevation of the aminotransferases. Although paracetamol metabolism is inhibited as patients develop severe liver failure, the absence of paracetamol in the blood does not exclude the diagnosis of paracetamol-induced severe liver failure. Very prolonged PT, aminotransferases >10 000, acidosis, and early renal failure are all characteristic clinical features of paracetamol poisoning. Acute viral hepatitis is excluded with the negative serology and other less common conditions such as Wilson's disease, pregnancy-associated conditions, and Budd–Chiari syndrome are excluded by the clinical features and negative investigations.

Diagnosis

Paracetamol-induced ALF.

Discussion

Currently paracetamol poisoning is the single most common cause of ALF in many parts of the world [1,2]; in contrast with other causes of ALF, paracetamol overdose characteristically follows a hyperacute clinical course with rapid onset of liver failure and HE. These patients can deteriorate very quickly, and it is essential that they are discussed at an early stage with a regional liver or transplant centre. In this particular case there are several worrying clinical features. First the patient has already presented with HE, the clinical features being those of grade I HE. She has a markedly prolonged PT and creatinine >300 μmol/L. Such clinical features should prompt referral to the regional liver transplant centre (Box 13.2).

Patient management

Initial management of this patient should include the following:
• This patient should be moved to an intensive care or high dependency unit, so that regular and frequent monitoring of her cardiovascular status, renal function, and neurological condition can be performed [5,6].
• Prompt access to endotracheal intubation and mechanical ventilation is essential. Indications for

---

Box 13.2 Criteria for transfer of patients after paracetamol (acetaminophen) poisoning to a regional liver transplant centre

Any grade of encephalopathy

Prothrombin time (PT) >50 s prolonged

Rising PT

PT (in s) greater or equal to the time in hours after paracetamol overdose

Hypoglycemia

Acidosis

Renal dysfunction

---

ventilation in this patient would include increasing coma (grade III HE) and respiratory failure.
• Transfer to the regional liver transplant unit should be arranged to allow further assessment for liver transplantation. Indications for transfer to a transplant centre are listed in Box 13.2. If the patient has any grade of HE this is likely to deteriorate during transfer, and ideally the patients should be transferred with both medical and nursing staff who are able to intubate the patient if necessary.
• Despite this patient's late presentation after paracetamol overdose, intravenous N-acetylcysteine should be given using the same regimen as for any paracetamol overdose that requires treatment. There are data to show that this can be beneficial even in patients who delay presentation, through limiting the progression of HE.
• Urgent psychiatric review should also be arranged, because it is very important to gain as much psychiatric and background information as possible before the patient's HE grade worsens and her conscious level decreases. Expedient assessment of the patient's psychiatric history while the patient is still conscious and coherent allows for a much more informed decision to be made by the liver transplant team should the patient deteriorate to the point of requiring liver transplantation. However, this review should not delay transfer to a liver transplant unit.
• Frequent monitoring of blood glucose should be performed (hourly BM stix). Other laboratory data should be collected. After paracetamol poisoning, hypophosphatemia is common and should be corrected. Blood gases, including arterial lactate concentration, are critical in determining prognosis and should be obtained even in the presence of significant coagulopathy. Recent evidence suggests that hyponatremia should be avoided and treated with intravenous hypertonic saline.
• Correction of the very prolonged PT should be avoided, unless there is clinical evidence of bleeding. Vitamin K administration is usually ineffective but may be indicated if the patient has been fasting or starving for some time before presentation (this also enhances the hepatotoxic effect of paracetamol). Low platelet counts are common after paracetamol poisoning. Routine correction of thrombocytopenia should be also avoided unless there is clinical hemorrhage.

Subsequent management of patients with severe liver failure secondary to paracetamol poisoning often requires close collaboration between physician and intensivist [5–7]. Multiorgan failure can develop rapidly and the opportunity for life-saving liver transplantation can be lost. Meticulous attention to monitoring organ dysfunction and early and goal-directed organ support is essential. The following complications require consideration:

- Cardiovascular: hypotension
- Respiratory:
  - pneumonia
  - non-cardiogenic pulmonary edema
  - adult respiratory distress syndrome (ARDS)
- Renal: acute tubular necrosis
- Neurological:
  - encephalopathy
  - raised intracranial pressure and cerebral edema
- Metabolic:
  - hypoglycemia
  - acidosis
  - hypophosphatemia
  - Hematological:
  - thrombocytopenia
  - prolonged PT
  - disseminated intravascular coagulation (DIC)
- Infection.

Transplantation

Survival after emergency liver transplantation in patients who have taken a paracetamol overdose is generally reduced compared with patients transplanted for chronic liver disease. There is an initial high mortality. Longer term there may be more problems with compliance and poor graft function compared with patients with chronic liver failure. However, patients with acute liver failure, especially when caused by paracetamol poisoning, have survival measured in days and so are usually afforded priority over patients with chronic liver disease. The decision about whether liver transplantation is indicated in patients with paracetamol-induced acute liver failure requires very careful consideration. Unfortunately, because of the unstable clinical state of the patient, these decisions have to be taken relatively quickly and often without the direct input of the patient. Initial psychiatric assessment before the onset of HE can be crucial. Consideration of the prognosis of the patient without transplantation is derived in the UK from the King's College criteria (Box 13.3). However, several medical and psychiatric contraindications to liver

transplantation are also considered before listing a patient for emergency liver transplantation (Box 13.4) The explanted liver shows classic centrilobular necrosis (Figure 13.1).

Liver support devices

Treatment strategies using liver support devices designed to help patients with ALF have either been those aimed at detoxifying the blood or those providing liver-derived factors [8]. The former includes charcoal hemoperfusion, plasmapheresis, and MARS (molecular adsorbent recirculating system), and the latter require liver cells. Early attempts utilized extracorporeal hepatic perfusion. However, incorporation of hepatocytes into a filtering system that contains a framework to physically support the cells (a bioreactor) as a bioartificial liver support device are currently being assessed. None of these liver support devices has proven to improve patient survival, but may be considered currently as a "bridge" to liver transplantation in very selected patients.

Box 13.3 King's College transplant criteria in use in the UK for listing patients with acute liver failure for emergency liver transplantation

Paracetamol (acetaminophen)

Arterial pH <7.25 or

Coexisting HE grade III or IV, creatinine >300 μmol/L, PT >100 s or

Two of three above with deterioration (and no sepsis) or

Lactate 24-h post-overdose >3.5 mmol/L on admission or >3.0 mmol/L after fluid resuscitation

Non-paracetamol

PT >100 s or

Three of the following: PT >50 s, age <10 or >40 years, jaundice to encephalopathy >7 days, bilirubin >300 μmol/L or etiology not HAV or HBV or

Acute Budd–Chiari syndrome or Wilson's disease with coagulopathy and HE

HAV, hepatitis A virus; HBV, hepatitis B virus; HE, hepatic encephalopathy; PT, prothrombin time.

Box 13.4 Medical and psychiatric contraindications to emergency liver transplantation

Medical

Untreated or progressive infection

Clinically apparent extrahepatic or metastatic malignancy

Progressive hypotension, resistant to vasopressor support

Clinically significant ARDS, FiO_2 >0.8

Fixed dilated pupils >1 h in the absence of thiopental

Severe coexistent cardiopulmonary disease, AIDS

Psychiatric

Multiple episodes of self-harm (>5) within an established pattern of behavior (especially if non-drug methods used)

Consistently stated wish to die, in the absence of established mental illness

Chronic refractory schizophrenia or other mental illness, resistant to therapy

Incapacitating dementia or learning disability

Active intravenous drug abuse or oral polydrug use

Alcohol dependence or abuse

Established pattern of non-compliance with treatment

AIDS, acquired immune deficiency syndrome; ARDS, adult respiratory distress syndrome; FiO_2, fraction of inspired oxygen.

Case 2: jaundice in a young male patient

Case presentation

A 24-year-old marine engineer presented with a 2-week history of nausea, vomiting, epigastric abdominal pain, and jaundice. He had pale stools and dark urine and was admitted under the care of the surgeons. Excluding obstructive jaundice, the patient was transferred to an infectious diseases hospital, where further blood testing showed worsening jaundice. Stool cultures identified salmonella infection and the patient was treated with a 1-week course of ciprofloxacin. However, the patient became progressively more jaundiced and intermittently drowsy. He was then transferred to the liver unit.

Past medical history was unremarkable. He had been on no medication before his admission to hospital. He smoked 10 cigarettes a day and drank

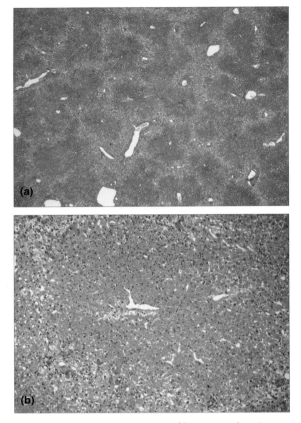

Figure 13.1 (a) Low power view of hepatic explant in patient transplanted for ALF secondary to paracetamol (acetaminophen) poisoning. Note the islands of eosinophilic necrotic centrilobular hepatocytes in areas of pale and injured surviving hepatocytes. (b) Higher power view of necrotic centrilobular area showing hemorrhagic necrosis after paracetamol poisoning.

alcohol in binges, drinking up to 10 pints of beer a day. There was no history of foreign travel, apart from a holiday to Portugal, 3 months before his presentation. He was single and heterosexual.

Examination showed a deeply jaundiced and clinically anemic patient. There was no hepatic fetor, but he was drowsy and disoriented. He had a flapping tremor. There was a single spider nevus, but no other cutaneous stigmata of chronic liver disease. His pulse was 76 beats/min in sinus rhythm, with normal blood pressure and cardiovascular examination. Examination of the chest was normal. Abdominal examination showed mild generalized tenderness, although this was most apparent in the right upper quadrant. There was no splenomegaly or ascites present. Examination of the central nervous system revealed no focal abnormality. His GCS score was 13.

Investigations (normal values in brackets)
Hb 5 (115–165) g/dL
WCC 14.4 (4.0–11.0) × 10⁹/L
Platelet count 194 (150–350) × 10⁹/L
MCV 107 (78–98) fL
Reticulocytes 8.0%
Coombs' test negative
PT 48 (control 15) s
Urea 12.8 (2.5–6.6) mmol/L
Creatinine 288 (60–120) μmol/L
Na⁺ 142 (135–145) mmol/L
K⁺ 3.4 (3.6–5.0) mmol/L
Bilirubin 796 (3–16) μmol/L
ALT 59 (10–50) U/L
ALP 31 (40–125) U/L
GGT 150 (5–35) U/L
Albumin 24 (35–50) g/L
HAV IgM negative
HCV negative
HBsAg negative
HB IgM anticore antibody negative
Ceruloplasmin undetectable
Ultrasonography: abnormal echogenic pattern to the hepatic parenchyma, moderate splenomegaly, no ascites or gallstones; biliary tree not dilated

Questions

- What is the diagnosis?
- What other tests may be helpful?
- How would you assess this patient's prognosis?
- What therapies are available?

Differential diagnosis

This case describes a relatively short history of non-specific gastrointestinal upset and jaundice in a young man. Clinical examination reveals findings consistent with mild HE, but no other clinical findings to suggest that the patient had chronic liver disease. The finding of splenomegaly, by ultrasound scan, suggests portal hypertension. This finding can occur in patients with ALF, but is uncommon. However, there are several clues in this patient's investigations that conform to a characteristic clinical pattern which leads the astute physician to an immediate diagnosis. The investigations are characterized by a Coombs' negative hemolytic anemia, and renal impairment without marked derangement of liver aminotransferases apart from an elevated bilirubin. The elevated bilirubin is a manifestation of the hemolytic anemia. Note is also made of the reduced alkaline phosphatase (ALP). These are classic findings of somebody who has ALF secondary to Wilson's disease. This is confirmed by a reduced or undetectable ceruloplasmin. Further clinical examination with a slit-lamp looking for Kayser–Fleischer rings may be helpful.

Occasionally, Wilson's disease may be difficult to diagnose. The finding of low or absent ceruloplasmin is not universally observed. Ceruloplasmin is an acute phase protein and can be artificially raised in ALF; up to 15% of cases with ALF due to Wilson's disease have a normal ceruloplasmin. Classically the patients develop a hemolytic anemia due to direct toxicity of circulating copper on red cell membranes. This produces very high serum bilirubin, which is out of keeping with the relatively normal serum aminotransferases. The ALP is often reduced, a ratio of ALP:bilirubin <2.0 was reported to differentiate ALF due to Wilson's disease from other causes. However, this ratio is not helpful in children and young adults due to bone-derived ALP.

Additional laboratory tests include measurement of the serum copper (which can be elevated in ALF due to Wilson's disease) and urinary copper, which is increased especially after penicillamine challenge. The latter can be misleading due to difficulties with urine collection – urine must be collected into a container with no preservative. The most commonly used preservative in urine collection containers interferes with heavy metal testing. The penicillamine challenge involves collecting a 24-hour urine sample, with penicillamine (500 mg) administered at the start of and 12 hours into the urine sampling. This test has been validated only in children. Occasionally a family history of Wilson's disease is obtained. Alternatively, ALF has been described in patients with Wilson's disease who are poorly compliant with chelation medication. Liver biopsy often shows non-specific changes and cirrhosis. Direct measurement of the liver copper content of the biopsy can be diagnostic, but histochemical staining of hepatic copper is not sensitive enough to be helpful in confirming Wilson's disease. These additional tests can take some time to collect or process. In the case described here the clinical and biochemical features are sufficiently typical to make the diagnosis of ALF due to Wilson's disease.

Diagnosis

ALF secondary to Wilson's disease.

Discussion

This patient has ALF secondary to Wilson's disease as shown by the development of HE. Up to a third of patients presenting with Wilson's disease present with ALF. He also has significant hemolytic anemia, prolongation of PT, and renal impairment. These patients do not respond well to penicillamine or other chelating treatments. In contrast with all other causes of ALF, such patients usually have pre-existing liver cirrhosis. However, the presence of HE predicts a poor prognosis and these patients are listed for emergency liver transplantation if they are to survive (see Box 13.3). The moderate splenomegaly noted on ultrasonography is suggestive of portal hypertension.

Wilson's disease is an autosomal recessive inherited defect of copper accumulation. It is an uncommon condition with a prevalence of 1 in 30000 in the general population. The primary defect is in a copper-transporting P-type ATPase, encoded by the *ATP7B* gene, located on the long arm of chromosome 13. There are numerous gene mutations affecting the *ATP7B* gene.

Although most patients with Wilson's disease present in their teens or 20s some unusual cases have been reported as presenting in their 70s. The phenotype of the condition mainly involves the liver and brain. Hepatic presentations of Wilson's disease can vary from asymptomatic abnormalities of liver function tests through to decompensated liver cirrhosis. Presentation of cerebral Wilson's disease usually occurs in older age groups compared with hepatic presentations. Disorders described most often include parkinsonism, and occasionally patients may present with primarily psychiatric or behavioral symptoms. These are clinically very distinct from the HE that defines ALF secondary to Wilson's disease. Other organ systems can be affected, including endocrine abnormalities such as hypoparathyroidism, renal

involvement may result in aminoaciduria, and nephrolithiasis, cardiomyopathy, and premature osteoporosis have also been reported.

Unfortunately, copper-chelating treatment such as D-penicillamine and trientine are ineffective in patients who present with ALF secondary to Wilson's disease. They take too long to become effective. Oral zinc, which reduces the intestinal absorption and promotes fecal excretion of copper, is also ineffective in these patients. There have been some reports of bridging patients to liver transplantation using liver assist devices. However, liver transplantation is the only effective treatment for the management of the patient with ALF due to Wilson's disease. Transplantation corrects the enzyme defect, and there is no requirement for chelation or zinc therapy post-liver transplantation. More difficult to define is the prognosis of patients presenting with decompensated cirrhosis due to Wilson's disease but who do not have HE. Several prognostic scores have been proposed utilizing variously bilirubin, serum aminotransferases, WCC, coagulation, and albumin. However, these scores have not been validated in either adult or large prospective series due to the relative rarity of the disorder.

In patients with Wilson's disease but no HE, therapy is directed at removing copper for the body. D-Penicillamine mobilizes and complexes with copper, inducing excretion of copper in the urine. Initial low doses are gradually increased up to a maintenance dose of 1.0–1.5 g/day. D-Penicillamine is combined with vitamin B_6, because pyridoxine deficiency has been reported with this drug. Unfortunately, other side effects are common; hypersensitivity and marrow dyscrasia are relatively frequent. Other D-penicillamine side effects can become apparent many years after initiating treatment; skin changes, arthropathy, and immune-mediated abnormalities such as proteinuria and nephrotic syndrome can occur. Trientine has been used both as initial therapy and as maintenance treatment in the presence of D-penicillamine side effects. It is associated with fewer side effects than D-penicillamine, but is a less effective copper chelator.

Zinc therapy acts via induction of intestinal cell metallothionine expression. This both reduces copper absorption and increases copper loss through shedding of intestinal cells. Zinc is most often used in asymptomatic individuals and is generally well tolerated. Unfortunately, it can be difficult to source. Oral chelation therapy is effective in most patients, with long-term responses observed. Although initial clinical responses may be observed within 6 weeks of starting treatment, normalization of liver function may take up to 1 year. Even with effective chelation treatment, up to 20% of compliant cases have persistently elevated serum aminotransferases. These elevations are usually mild and benign, but discontinuing chelation therapy may precipitate ALF and needs to be avoided.

Liver transplantation as discussed above corrects the gene defect. Transplantation is used in those with ALF and others who have failed to respond to chelation therapy. Relative frequency in published series suggests that the former is the more common indication for transplantation in Wilson's disease. However, patient survival post-transplantation is reduced in patients with ALF compared with patients with decompensated chronic liver disease due to Wilson's disease.

Case 3: nausea and jaundice in a young female patient

Case presentation

A 25-year-old hairdresser presented with a 1-month history of intermittent nausea and vomiting. She had developed anorexia and lost 4 lb (1.8 kg) in weight over this 4-week period. Two weeks before her admission she noticed jaundice, accompanied by dark urine, but normal colored stools. She had no abdominal pain. The jaundice worsened and she presented to hospital when her family noticed that she was mildly confused.

There was no past medical history apart from a short admission to the local psychiatric hospital 5 years previously with a psychotic episode associated with cannabis use. She had never used illicit drugs since, and was taking no prescription or over-the-counter medications. She smoked 10 cigarettes a day and drank up to 3 bottles of wine a week. This level of alcohol consumption was variable; some weeks she would drink no alcohol at all. She was unmarried, but lived with a partner who was known to use intravenous drugs. She had met him relatively recently. There was no history of foreign travel.

Examination on admission was as follows:
Pulse 105 beats/min
Blood pressure 158/80 mmHg
Temperature 36.1°C
Respiratory rate 16/min
She was drowsy, and disoriented to time and place, but not to people. Her GCS score was 12. She had no hepatic fetor but there was a gross flapping tremor. There were no stigmata of chronic liver disease, but the patient was deeply jaundiced. Examination of the cardiovascular and respiratory systems was normal. Abdominal examination revealed a soft non-tender abdomen with no organomegaly or ascites and the bowel sounds were normal. Examination of the central nervous system revealed no focal abnormality.

Investigations (normal values in brackets)
Hb. 10.9 g/dL (115–165)
WCC. 11.8 (4.0–11.0) $\times 10^9$/L
Platelet count 246 (150–350) $\times 10^9$/L
MCV 118 (78–98) fL
PT 26 (control 9) s
Urea 1.4 (2.5–6.6) mmol/L
Creatinine 89 (60–120) μmol/L
Na$^+$ 139 (135–145) mmol/L
K$^+$ 3.3 (3.6–5.0) mmol/L
Bilirubin 591 (3–16) μmol/L
ALT 1650 (10–50) U/L
ALP 153 (40–125) U/L
GGT 28 (5–35) U/L
Albumin 26 (35–50) g/L
Total protein 49 (60–80) g/L
Ceruloplasmin 0.23 (0.20–0.60) g/L
IgA 4.7 (0.8–4.5) g/L
IgG 13.6 (6.0–15.0) g/L
IgM 1.5 (0.35–2.9) g/L
HAV IgM negative
HCV negative
HBsAg positive
HB IgM anticore positive
HBe Ag negative
HBe antibody positive
Hepatitis δ (HDV) IgM positive
HIV negative
Ultrasonography: mild hepatomegaly with altered hepatic echo texture; no focal abnormality; patent hepatic and portal veins; gross splenomegaly (15 cm), contracted gallbladder; no ascites

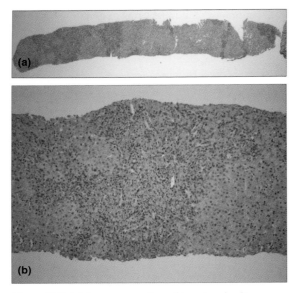

Figure 13.2 (a) Low power view of transjugular liver biopsy from patient with HBV/HDV coinfection stained with Sirius red. Note should be made of the densely staining areas of hepatic collapse. (b) Higher power view showing areas of hepatic collapse, with loss of hepatic architecture, inflammatory cell infiltrate, and edema.

Transjugular biopsy (Figure 13.2): hepatic collapse with loss of hepatic architecture and inflammatory cell infiltrate and edema; no significant fibrosis

Questions

• How would you interpret the hepatitis virology?
• What is the patient's prognosis?
• What treatments are available?

Differential diagnosis

This case describes a young woman with a 1-month history of gastrointestinal upset, with weight loss. This was followed by the development of jaundice and confusion. The only other feature of note in the clinical history was the relatively new sexual partner, who had been known to use intravenous drugs. Clinical examination revealed features consistent with HE in the absence of any other features of chronic liver disease.

Laboratory investigations show a prolonged PT, normal renal function, hyperbilirubinemia, and increased aminotransferases. There is a slightly reduced ceruloplasmin. There are polyclonal increases in the immunoglobulins. She is hepatitis A and C negative. Hepatitis B virology shows that she is HBsAg positive. In addition to being HBV IgM anti-core antibody positive, she is also hepatitis δ IgM positive.

These would be the clinical features, examination, and laboratory findings one would expect in patients who had an acute infection with hepatitis B and hepatitis δ.

Gross splenomegaly was noted on ultrasonography with mild hepatomegaly, which may indicate portal hypertension. This is noted occasionally in patients with ALF, especially if there has been a prolonged clinical course as occurs in ALF due to causes other than paracetamol. Collapse of the liver parenchyma can be associated with increased portal pressure, splenomegaly, and the development of acute varices (see Figure 13.2). Very occasionally these acute varices can bleed. The presence of splenomegaly in patients with fulminant liver failure should prompt the physician or radiologist to look carefully for the presence of ascites and blood flow in the hepatic veins. If the latter is absent, this may indicate that the patient has an acute presentation of Budd–Chiari syndrome.

Diagnosis

ALF due to HBV and HDV coinfection.

Discussion

HDV was first identified by Rizzetto and colleagues in 1977 in patients chronically infected with hepatitis B [9]. HDV is a unique virus affecting animals with a single-strand-minus circular RNA. Viral RNA is replicated in host hepatocytes by host RNA-dependent RNA polymerases, without production of any DNA intermediate. HDV viroids are composed of an outer envelope of HBsAg proteins and host lipids surrounding an inner nucleocapsid of HDV antigen and viral RNA genome of approximately 1700 nucleotides. The HDV antigen is the only identified viral protein product, which exists in two forms depending on the protein sequence. Large and small HDV antigens are products of the same open reading frame and differ in only 19–20 amino acids added to the large HDV antigen.

Globally, approximately 5% of HBV-infected individuals are also infected with HDV. Studies from the UK suggested an increasing frequency of HDV infection in those with HBV; currently about 8% of HBV infected individuals are also HDV infected. High-risk groups for both HBV and HDV infection include parenteral drug users, male and female prostitutes, and immigrants from high-risk endemic areas. These groups reflect the potential modes of transmission, which include intravenous drug use and sexual contact; clusters in family members are also reported, but perinatal transmission is very rare. Interestingly the geographical distribution of HDV does not closely mirror that of HBV; some areas of high HBV prevalence have very low rates of HDV positivity. In contrast others, such as Italy, some parts of South America, Pakistan, and western Asia, have a high prevalence of both HBV and HDV infection.

Acute HDV infection can occur simultaneously with acute HBV infection (coinfection) or in a patient already infected with HBV (superinfection). Coinfection is said to result in a biphasic elevation of the serum aminotransferase associated with replication of HBV and HDV. Rarely coinfected patients present with severe hepatitis or ALF (<1% infected individuals). The relationship between HDV factors and clinical course is unclear. HDV has seven major genotypes: genotype 3, exclusively found in Columbia, Venezuela and Peru, is associated with severe and fulminant forms of hepatitis and with coinfection with HBV genotype F. HDV genotype 2, common in Japan and Taiwan, is associated with milder clinical disease and low levels of circulating virus. Resolution is the most common clinical outcome after coinfection; less than 2% develop chronic infection.

In contrast with coinfected individuals, patients with chronic HBV infection superinfected with HDV often develop chronic HDV infection. Patients with chronic HBV and HDV infection have more rapid progression to cirrhosis and hepatocellular carcinoma compared with patients infected with HBV alone. In addition, superinfection reportedly results in more severe hepatitis compared with coinfected patients, and is an important cause of outbreaks of ALF in populations with high incidence of both HBV and HDV infections, such as in South America.

Laboratory diagnosis of HDV infection relies on the identification of both viral products and the host's immune reaction. HDV RNA is detectable in serum early and transiently in the clinical course, HDV can also be identified in liver tissue if available. Coexistent appearance of HDV antigen in serum and liver may be detectable, but is technically challenging. Later in the clinical course anti-HDV antibody appears, initially of the IgM type. These laboratory findings are also associated with positive markers of HBV infection. In coinfected individuals HBsAg is positive in the early stages and clears in association with the appearance of HBV anticore antibody, initially IgM type. Recovery from HBV and HDV coinfection is associated with the appearance of anti-HBsAb and declining titers of IgM anti-HDV antibody. In superinfected individuals HBV IgM anticore antibody is negative, high levels of HDV virus, antigen, and anti-HDV antibodies are detectable, titers of HBsAg and HBV DNA fall, and there is often associated seroconversion from HBeAg to anti-HBeAg. It is recommended that all patients with severe hepatitis or ALF secondary to acute HBV be screened for HDV coinfection by measuring anti-HDV antibody.

Acute coinfection with HBV and HDV is usually associated with spontaneous viral clearance and clinical recovery. These patients (and patients with ALF due to HAV infection) usually have a better prognosis compared with other non-paracetamol causes of ALF (see Box 13.3). There are few data available about antiviral treatment in coinfected or superinfected individuals. In patients with chronic HDV infection, interferon therapy may be effective, but antiviral treatment has produced disappointing results. Prevention of HDV infection is through HBV immunization.

ALF may occur in patients with chronic HBV infection, unrelated to HDV infection, through reactivation of HBV replication [10]. This can occur in patients who are HBsAg positive, HBeAg negative, anti-HBeAb positive with low levels of HBV DNA (healthy carriers), but has also been reported in HBsAg negative, anti-HBc and anti-HBs antibody-positive (occult HBV) individuals after infection with HIV or drug therapy with either immunosuppressive drugs or cytotoxic chemotherapy. Occasionally no identifying precipitating factor can be implicated. The classic clinical picture occurs in a patient with previous HBV infection (or known to be HBsAg positive) with rapid increasing HBV DNA levels and positive HBV IgM anticore antibody. The prevention of reactivation of HBV infection during immunosuppressive or cytotoxic chemotherapy requires antiviral therapy with lamivudine or other antiviral agents, which can also be used to treat clinically apparent reactivation.

Although this patient has HE, she does not fulfill any of the other poor prognostic criteria for somebody with an acute presentation of hepatitis B (see Box 13.2) [1]. There is some evidence that antiviral treatment may be beneficial in patients with ALF due to HBV irrespective of their HDV status and she was treated with antiviral drugs with good effect.

Conclusions

ALF is an uncommon condition affecting the liver. Sudden severe liver injury results in a profound loss of liver functions, the most important clinical manifestation of which is the development of HE. However, many patients present with acute hepatitis induced by drugs, viruses, or toxins, and do not develop HE; hence they do not fulfill the definition of ALF. The most common cause of ALF in the UK, the USA, and many countries in Europe is paracetamol poisoning, either through suicide attempt or accidental consumption of excessive amounts of paracetamol (see Box 13.1) [1]. However, paracetamol poisoning as a cause of ALF is rarely encountered in other countries such as Australia, Spain, and India. Patients with ALF due to paracetamol poisoning follow a hyperacute clinical course and have recovered spontaneously, died, or been transplanted within 2 weeks of ingesting the drug. In contrast, other causes of ALF produce a more slowly developing clinical picture. This is most commonly due to viral hepatitis, which, on a worldwide basis, is usually due to either HBV or HAV, or idiosyncratic drug reactions. Of note is the relative lack of reports linking acute HCV infection with ALF. However, in many patients the cause of ALF is unknown; these patients are described as having non-A–E hepatitis, which has also been termed "seronegative or cryptogenic hepatitis." Non-A–E hepatitis is often the second single most common cause of ALF reported in series at least from the UK and USA. Idiosyncratic drug reactions are most commonly caused by antibiotics and anticonvulsants, and have been reported with herbal remedies and non-

prescribed medications such as ecstasy and cocaine. Less common causes reported include fatty liver of pregnancy and hemolysis, elevated liver enzymes, and low platelets (HELLP syndrome). Wilson's disease as described above produces a characteristic but relatively rare clinical picture. In Budd–Chiari syndrome, patients often present with abdominal pain and ascites as well as ALF.

Careful clinical examination to exclude the presence of signs of chronic liver disease is essential. Further investigation including ultrasonography or CT may show splenomegaly, as in the case of acute hepatitis B/D discussed above or in patients with Budd–Chiari syndrome, who may also develop ascites (Figures 13.3 and 13.4). Such findings on ultrasonog-

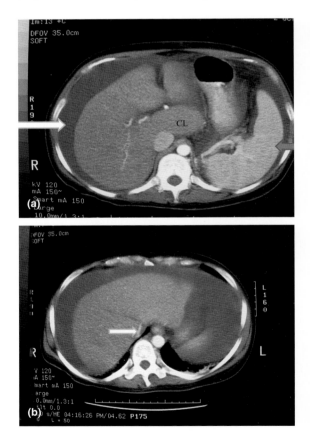

Figure 13.3 CT scan of patient with Budd–Chiari syndrome demonstrating: (a) caudate lobe (CL) hypertrophy, ascites (white arrow) and splenomegaly (gray arrow); and (b) compression of the inferior vena cava by the swollen liver (white arrow).

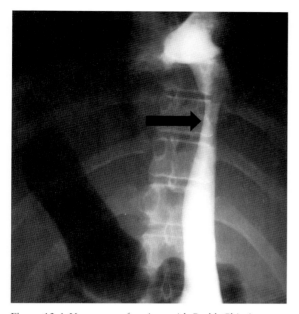

Figure 13.4 Venogram of patient with Budd–Chiari syndrome demonstrating inferior vena cava compression (black arrow) by the hypertrophied caudate lobe.

raphy therefore do not exclude ALF. Some patients may require a liver biopsy, which often has to be performed via the transjugular route in view of the patient's coagulopathy. This may provide both diagnostic and prognostic information on the patient (see Figures 13.1 and 13.2).

Once the cause of ALF has been defined, specific treatment may benefit early cases such as antiviral treatment in the case of acute hepatitis B or delivery of the infant in pregnancy-associated ALF. However, in many cases, specific treatment is either not available or ineffective. In these cases general supportive medical therapy is key in achieving optimal survival, as discussed in the case of paracetamol poisoning

[11,12]. This may include emergency liver transplantation. The most common indicators for emergency liver transplantation adopted in the UK are the King's College criteria (see Boxes 13.3 and 13.4). Other criteria are used in other parts of the world. In general the results of liver transplantation in patients with ALF are less good compared with patients with chronic liver disease. However, in selected cases survival rates of 60–70% at 5 years are achievable.

References

1 Craig DG, Lee A, Hayes PC, Simpson KJ. Review article: the current management of acute liver failure. *Aliment Pharmacol Ther* 2010;**31**:345–58.
2 Bernal W, Auzinger G, Dhawan A, Wendon J. Acute liver failure. *Lancet* 2010;**376**:190–201.
3 Stravitz RT, Kramer DJ. Medscape. Management of acute liver failure. *Nat Rev Gastroenterol Hepatol* 2009;**6**:542–53.
4 Polson J. Assessment of prognosis in acute liver failure. *Semin Liver Dis* 2008;**28**:218–25.
5 Schilsky ML, Honiden S, Arnott L, Emre S. ICU management of acute liver failure. *Clin Chest Med* 2009;**30**:71–87.
6 Bernal W, Auzinger G, Sizer E, Wendon J. Intensive care management of acute liver failure. *Semin Liver Dis* 2008;**28**:188–200.
7 Stravitz RT. Critical management decisions in patients with acute liver failure. *Chest* 2008;**134**:1092–102.
8 Phua J, Lee KH. Liver support devices. *Curr Opin Crit Care* 2008;**14**:208–15.
9 Rizzetto M. Hepatitis D: thirty years after. *J Hepatol* 2009;**50**(5):1043–50.
10 Mutimer D. Review article: hepatitis B and liver transplantation. *Aliment Pharmacol Ther* 2006;**15**;23(8):1031–41.
11 Larsen FS, Wendon J. Prevention and management of brain edema in patients with acute liver failure. *Liver Transpl* 2008;**14**(suppl 2):S90–6.
12 Larson AM. Diagnosis and management of acute liver failure. *Curr Opin Gastroenterol* 2010;**26**:214–21.

14 The Chronic Liver Disease Patient

Joanna K. Dowman and Phil N. Newsome

NIHR Biomedical Research Unit and Centre for Liver Research, Queen Elizabeth Hospital, University of Birmingham, UK

Case 1: abnormal liver function tests in a diabetic patient

Case presentation

A 45-year-old Caucasian bus driver was found to have abnormal liver function tests (LFTs) during the course of routine diabetes investigations. Type 2 diabetes had been diagnosed 9 years earlier and was tablet controlled with metformin. His other past medical history was of hypertension, hyperlipidemia, asthma, and obesity.

He reported drinking one 500 mL bottle of beer twice a week and denied ever having been a heavy drinker. He had never smoked. There was no personal or family history of liver disease although his mother had been diagnosed with diabetes.

There was no history of foreign travel other than a trip to Africa at the age of 21. Current medications included metformin, ramipril, omeprazole, and various inhalers.

Examination revealed the following:

Height 1.9 m
Weight 122 kg
BMI 33.8
No stigmata of chronic liver disease
Cardiovascular: pulse 90 beats/min; BP 131/72 mmHg. Heart sounds normal with no added sounds.
Respiratory: normal examination
Gastrointestinal: abdominal obesity but no tenderness, organomegaly or shifting dullness.

Investigations were as follows (normal values in brackets)
Hb 10.7 (13.5–17.5) g/dL
WCC 6.9 (4–11) × 10^9/L
Platelets 160 (150–400) × 10^9/L
MCV 99 (76–98) fl
AST 30 (10–40) IU/L
ALT 31 (5–30) IU/L
GGT 150 (5–30) IU/L
Albumin 38 (35–55) g/L
INR 1.3 (0.9–1.2)
Bilirubin 20 (2–17) µmol/L
ALP 264 (30–130) IU/L
Urea 9.1 (2.5–6.5) mmol/L
Creatinine 132 (50–120) µmol/L
Na^+ 137 (135–145) mmol/L
K^+ 5.6 (3.5–5.0) mmol/L
Cholesterol 6.4 (<5.2) mmol/L
Triglycerides 4.8 (0–1.5) mmol/L
Glucose 8.2 (3.5–5.5) mmol/L
HbA1c 8.5 (4–6)%
TSH 1.8 (0.17–3.2) mU/L
Free T_4 15.3 (11–22) pmol/L
Ferritin 361 (20–250) µg/L
Transferrin saturation 26.6 (22–40)%
Ceruloplasmin 0.31 (<0.35) g/L
$α_1$-Antitrypsin 1.7 (1.5–3.5) g/L
$α_1$-AT phenotype PiMS
AFP 3 (<7.0) µg/L
IgM 2.8 (0.5–2.0) g/L

Problem-based Approach to Gastroenterology and Hepatology, First Edition. Edited by John N. Plevris, Colin W. Howden.
© 2012 Blackwell Publishing Ltd. Published 2012 by Blackwell Publishing Ltd.

IgA 6.3 (1.0–4.0) g/L
IgG 16.8 (5–16) g/L
ANA 1:160
ANCA negative
Anti-Sm negative
Anti-LKM negative
AMA negative
HBsAg negative
HBsAb positive
HCVAb negative

Abdominal ultrasound scan report
Liver appearance is unremarkable with no obvious focal abnormality seen within the liver but limited views obtained. No biliary dilation. No stones in the gallbladder. Spleen is 13 cm in diameter; pancreas normal; no ascites.

In view of these results, a liver biopsy was performed to definitively assess disease stage and facilitate appropriate management and follow-up.

Liver biopsy
Hepatic architecture distorted by cirrhosis, more predominant in zone 3. Mild steatosis, with some lobular inflammation and ballooned hepatocytes containing Mallory-Denk hyaline.

Questions

• What is the likely cause of cirrhosis in this patient?
• How would you interpret the immunoglobulin levels and auto-antibody titers in this patient?
• What methods could be used to assess the prognosis and aid decisions on further management?

Differential diagnosis

The main causes of chronic liver disease that need to be excluded are shown in Table 14.1.

In many cases the clinical history will point to a diagnosis but it is still essential to exclude any of the above pathologies that may coexist.

If the diagnosis cannot be determined adequately from the history and appropriate serological and radiological investigations, a liver biopsy may be indicated. However, liver biopsy may be unhelpful in end-stage liver disease when the liver is shrunken and cirrhotic, and characteristic disease features may no longer be present. Biopsy of the cirrhotic liver is asso-

Table 14.1 Main causes of chronic liver disease

Viral	Autoimmune
Chronic hepatitis B	Autoimmune hepatitis
Chronic hepatitis C	Primary biliary cirrhosis
	Primary sclerosing cholangitis
Miscellaneous	Metabolic
Alcoholic liver disease	α_1-Antitrypsin deficiency
Budd–Chiari syndrome (hepatic vein thrombosis)	Hemochromatosis
Drug induced	Non-alcoholic steatohepatitis
Secondary biliary cirrhosis	Wilson's disease
Congestive (chronic right heart failure)	
Cryptogenic cirrhosis	

ciated with an increased risk of morbidity and mortality, so there needs to be a clear rationale for undertaking it. A liver biopsy can also provide information on the severity of liver disease.

Diagnosis

The clinical picture is in keeping with non-alcoholic steatohepatitis (NASH), although the 1:160 titer of ANA with elevated immunoglobulins raises the possibility of autoimmune liver disease. This finding is seen infrequently, but does not always indicate the presence of autoimmune disease [1]. Although a polyclonal elevation in immunoglobulin levels was seen, this is frequently observed in cirrhosis of any cause, and not indicative of autoimmune disease in the absence of associated liver-specific autoantibodies. Other causes of chronic liver disease were excluded by the investigations presented above. Hepatitis B and C were excluded by negative serology. Ferritin was raised but hemochromatosis was excluded by the normal transferrin saturation. There are no features to support PSC. The metabolic diseases α_1-antitrypsin

(α_1-AT) deficiency and Wilson's disease are rare. Furthermore, his phenotype, PiMS, is not associated with liver disease, and he has a normal serum ceruloplasmin [2].

He is overweight, denies excessive alcohol consumption, and has evidence of hepatic steatosis. Provided that his alcohol history can be verified by speaking to other family members or his GP, alcohol can be excluded as the likely cause. He fulfils sufficient criteria to have the metabolic syndrome, which is commonly associated with NASH [3]. The metabolic syndrome is a cluster of metabolic abnormalities characterized by abdominal obesity, insulin resistance, impaired glucose metabolism, hypertension, and dyslipidemia. NASH is now recognized as the hepatic manifestation of this syndrome. The rapidly increasing prevalence of obesity and the metabolic syndrome in the general population is therefore leading to a large increase in incidence of non-alcoholic fatty liver disease (NAFLD) and its complications.

Our patient has several features of the metabolic syndrome including obesity, insulin resistance, diabetes, hypertension, and dyslipidemia. NAFLD encompasses a spectrum of disease from simple steatosis through steatohepatitis to fibrosis and cirrhosis. A greater number of features of the metabolic syndrome are associated with a higher risk of disease progression [4].

Generally recognized indications for biopsy in NASH include establishing the diagnosis and staging the disease, but no strict consensus or guidelines have yet been formulated as to which patients with NAFLD should be biopsied [5].

Characteristic histological findings in NASH are steatosis, hepatocyte ballooning, and lobular inflammation, with development of fibrosis and cirrhosis at later stages of disease (Figure 14.1). In established cirrhosis, typical histological features may no longer be recognizable and diagnosis can be challenging [6]. NASH and ASH (alcoholic steatohepatitis) share many histological features and it can be impossible to distinguish the two conditions. However, there are a number of features that are more common in one or the other of these diagnoses. For example, histological changes more suggestive of NASH are higher levels of steatosis and nuclear vacuolization, with fibrosis often starting in the zone 3 region. Mallory hyaline and periportal fibrosis are features more commonly seen in ASH.

Several non-invasive scoring systems and radiological modalities have been developed as an alternative to liver biopsy. The NAFLD fibrosis score is an equation that generates a numerical value based on six variables of age, hyperglycemia, BMI, platelet count, albumin, and AST:ALT (aspartate aminotransferase:alanine aminotransferase) ratio. A score <-1.455 excludes the presence of significant

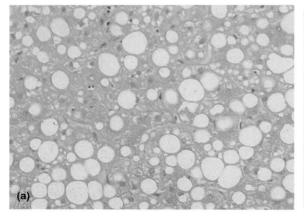

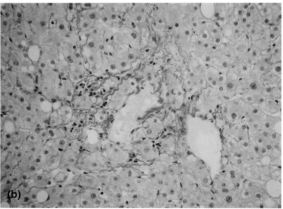

Figure 14.1 Non-alcoholic steatohepatitis on liver biopsy: (a) marked macrovesicular steatosis; (b) the presence of a low-grade, mixed neutrophilic and mononuclear infiltrate, with fibrosis, which is typically perisinusoidal (pericellular). (Images courtesy of Dr Desley Neil.)

fibrosis with a negative predictive value of 93%, whereas a score >0.676 predicts the presence of advanced fibrosis with a positive predictive value of 90% [7]. The NAFLD fibrosis score thus allows the identification of patients with more advanced disease who need ongoing follow-up, and considerably reduces the requirement for liver biopsy in the minority of patients with an indeterminate score.

Transient elastography (Fibroscan®) is a non-invasive method of assessing liver fibrosis which can be performed at the bedside or in the outpatient clinic. It employs ultrasound-based technology to measure liver stiffness (LS), and is currently validated for use in chronic hepatitis C, HIV/HCV coinfection and cholestatic liver diseases [8]. Although Fibroscan is less well validated in NAFLD, a recent study demonstrated good accuracy for the diagnosis of fibrosis in such patients, with areas under the receiver operating curve (AUROCs) of 0.84, 0.93, and 0.95 for diagnosing moderate fibrosis (F $\geq$ 2), bridging fibrosis (F $\geq$ 3), and cirrhosis (F 4) respectively [9]. In this study the best LS cut-off scores for predicting F $\geq$ 2, $\geq$3, and 4 were 7.0 kPa, 8.7 kPa, and 10.3 kPa respectively. Transient elastography thus represents a useful tool for the rapid, non-invasive assessment of liver fibrosis and determination of the need for biopsy.

Patient management

With no proven specific treatment available for NAFLD/NASH, management is usually directed at improving the various components of the metabolic syndrome. As insulin resistance and obesity are key features in the pathogenesis of NASH, weight loss is likely the most effective intervention.

Diets aimed at achieving a 10% weight reduction have been shown to improve both metabolic and histological abnormalities in NAFLD. Regular exercise has a synergistically beneficial effect on metabolic profiles and should accompany dietary manipulation [10,11]. Dieting is not always successful, and thus other means of trying to reduce weight are often required. This can include the use of drugs such as Orlistat, which inhibits fat malabsorption, or surgical approaches such as gastric bypass surgery to reduce the functional gastric volume. Although Orlistat has been demonstrated to result in weight loss [12], the effects are modest and are lost when the drug is dis-continued. Consequently, greater attention has been directed at surgery which has been shown to improve both metabolic and hepatic abnormalities [13].

Pharmacological interventions include insulin sensitizers and lipid-lowering agents. The strong relationship between insulin resistance and NAFLD suggests that insulin-sensitizing agents may be effective in the treatment of NASH. Metformin is already a first-line agent for the treatment of type 2 diabetes and obesity, and in recent trials has been shown to improve both liver biochemistry and histological findings in NASH [14]. However, no large clinical trials have yet established metformin to be a safe and effective therapy for NASH. The other main class of insulin-sensitizing agents is the thiazolidinediones, such as rosiglitazone and pioglitazone, which bind to the peroxisome proliferator-activated receptor-γ (PPARγ), leading to improved insulin sensitivity and redistribution of adipose tissue [15]. Rosiglitazone has now been suspended by the European Medicines Agency due to an increased risk of cardiovascular events, but pioglitazone does not appear to be associated with such risks. Both biochemical and histological improvements in NASH have been demonstrated with this class of drugs although their side-effect profile, which includes significant weight gain, is of concern in this group of patients [16,17]. The recent PIVENS randomized, double-blind, placebo-controlled trial evaluated 96 weeks of pioglitazone versus vitamin E therapy in non-diabetic patients with biopsy-proven NASH, and demonstrated improvements in liver enzymes, steatosis and inflammation in both treatment arms, although no improvement in fibrosis [18]. However, the primary endpoint of a prespecified improvement in liver histology was achieved only in the vitamin E arm, which has led to increased interest in the use of this antioxidant therapy in NAFLD, although more evidence is required on the efficacy and long-term safety of vitamin E.

The FLIRT trial suggested that the benefits of ros-iglitazone on liver histology in NASH are limited to the first year of treatment, with no further benefits observed with a longer duration of therapy [19], and in other studies the improvements in aminotrans-ferases, insulin resistance, and histology with thiazolidinedione therapy have been shown to disappear on discontinuation of therapy, suggesting that lifelong treatment may be required [20].

Lipid-lowering agents such as statins improve the dyslipidemia, which is an important component of the metabolic syndrome, and can be safely used in NAFLD/NASH, although a beneficial effect on liver histology remains to be established [21]. The glucagon-like peptide-1 (GLP-1) analogues, exenatide and liraglutide, represent a promising treatment option in overweight patients with NAFLD. These agents increase insulin secretion, suppress glucagon secretion, slow gastric emptying, and increase satiety [22], and have been shown to induce significant weight loss in addition to improved glycemic control [23].

Treatment of hypertension as another component of the metabolic syndrome is also important. Studies suggest that the renin–angiotensin system (RAS) antagonists may be particularly beneficial in NASH, with trials demonstrating improvements in markers of hepatic fibrosis and serum AST with the angiotensin receptor blocker losartan [24].

If treatment is started before the development of significant fibrosis or cirrhosis, successful weight loss and control of metabolic parameters should prevent progression of disease. However. once cirrhosis has developed treatment strategies become more focused on preventing and controlling the manifestations of advanced liver disease such as ascites, variceal bleeding. and the development of encephalopathy. Surveillance for hepatocellular carcinoma (HCC) is also important for these patients because NAFLD is emerging as an important factor in its development.

Ultimately, in the presence of decompensated cirrhosis liver transplantation may be the only remaining option, and NASH cirrhosis is becoming an increasingly common indication for this treatment.

Case 2: jaundice and abdominal swelling

Case presentation

A 38-year-old woman presented with a 3-week history of jaundice and abdominal swelling. She had been drinking heavily for the past 7 years, with an average daily consumption of 1 L vodka. Her jaundice and abdominal swelling had developed over 2–3 days, and was accompanied by right upper quadrant (RUQ) pain and some ankle swelling. She was nauseated with frequent vomiting. She was opening her bowels approximately every 2 days, and her stool was slightly pale with normal consistency. Her urine had become dark and decreased in volume.

The patient had been staying in an alcohol rehabilitation centre for the past 2 months, before which she had been living alone. She had never smoked but admitted to a poor diet. She would often go several days without eating, and consumed only very small amounts when she did eat, preferring to drink alcohol instead.

There was no significant past medical history other than her excessive alcohol intake, and she had no previous hospital admissions. Her only medications were thiamine and Vitamin B Complex-Strong, prescribed by her GP. There was a family history of cardiovascular disease but not of liver disease.

Examination revealed the following:

Cachectic and deeply jaundiced; tremulous but no flap; alert and oriented

Palmar erythema and spider nevi present

Temperature 37.7°C

Cardiovascular: pulse 120 beats/min, regular; BP 115/82 mmHg; heart sounds normal; peripheral pitting edema

Respiratory: normal examination

Gastrointestinal: abdomen grossly distended with shifting dullness

No organomegaly palpable but examination difficult due to abdominal distension; tender in RUQ

Investigations were as follows (normal values in brackets)

Hb 10.0 (11.5–15.5) g/dL

WCC 13.6 (4–11) $\times$ 10^9/L

Platelets 232 (150–400) $\times$ 10^9/L

MCV 100 (76–98) fL

AST 109 (10–40) IU/L

ALT 13 (5–30) IU/L

GGT 1047 (5–30) IU/L

Albumin 30 (35–55) g/L

INR 2.1 (0.9–1.2)

Bilirubin 261 (2–17) µmol/L

ALP 238 (30–130) IU/L

Urea 1.3 (2.5–6.5) mmol/L

Creatinine 71 (50–120) µmol/L

Na^+ 136 (135–145) mmol/L

K^+ 2.6 (3.5–5.0) mmol/L

Cholesterol 5.4 (<5.2) mmol/L

Triglycerides 6.8 (0–1.5) mmol/L

THE CHRONIC LIVER DISEASE PATIENT

Glucose 3.2 (3.5–5.5) mmol/L
HbA1c 4.8 (4–6)%
TSH 2.2 (0.17–3.2) mU/L
Free T$_4$ 13.1 (11–22) pmol/L
Ferritin 1035 (20–250) µg/L
Transferrin saturation 32.0 (22–40)%
Ceruloplasmin 0.28 (<0.35) g/L
α$_1$-Antitrypsin 2.36 (1.5–3.5 g/L)
α$_1$-AT phenotype PiMM
AFP 1 (<7.0) µg/L
IgM 2.0 (0.5–2.0) g/L
IgA 4.2 (1.0–4.0) g/L
IgG 14.0 (5–16) g/L
ANA negative
ANCA negative
Anti-Sm negative
Anti-LKM negative
AMA negative
HBsAg negative
HBsAb negative
HCVAb negative

Abdominal ultrasound scan report
The liver is large and echobright with a coarse, abnormal texture. No focal liver abnormality; no biliary dilation; portal vein and hepatic vessels patent; large amount of ascites present.

Ascitic fluid aspirate
Neutrophil polymorphs 80/mm^3
Mononuclear cells 40/mm^3
RBCs 380/mm^3
No significant growth of organisms in culture

Questions

• What is the likely cause of her recent deterioration?
• How would you assess her prognosis?
• How should this patient be managed?

Differential diagnosis

The patient has signs of chronic liver disease and a history of heavy alcohol intake for several years. Her liver screen has not revealed any other causes of liver disease. She has a recent and fairly sudden onset of symptoms of jaundice, ascites, and RUQ pain, and is pyrexial. Her LFTs show a moderate transaminitis,

hyperbilirubinemia, and coagulopathy. CBC shows a raised WCC and macrocytic anemia.

As with the first case consideration has to be given to all the causes of chronic liver disease, even though there is a strong clue as to the etiology. Her elevated ferritin raises suspicion of a contribution of iron overload, but as ferritin is an acute phase protein its elevation does not always imply iron overload.

The likely differential diagnosis of an enlarged liver in the context of chronic liver disease includes further acute injury (such as alcoholic hepatitis) or the development of an HCC.

Spontaneous bacterial peritonitis was excluded by a negative ascitic fluid tap, and this is an essential investigation in any patient admitted with ascites due to liver disease. Other causes of a sudden deterioration which should be excluded include toxicity from paracetamol (acetaminophen) or other drugs.

Diagnosis

In view of the history and the results of the liver screen, alcoholic hepatitis is the most likely diagnosis.

The key signs and symptoms that should prompt consideration of a diagnosis of alcoholic hepatitis are jaundice, leukocytosis, fever, and encephalopathy associated with a history of chronic alcohol abuse [25]. Most patients who present with alcoholic hepatitis either already have cirrhosis or progress to develop it in the near future [26].

Investigation of alcoholic hepatitis often utilizes standard laboratory tests, but some groups argue that it is important to obtain histological confirmation of the diagnosis as the clinical syndrome of alcoholic hepatitis overlaps significantly with sepsis. One of the treatment options for alcoholic hepatitis, steroid therapy, is contraindicated in sepsis and thus histological confirmation of alcoholic hepatitis can be reassuring. This has to be weighed against the risks of liver biopsy in a patient who is ill, with coexisting cirrhosis and coagulopathy. Consequently the biopsy needs to be performed by the transjugular route which can result in suboptimal specimens being collected.

Liver biopsy can be useful to definitively confirm the presence of hepatitis. Histologically, the liver exhibits characteristic centrilobular ballooning necrosis of hepatocytes, neutrophilic infiltration, megamitochondria, and Mallory–Denk hyaline inclusions

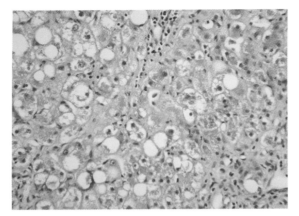

Figure 14.2 Alcoholic hepatitis on liver biopsy. Image demonstrates ballooned hepatocytes with Mallory–Denk hyaline bodies. There is also a mixed inflammatory infiltrate including several neutrophil polymorphs. (Image courtesy of Professor Stefan Hubscher.)

(Figure 14.2). Steatosis (fatty liver) and cirrhosis frequently accompany alcoholic hepatitis. Biopsy can also be useful in determining whether or not there is concomitant cirrhosis, which is associated with a significantly higher 1- and 5-year mortality than alcoholic hepatitis alone [27].

Although there are data demonstrating a genetic association with alcoholism, the role of such factors in determining susceptibility to alcoholic liver injury is not proven. Most people who drink excessively do not develop severe or progressive liver injury.

A recent meta-analysis of 50 studies looked at the association of alcoholic liver disease and genetic polymorphisms and did not find any robust association [28]. Given that only a small fraction of even heavy drinkers develop cirrhosis, further studies investigating the genetic basis of alcohol-induced liver disease are required.

The genetic factor that most clearly affects susceptibility is gender. The estimated minimum daily alcohol intake required for the development of cirrhosis is 40 g for men and 20 g for women older than 15–20 years. Possible reasons for this include a higher prevalence of liver autoantibodies found in female drinkers compared with male drinkers, although there is no overt evidence of autoimmune hepatitis,

and lower gastric mucosal ADH (antidiuretic hormone) content in women possibly leading to less first-pass clearance of alcohol in the stomach.

Although the histology of alcoholic hepatitis is well characterized, the pathogenesis is not fully understood. Both hepatocellular and inflammatory processes are involved and the immune response is thought to be intimately involved. The basis of treatment interventions is therefore based on blocking cytokine release and other aspects of the inflammatory response [29].

Patient management

The treatment of alcoholic hepatitis remains a controversial area. Abstinence from alcohol is essential, and hospitalized patients should usually receive alcohol withdrawal prophylaxis. Alcoholic hepatitis induces a profound catabolic state, and malnutrition contributes to the high mortality rate associated with this condition. Nutritional support is therefore a key aspect of management [25].

A course of parenteral thiamine (Pabrinex) should be given during the first few days of detoxification to prevent the development of Wernicke's encephalopathy and chronic memory deficits. Patients with chronic alcohol abuse are already chronically thiamine deficient. Wernicke-type brain damage is highly prevalent in patients with alcohol problems, together with the associated memory deficits that can lead to permanent disability [30]. The administration of glucose for the treatment of hypoglycemia may exacerbate the acute loss of thiamine (vitamin B_1) even further in the detoxifying patient, and it is essential that parenteral thiamine be administered before the glucose load, because oral thiamine preparations may be poorly absorbed in such patients.

Several other therapies have been trialed in alcoholic hepatitis, but only corticosteroids and pentoxifylline have been shown to be of significant benefit. Pentoxifylline is a partial tumor necrosis factor α (TNFα) antagonist which has been shown to significantly reduce the incidence of hepatorenal syndrome and associated mortality in patients with severe alcoholic hepatitis. The reduction in mortality in this randomized controlled trial appeared to be due to a reduction in hepatorenal syndrome in these patients [31].

Corticosteroid therapy has been studied in multiple studies with conflicting results. Meta-analysis does suggest that steroid therapy, in selected patients, leads to an improvement in liver function and mortality [32]. High-dose steroid therapy is a potent immunosuppressant, in contrast to pentoxifylline, and thus the clinician needs to be vigilant to the possibility of sepsis.

There are several scoring systems available to predict survival in alcoholic hepatitis.

The modified Maddrey Discriminant Function (mDF) score is calculated using the variables of admission prothrombin time (PT) and serum bilirubin. An mDF score ≥32 is associated with a 68% 28-day survival in the absence of steroid treatment, in contrast with 93% in those with a mDF <32 [33]. Based on data from several randomized-clinical trials the mDF has therefore been recommended as a tool to assess the severity of alcoholic hepatitis with a threshold of 32 used to consider corticosteroid therapy [34].

The mDF is calculated as follows:

$$4.6 \, (\text{patient's PT [s]} - \text{control time}) + \text{serum bilirubin (mg/dL)}.$$

Concerns about the low specificity of the mDF led to the introduction of the Glasgow alcoholic hepatitis score (GAHS). Evidence suggests that the GAHS may select better those patients most likely to benefit from corticosteroid therapy [35]. It is also more accurate than the mDF in predicting outcome at 28 and 84 days after admission, and more specific for predicting death [36]. The GAHS (Table 14.2) is calculated using five variables and is much more amenable to use at the bedside than the mDF. A score is given for each variable producing a combined score of between 5 and 12.

A GAHS of ≥9 is associated with a poor prognosis and recent studies have demonstrated that this is an appropriate cut-off for the use of corticosteroid therapy. When the GAHS is <9, there is no survival benefit between untreated and corticosteroid-treated patients. For patients with a GAHS ≥9, corticosteroid treatment significantly improves both the 28- and 84-day survival [35]. For patients in whom steroid therapy is indicated, most studies have used 40 mg prednisolone daily for up to 28 days.

Our current patient has a GAHS of 9 (age = 1, WCC = 1, urea = 1, INR = 3, bilirubin = 3), predictive of a poor prognosis. She was managed with chlordiazepoxide to prevent withdrawal, nutritional supplements, and vitamins. As her GAHS was 9, she also received 40 mg prednisolone daily for 28 days.

The patient remained in hospital for 14 days and was discharged on oral vitamins and corticosteroid therapy for a further 14 days. Her longer-term prognosis will depend on whether she manages to remain abstinent from alcohol in the future.

Case 3: abnormal liver function tests in a patient from Ghana

Case presentation

A 35-year-old male construction worker of Ghanaian origin was found by his GP to have abnormal liver function tests. Examination revealed him to be clinically well with no signs of chronic liver disease. He was asymptomatic other than complaining of intermittent RUQ pain.

Investigations were as follows (normal values in brackets):
Hb 10.9 (13.5–17.5) g/dL
WCC 6.3 (4–11) × 10^9/L
Platelets 61 (150–400) × 10^9/L
MCV 88 (76–98) fL
Albumin 32 (35–55) g/L
AST 236 (10–40) IU/mL
ALT 417 (5–30) IU/mL
GGT 267 (5–30) IU/mL
INR 1.7 (0.9–1.2)
Bilirubin 42 (2–17) μmol/L
ALP 192 (30–130) IU/L
Urea 2.8 (2.5–6.5) mmol/L

Table 14.2 Glasgow Alcoholic Hepatitis Score (GAHS)

Score given	1	2	3
Age (years)	<50	≥50	
WCC (× 10^9/L)	<15	≥15	
Urea (mmol/L)	<5	≥5	
PT ratio or INR	<1.5	1.5–2.0	>2.0
Bilirubin (μmol/L)	<125	125–250	>250

INR, international normalized ratio; PT, prothrombin time; WCC, white cell count.

Creatinine 92 (50–120) µmol/L
Cholesterol 4.8 (<5.2) mmol/L
Triglycerides 1.2 (0–1.5) mmol/L
Na^+ 134 (135–145) mmol/L
K^+ 4.6 (3.5–5.0) mmol/L
Glucose 5.0 (3.5–5.5) mmol/L
TSH 0.8 (0.17–3.2) mU/L
Free T_4 18.2 (11–22) pmol/L
Ferritin 120 (20–250) µg/L
Transferrin saturation 26.6 (22–40)%
Ceruloplasmin 0.3 (<0.35) g/L
α_1-Antitrypsin 0.93 (1.5–3.5) g/L
α_1-AT phenotype PiMS
AFP 3 (<7.0) µg/L
IgM 1.5 (0.5–2.0) g/L
IgA 2.8 (1.0–4.0) g/L
IgG 15.2 (5–16) g/L
ANA 1:40
ANCA negative
Anti-Sm negative
Anti-LKM negative
AMA negative
HCVAb negative
Hepatitis B serology was as follows:
HBsAg positive
HBcAb positive
HBcAb IgM negative
HBeAg negative
HBV DNA 25 000 IU/mL

Ultrasound scan report
Heterogeneously coarse, nodular liver, with normal spleen and no ascites. Portal vein and hepatic vessels patent.

Liver biopsy
Chronic hepatitis with mild activity, marked bridging and regenerative nodules, Ishak stage 5/6.

Questions

- How should this patient be managed?
- What are the main complications that this patient may develop?
- How should these complications be prevented/monitored?
- What is the differential diagnosis?
- How should this be investigated further?

Initial management

Liver biopsy reported above revealed evidence of chronic hepatitis B cirrhosis with regeneration. The elevated HBV DNA levels and ALT indicated the presence of ongoing inflammation. He was therefore started on entecavir 0.5 mg daily. Entecavir has a very low resistance profile in comparison to lamivudine, and is therefore more suitable for patients with cirrhosis in whom viral breakthrough could induce decompensation [36,37]. In view of the biopsy and ultrasound evidence of cirrhosis, HCC surveillance was commenced with 6-monthly ultrasound scan and α-fetoprotein (AFP) measurements.

Two years later his ALT had reduced to 57 and HBV DNA levels were undetectable. Entecavir was continued indefinitely to maintain viral suppression.

A routine surveillance abdominal ultrasound scan was reported as follows: The liver has a diffusely abnormal nodular echotexture. There is an 11×18 mm hypoechoic focal structure within the right lobe, which appears more prominent than the other nodules. Portal vein patent. Spleen not enlarged. No ascites.

The AFP level was 2.

Differential diagnosis

The differential diagnosis of a hepatic nodule in a cirrhotic liver includes two major lesions: regenerative lesions and dysplastic or neoplastic lesions [38].

Regenerative nodules result from localized proliferation of hepatocytes and their supporting stroma. In the context of cirrhosis, regenerative lesions include regenerative and cirrhotic nodules. A regenerative nodule is a well-defined region of parenchyma that has enlarged in response to necrosis, altered circulation, or other stimulus. It may contain one (monoacinar) or multiple (multiacinar) portal tracts. The diameter of monoacinar nodules is usually 0.1–10 mm, and that of multiacinar nodules should be at least 2 mm, with large multiacinar nodules being 5–15 mm in diameter.

Cirrhotic nodules are regenerative nodules that are largely or completely surrounded by fibrous septa. Macronodular cirrhosis contains nodules >3 mm in diameter.

Dysplastic or neoplastic lesions are composed of hepatocytes that show histological characteristics of abnormal growth caused by a presumed or proven genetic mutation. Dysplastic or neoplastic nodules include hepatocellular adenoma, dysplastic nodules, and HCC.

A dysplastic nodule is defined as a nodular region of hepatocytes >1 mm in diameter with dysplasia but no definite histological criteria for malignancy. These nodules are usually found in cirrhotic livers. Dysplasia indicates the presence of nuclear and cytoplasmic changes, such as minimal to severe nuclear atypia and an increased amount of cytoplasmic fat or glycogen, within the cluster of cells that compose the nodule. Dysplastic nodules can be low grade (increased number of cells with an increased nuclei:cytoplasm ratio) or high grade (increased thickness of the layers of hepatocytes, which contain nuclei that are variable in size and shape). HCC is a malignant neoplasm composed of cells with hepatocellular differentiation.

A small HCC is defined as ≤2 cm in diameter. The criteria used to distinguish HCC from high-grade dysplastic nodules are not clearly defined but factors which would be in favor of malignancy include:
• prominent nuclear atypia
• a high nuclear cytoplasmic ratio with nuclear density twice as great as normal
• plates three or more cells thick, numerous unaccompanied arteries
• mitoses in moderate numbers
• invasion of the stroma or portal tracts.
Most small HCCs cannot be distinguished histologically from dysplastic nodules with certainty and, furthermore, foci of carcinoma can be found in otherwise benign dysplastic nodules.

Diagnosis

The patient then proceeded to CT and MRI.

A triple phase contrast CT (including arterial, portal venous, and delayed phases) of the liver was performed. This was reported as showing a 1.9 cm homogenously hypervascular lesion high in segment 4, which remained slightly hyperintense on the portal venous phase. No other abnormalities were noted.

Contrast MRI was then performed using gadolinium and Resovist. This measured the nodule at 2.5 cm.

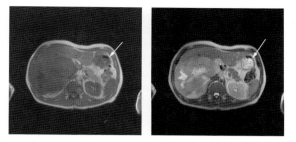

Figure 14.3 MRI of hepatocellular carcinoma. These images demonstrate the presence of a large right lobe of liver lesion measuring 15 × 16 cm up to and displacing anteriorly the right portal vein and main portal vein without definite invasion, and extending into the caudate lobe. The mass is generally irregular, with central necrosis, and perhaps some fibrous areas. It is generally lobular in appearance and breaches the liver capsule posteriorly and is up against the diaphragm. It extends inferiorly to displace the right kidney a little. Conclusion: likely primary liver tumor.

It was hypervascular with early washout and did not take up Resovist, consistent with a diagnosis of HCC. Resovist consists of superparamagnetic iron oxide (SPIO) particles coated with carboxydextran, which accumulate in cells of the reticuloendothelial system of the liver, but are not retained in tumor tissue [39]. There was no evidence of vascular invasion or other focal lesions. Figure 14.3 illustrates the appearance of HCC on MRI.

The radiological investigations were reviewed at a multidisciplinary meeting where there was agreement that the nodule was an HCC.

The signal intensity and enhancement characteristics of dysplastic nodules are not yet well established. There is most likely a stepwise transition from a regenerative nodule to a low-grade dysplastic nodule, a high-grade dysplastic nodule, and eventually a HCC, and consequently the hepatocytes within hepatic nodules undergo numerous changes. These may not be reflected in their signal intensity or vascularity, and thus, current MRI sequences might not allow differentiation of regenerative nodules from dysplastic nodules with a high level of certainty.

Typically, regenerative nodules show low signal intensity on T2-weighted images, variable signal intensity on T1-weighted images, and no enhancement on arterial phase, dynamic, gadolinium-enhanced images. Distinguishing between dysplastic nodules and small HCCs in a patient with cirrhosis is also of clinical importance. Early detection of HCC is critical because treatment options differ and in general treatment of HCC is most effective when the tumor is small.

Dysplastic nodules are generally hypo- or hyperintense on T1-weighted images and iso- or hypointense on T2-weighted images. HCC may be hypo-, iso-, or hyperintense on T1-weighted images and iso- or hyperintense on T2-weighted images. A feature that can be helpful in distinguishing a dysplastic nodule from HCC at unenhanced MRI is the fact that dysplastic nodules are almost never hyperintense on T2-weighted images. The main blood supply of dysplastic nodules is from the portal venous system and that of HCC is from the hepatic arterial system. Using this, HCC can often be distinguished from dysplastic nodules by dynamic, gadolinium-enhanced MRI on the basis of identification of hepatic arterial phase enhancement, whereas dysplastic nodules do not generally enhance during the arterial phase.

Although the pathophysiology of hepatic arterial phase enhancement of dysplastic nodules is unclear, one hypothesis is that these lesions contain increased numbers of unpaired arteries (i.e. arteries unaccompanied by bile ducts) compared with regenerative nodules. Thus, abnormal angiogenesis may account for hepatic arterial phase enhancement of some dysplastic nodules.

Management of HCC

Surveillance for HCC

Current guidelines recommend 6-monthly ultrasonography and AFP measurements for cirrhotic patients, which is in part based on our knowledge of tumor doubling times [40]. The AFP alone is an inadequate screening test.

A receiver operating characteristic (ROC) curve analysis of AFP used as a diagnostic test suggests that a value of 20 ng/mL provides the optimal balance between sensitivity and specificity [40]. However, at this level sensitivity is only 60%, meaning that 40% of tumors would be missed if AFP alone were used to determine the need for further assessment. AFP measurement does have a role in the diagnosis of HCC. In cirrhotic patients a persistently elevated AFP is a definite risk factor for HCC, and a level >200 ng/mL in association with a mass in the liver is considered diagnostic of HCC for treatment purposes [40].

When a nodule is found on ultrasonography in a cirrhotic liver, further investigations depend on the size of the lesion.

Size of lesion

- <1 cm: repeat ultrasonography at 3- to 6-monthly intervals. If no growth after 18–24 months revert to normal surveillance. If enlarging, proceed according to lesion size.
- 1–2 cm: investigate further with two dynamic imaging studies, either CT, contrast ultrasonography, or contrast MRI. If appearances are typical of HCC (i.e. hypervascular with washout in the portal/venous phase) with two techniques the lesion should be treated as HCC. If findings not characteristic or vascular profile differs between imaging techniques the lesion should be biopsied.
- >2 cm: typical features on a single dynamic imaging technique or AFP >200 ng/mL is considered diagnostic. Biopsy is required only if vascular profile on imaging is not diagnostic or the nodule is detected in a non-cirrhotic liver [40].

Cirrhosis of any cause is associated with an increased risk of developing HCC [41]. This risk is particularly high in patients with chronic hepatitis B infection, in whom it may develop even in those without cirrhosis. HCC has a tendency to occur at a younger age in patients of African or Asian origin [40]. HCC surveillance is currently recommended for all patients with cirrhosis, and potentially for certain groups of non-cirrhotic patients with hepatitis B.

The Barcelona Clinic Liver Cancer (BCLC) staging system is widely used and validated in the management of patients with HCC. It includes variables related to tumor stage, liver function (Child–Pugh score), performance status, and cancer-related symptoms. It links staging with treatment modalities and with an estimation of life expectancy based on known response rates to the various treatments (Figure 14.4).

Surgical resection is the treatment of choice for HCC in non-cirrhotic patients, but this only accounts for 5% of cases in western countries and 40% in Asia. Cirrhotic patients should undergo anatomical resection only if they have well-preserved liver function, normal bilirubin, and hepatic venous pressure gradi-

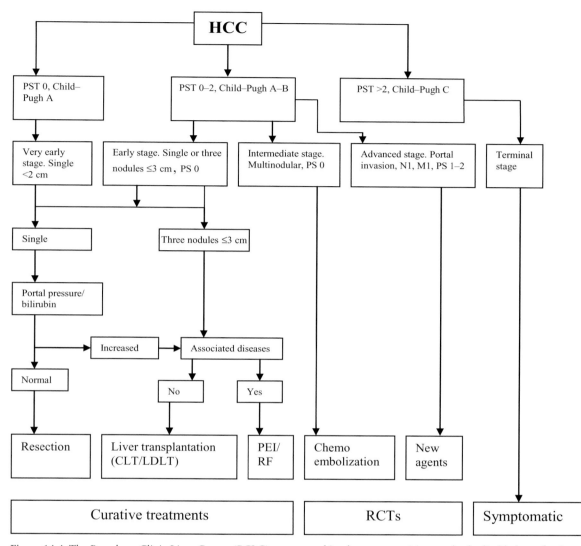

Figure 14.4 The Barcelona Clinic Liver Cancer (BCLC) staging system [40]. Stage 0 is fully active, no symptoms; stage 1 is minor symptoms, able to do light activity; stage 2 is capable of self-care but unable to carry out work: up for more than 50% waking hours; stage 3 is limited self-care capacity: confined to bed or chair >50% of waking hours; stage 4 is completely disabled: confined to bed or chair. CLT, cadaveric liver transplantation; HCC, hepatocellular carcinoma; LDLT, living donor liver transplantation; PEI, percutaneous ethanol injection; PST, World Health Organization Performance Status; RCTs, randomized controlled trials; RF, radiofrequency.

ent <10 mmHg (i.e. no evidence of portal hypertension), because patients with more advanced disease have a significant risk of decompensation after surgery [40]. In well-selected cases, the 5-year survival rate post-resection exceeds 70%, although the risk of tumor recurrence also exceeds 70% 5 years post-resection (both recurrent and new tumors) [40].

Liver transplantation is an option for patients with liver disease exceeding the above criteria, or for those with a larger tumor burden that precludes resection.

The Milan criteria used for selecting those patients with HCC who would be suitable candidates for liver transplantation have recently been expanded, and potential transplant candidates now include those with (1) a single tumor ≤5 cm, (2) up to three nodules <3 cm, or (3) a single tumor >5 cm and ≤7 cm diameter where there has been no evidence of tumor progression, extrahepatic spread, or new nodule formation over a 6-month period [42].

Percutaneous ablation therapies include ethanol injection and radiofrequency ablation therapy. These treatments are best for patients with early stage HCC who are not suitable for resection or transplantation, or as a bridge to transplantation. Child–Pugh A patients with successful tumor necrosis after percutaneous ablation therapy may achieve a 50% 5-year survival rate [40].

Non-curative options include transarterial chemoembolization (TACE) for non-surgical patients with large or multifocal tumors that do not have vascular invasion or extrahepatic spread. This treatment is considered only in patients with compensated cirrhosis. The improvement in survival after TACE ranges from 20% to 60% [40]. TACE is also used to downstage HCC before transplantation [43], although other biological characteristics of the tumor may be more important than size and number in predicting tumor aggressiveness and recurrence risk [44].

Sorafenib is a multi-kinase inhibitor that is the first oral agent to show any significant benefit in advanced HCC, increasing survival by approximately 37% [45], which equates to an increased survival of approximately 3 months. Further studies will address its role in earlier forms of HCC.

In this case there was a high level of certainty that he had an HCC, and as such liver transplantation was felt to be the most appropriate treatment option. With increasing demand for donor organs there is a suggestion that in the future surgery or ablative modalities may be undertaken without immediate recourse to liver transplantation. This patient was listed for liver transplantation after a satisfactory assessment, and underwent a successful orthotopic liver transplantation 2 months later. The explanted liver histology showed established cirrhosis with a moderately differentiated HCC. The tumor had been completely excised with no evidence of vascular invasion.

Discussion

These cases highlight some of the principal ways in which patients with chronic liver disease present. The first case highlights the importance of screening for the different causes of liver disease, and the issues associated with performing liver biopsy in a cirrhotic patient. NAFLD is rising in incidence and is predicted to become the most common cause of liver disease in the western world. Radical new strategies will be required to tackle the obesity epidemic, which is at the heart of this condition. More aggressive management of obesity by means of drugs such as Orlistat or the use of gastric surgery will be necessary. In addition, there are numerous phase 2/3 trials currently under way studying the use of pharmacological agents that aim to reduce steatohepatitis.

The second case reflects another very common presentation, alcoholic hepatitis, which is becoming more common in women of younger age than previously seen. The key is taking a careful history and being aware of the non-specific manner with which it can present. Often patients do not have evidence of liver decompensation and the diagnosis is made on the basis of systemic symptoms such as pyrexia and elevated WCC, with often minimal changes to LFTs. Although the mainstay of treatment in such patients is conservative management, there is a compelling need for more effective and safe anti-inflammatory agents. It should be appreciated that many of these patients either have, or go on to develop, cirrhosis as well.

The third case demonstrates the evolution of management of patients with HCC, which is increasing in incidence worldwide. Further developments in therapy can be expected, with the earlier use of tyrosine kinase inhibitors such as sorafenib carrying particular promise. Concerns that patients in whom transplantation would offer an acceptable outcome are being excluded from such treatment have already led to expansion of the criteria for liver transplantation, although there remains controversy about a scheme that increases the number of potential recipients at a time when the number of donors is reducing or remaining static. It is likely, in the face of restricted access to liver transplantation, that patients with small single tumors will be initially considered for resection or ablative therapy with recourse to transplantation being taken when there is relapse. As such the development of agents that reduce or delay the recurrence of HCCs will play an important role in the management of such patients.

References

1 Adams LA, Lindor KD, Angulo P. The prevalence of autoantibodies and autoimmune hepatitis in patients with nonalcoholic Fatty liver disease. *Am J Gastroenterol* 2004;**99**:1316–20.

2 Merle U, Schaefer M, Ferenci P, et al. Clinical presentation, diagnosis and long-term outcome of Wilson's disease: a cohort study. *Gut* 2007;**56**:115–20.

3 Day C. Metabolic syndrome, or What you will: definitions and epidemiology. *Diab Vasc Dis Res* 2007;**4**: 32–8.

4 Hamaguchi M, Kojima T, Takeda N, et al. The metabolic syndrome as a predictor of nonalcoholic fatty liver disease. *Ann Intern Med* 2005;**143**:722–8.

5 Neuschwander-Tetri BA, Caldwell SH. Nonalcoholic steatohepatitis: summary of an AASLD Single Topic Conference. *Hepatology* 2003;**37**:1202–19.

6 Yeh MM, Brunt EM. Pathology of nonalcoholic fatty liver disease. *Am J Clin Pathol* 2007;**128**:837–47.

7 Angulo P, Hui JM, Marchesini G, et al. The NAFLD fibrosis score: a noninvasive system that identifies liver fibrosis in patients with NAFLD. *Hepatology* 2007;**45**:846–54.

8 de L, V, Vergniol J. Transient elastography (FibroScan). *Gastroenterol Clin Biol* 2008;**32**(6 suppl 1):58–67.

9 Wong VW, Vergniol J, Wong GL, et al. Diagnosis of fibrosis and cirrhosis using liver stiffness measurement in nonalcoholic fatty liver disease. *Hepatology* 2010;**51**:454–62.

10 Harrison SA, Day CP. Benefits of lifestyle modification in NAFLD. *Gut* 2007;**56**:1760–9.

11 Promrat K, Kleiner DE, Niemeier HM, et al. Randomized controlled trial testing the effects of weight loss on nonalcoholic steatohepatitis. *Hepatology* 2010;**51**: 121–9.

12 Hussein O, Grosovski M, Schlesinger S, et al. Orlistat reverse fatty infiltration and improves hepatic fibrosis in obese patients with nonalcoholic steatohepatitis (NASH). *Dig Dis Sci* 2007;**52**:2512–9.

13 Klein S, Mittendorfer B, Eagon JC, et al. Gastric bypass surgery improves metabolic and hepatic abnormalities associated with nonalcoholic fatty liver disease. *Gastroenterology* 2006;**130**:1564–72.

14 Bugianesi E, Gentilcore E, Manini R, et al. A randomized controlled trial of metformin versus vitamin E or prescriptive diet in nonalcoholic fatty liver disease. *Am J Gastroenterol* 2005;**100**:1082–90.

15 Shadid S, Jensen MD. Effects of pioglitazone versus diet and exercise on metabolic health and fat distribution in upper body obesity. *Diabetes Care* 2003;**26**:3148–52.

16 Aithal GP, Thomas JA, Kaye PV, et al. Randomized, placebo-controlled trial of pioglitazone in non-diabetic subjects with nonalcoholic steatohepatitis. *Gastroenterology* 2008;**135**:1176–84.

17 Belfort R, Harrison SA, Brown K, et al. A placebo-controlled trial of pioglitazone in subjects with nonalcoholic steatohepatitis. *N Engl J Med* 2006;**355**: 2297–307.

18 Sanyal AJ, Chalasani N, Kowdley KV, et al. Pioglitazone, vitamin E, or placebo for nonalcoholic steatohepatitis. *N Engl J Med* 2010;**362**:1675–85.

19 Ratziu V, Charlotte F, Bernhardt C, et al. Long-term efficacy of rosiglitazone in nonalcoholic steatohepatitis: Results of the fatty liver improvement by rosiglitazone therapy (FLIRT 2) extension trial. *Hepatology* 2009;**51**:445–53.

20 Lutchman G, Modi A, Kleiner DE et al. The effects of discontinuing pioglitazone in patients with nonalcoholic steatohepatitis. *Hepatology* 2007;**46**(2):424–9.

21 Nelson A, Torres DM, Morgan AE, et al. A pilot study using simvastatin in the treatment of nonalcoholic steatohepatitis: a randomized placebo-controlled trial. *J Clin Gastroenterol* 2009;**43**:990–4.

22 Iltz JL, Baker DE, Setter SM, et al. Exenatide: an incretin mimetic for the treatment of type 2 diabetes mellitus. *Clin Ther* 2006;**28**:652–65.

23 Astrup A, Rossner S, Van GL, et al. Effects of liraglutide in the treatment of obesity: a randomised, double-blind, placebo-controlled study. *Lancet* 2009;**374**:1606–16.

24 Yokohama S, Yoneda M, Haneda M, et al. Therapeutic efficacy of an angiotensin II receptor antagonist in patients with nonalcoholic steatohepatitis. *Hepatology* 2004;**40**:1222–5.

25 Crosse KI, Anania FA. Alcoholic hepatitis. *Curr Treat Options Gastroenterol* 2002;**5**:417–23.

26 Mathurin P, Beuzin F, Louvet A, et al. Fibrosis progression occurs in a subgroup of heavy drinkers with typical histological features. *Aliment Pharmacol Ther* 2007;**25**:1047–54.

27 Orrego H, Blake JE, Blendis LM, et al. Prognosis of alcoholic cirrhosis in the presence and absence of alcoholic hepatitis. *Gastroenterology* 1987;**92**:208–14.

28 Zintzaras E, Stefanidis I, Santos M, Vidal F. Do alcohol-metabolizing enzyme gene polymorphisms increase the risk of alcoholism and alcoholic liver disease? *Hepatology* 2006;**43**:352–61.

29 Rongey C, Kaplowitz N. Current concepts and controversies in the treatment of alcoholic hepatitis. *World J Gastroenterol* 2006;**12**:6909–21.

30 Ambrose ML, Bowden SC, Whelan G. Thiamin treatment and working memory function of

alcohol-dependent people: preliminary findings. *Alcohol Clin Exp Res* 2001;**25**(1):112–6.

31 Akriviadis E, Botla R, Briggs W, et al. Pentoxifylline improves short-term survival in severe acute alcoholic hepatitis: a double-blind, placebo-controlled trial. *Gastroenterology* 2000;**119**:1637–48.

32 Mathurin P, Mendenhall CL, Carithers RL, et al. Corticosteroids improve short-term survival in patients with severe alcoholic hepatitis (AH): individual data analysis of the last three randomized placebo controlled double blind trials of corticosteroids in severe AH. *J Hepatol* 2002;**36**:480–7.

33 Carithers RL Jr, Herlong HF, Diehl AM, et al. Methylprednisolone therapy in patients with severe alcoholic hepatitis. A randomized multicenter trial. *Ann Intern Med* 1989;**110**:685–90.

34 McCullough AJ, O'Connor JF. Alcoholic liver disease: proposed recommendations for the American College of Gastroenterology. *Am J Gastroenterol* 1998;**93**: 2022–36.

35 Forrest EH, Morris AJ, Stewart S, et al. The Glasgow alcoholic hepatitis score identifies patients who may benefit from corticosteroids. *Gut* 2007;**56**:1743–6.

36 Forrest EH, Evans CD, Stewart S, et al. Analysis of factors predictive of mortality in alcoholic hepatitis and derivation and validation of the Glasgow alcoholic hepatitis score. *Gut* 2005;**54**:1174–9.

37 EASL Clinical Practice Guidelines: management of chronic hepatitis B. *J Hepatol* 2009;**50**:227–42.

38 International Working Party. Terminology of nodular hepatocellular lesions. *Hepatology* 1995;**22**:983–93.

39 Tanimoto A, Kuribayashi S. Application of superparamagnetic iron oxide to imaging of hepatocellular carcinoma. *Eur J Radiol* 2006;**58**:200–16.

40 Bruix J, Sherman M. Management of hepatocellular carcinoma. *Hepatology* 2005;**42**:1208–36.

41 Leong TY, Leong AS. Epidemiology and carcinogenesis of hepatocellular carcinoma. *HPB (Oxford)* 2005;**7**(1): 5–15.

42 NHSBT Liver Advisory Group: *Protocols and Guidelines for Adults undergoing deceased donor liver transplantation in the UK*. 2009.

43 Chapman WC, Majella Doyle MB, et al. Outcomes of neoadjuvant transarterial chemoembolization to downstage hepatocellular carcinoma before liver transplantation. *Ann Surg* 2008;**248**:617–25.

44 Silva MF, Wigg AJ. Current controversies surrounding liver transplantation for hepatocellular carcinoma. *J Gastroenterol Hepatol* 2010;**25**:1217–26.

45 Zhang T, Ding X, Wei D, et al. Sorafenib improves the survival of patients with advanced hepatocellular carcinoma: a meta-analysis of randomized trials. *Anticancer Drugs* 2010;**21**:326–32.

15 Portal Hypertension: A Management Problem

Norma C. McAvoy and Peter C. Hayes

Centre for Liver & Digestive Disorders and Academic Hepatology, Clinical and Surgical Sciences, The Royal Infirmary of Edinburgh, Edinburgh, UK

Case 1: hematemesis in alcoholic liver disease

Case presentation

A 49-year-old teacher presented to A&E after vomiting some blood. His wife reported that he complained of nausea and then vomited large amounts of fresh blood with clots. She stated that he collapsed on to the bathroom floor but no loss of conscious was reported. He denied any similar episodes or any associated melena.

He had no significant past medical history and was not on any regular medication. He reported that for the last 15 years his alcohol intake consisted of a bottle of wine and a few whiskies per night. For the last 18 months, however, he reported that he had been under stress and had been drinking a bottle of whiskey per night. He was a smoker of 20 cigarettes per day. There was no family history of liver disease. He currently was on sick leave from his teaching post.

Clinical examination: he was mildly jaundiced with multiple spider nevi across his upper chest wall. Finger clubbing was present with nicotine staining. He was tremulous but no flapping tremor

Cardiovascular: heart rate 126 beats/min sinus rhythm; BP 90/50 mmHg; heart sounds were normal; there was mild peripheral edema

Respiratory: good air entry bilaterally with no focal signs

Abdomen: soft but tender epigastrium; liver edge palpable 2 cm below costal margin; no ascites;

bowel sounds normal; rectal examination – soft black feces; strongly FOB (fecal occult blood) positive

CNS: alert and oriented

Investigations (normal values in brackets)
Bilirubin 58 (3–16) µmol/L
Hb 84 (130–180) g/L
Na$^+$ 137 (135–145) mmol/L
K$^+$ 3.2 (3.5–5.0) mmol/L
ALT 55 (10–50) U/L
MCV 102 (78–98) fL
Bicarbonate 24 (22–30) mmol/L
ALP 125 (40–125) U/L
WCC 10.7 (4–11) × 10^9/L
Urea 13.7 (2.5–6.6) mmol/L
GGT 1260 (5–35) U/L
Platelets 75 (150–350) × 10^9/L
Creatinine 80 (60–120) µmol/L
Albumin 29 (35–50) g/L
PT 17 (10.2–12.7) s
ECG sinus tachycardia.
Chest and abdominal radiographs normal

Questions

- What is your differential diagnosis?
- How would you initially manage this patient?
- What is your subsequent management of this patient?

Problem-based Approach to Gastroenterology and Hepatology, First Edition. Edited by John N. Plevris, Colin W. Howden.
© 2012 Blackwell Publishing Ltd. Published 2012 by Blackwell Publishing Ltd.

Differential diagnosis

This man has chronic liver disease secondary to alcohol as indicated from the history and the presence of high mean corpuscular volume (MCV) and γ-glutamyltransferase (GGT), low platelet count, low albumin, and prolonged prothrombin (PT) time. In any patient with suspected chronic liver disease and fresh hematemesis, variceal hemorrhage (from esophageal, gastric, or ectopic varices) should always be actively excluded. Bleeding from a peptic ulcer, Mallory–Weiss tear, or Dieulafoy's lesion is less likely.

Variceal hemorrhage is the most likely diagnosis in this case and a medical emergency with a high mortality. Early diagnosis and treatment by endoscopy, following adequate resuscitation in a critical care unit, are very important to improve outcome. If active bleeding from esophageal varices is seen at endoscopy, or if varices with recent stigmata of bleeding are seen and no other source of bleeding identified, endoscopic band ligation of varices should be undertaken.

Bleeding from gastric or ectopic varices is a less common occurrence, but important to identify because the bleeding can be very difficult to control and banding as a means of achieving hemostasis is less effective or even contraindicated. This is because, unlike esophageal varices which represent mucosal folds with superficial dilated vessels perforating through the muscularis into the mucosal layer of the esophagus, gastric varices are more likely to be true veins; banding of such vessels can cause secondary severe bleeding once the bands detach.

The endoscopic treatment of choice for gastric or ectopic varices is sclerotherapy with cyanoacrylate (acrylic glue) or thrombin. Ectopic varices are more common in patients with non-cirrhotic portal hypertension such as portal vein thrombosis, or as a new presentation in a patient with cirrhosis who develops portal vein thrombosis commonly secondary to the development of hepatocellular carcinoma.

Bleeding from non-variceal sources in the patient with cirrhosis should be treated with epinephrine injection, clips, and/or heater probe. Attention should be given to correction of coagulopathy.

Patient management

The patient had two grey venflons inserted for large-bore intravenous access and aggressive fluid resuscitation with colloid, initially, then cross-matched blood (Figure 15.1).

Reversal of coagulopathy was achieved by administering intravenous vitamin K and fresh frozen plasma. Upper gastrointestinal (GI) endoscopy was performed after adequate fluid resuscitation in a high dependency unit without delay. Large (grade 3) esophageal varices were identified in the distal esophagus with numerous red signs. They were not actively bleeding but no alternate bleeding site was identified (Figure 15.2).

The varices in the lower 5 cm of the esophagus were treated with band ligation. Ceftriaxone 2 g was given intravenously and intravenous terlipressin was also administered.

Three hours after the original endoscopy the patient had a further large hematemesis associated with hemodynamic instability. Despite aggressive fluid resuscitation and correction of coagulopathy, bleeding continued.

A Minnesota tube (i.e. a modified Stenstaken–Blakemore tube with esophageal aspiration ports) was inserted by an experienced operator, with the gastric balloon being inflated with 300 mL air and then pulled back to exert adequate pressure to the esophagogastric junction and secured. The patient was ventilated to protect his airway and transferred to the radiology intervention laboratory where a transjugular intrahepatic portosystemic stent (TIPSS) was inserted (Figure 15.3). TIPSS was successful in lowering his portal pressure gradient (PPG) from 21 mmHg to 4 mmHg. After an overnight stay in intensive care, the patient was transferred to the ward for rehabilitation and made a full recovery.

Discussion

Portal hypertension is evaluated by the pressure gradient between the portal vein and the inferior vena cava. This gradient is estimated by subtracting the free from the wedged hepatic venous pressure in the hepatic veins to obtain a hepatic venous pressure gradient (HVPG). The normal HVPG should be <5 mmHg. Portal hypertension is clinically manifest when patients develop ascites or variceal hemorrhage and generally occurs when the PPG is >10 mmHg.

Esophageal varices are present in up to 60% of patients at the time of diagnosis of cirrhosis [1].

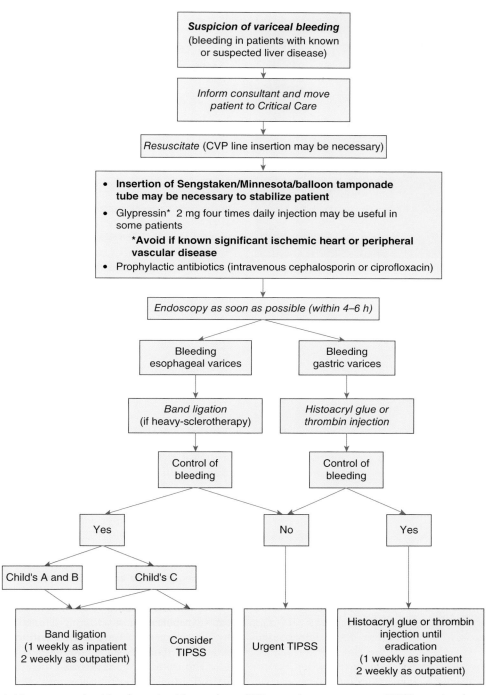

Figure 15.1 Management algorithm for variceal hemorrhage. CVP, central venous pressure; TIPSS, transjugular intrahepatic portosystemic stent.

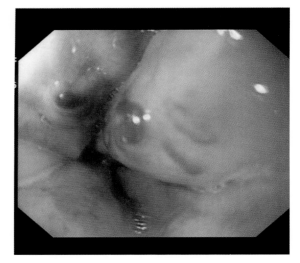

Figure 15.2 Upper gastrointestinal endoscopy revealed esophageal varices with red signs.

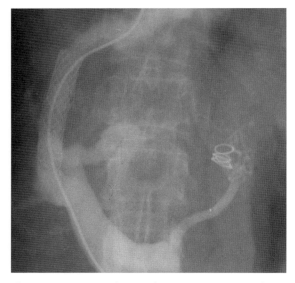

Figure 15.3 Transjugular intrahepatic portosystemic shunt (Palmaz stent). A coil that can be used to embolize bleeding vessels is also seen in this radiograph.

Thirty percent of patients with cirrhosis and varices will bleed with up to a 50% mortality rate associated with the first bleed [2].

Risk factors for variceal bleeding [3] include the following:

Table 15.1 Classification of esophageal varices

Grade 1	Small varices that flatten fully on air insufflation
Grade 2	Moderate varices that do not flatten completely with air insufflation
Grade 3	Large varices that do not flatten with air insufflation and protrude >50% into lumen

• **Portal pressure**: it has been demonstrated that esophageal variceal rupture generally occurs when the HVPG exceeds the critical threshold of 12 mmHg but this value is not absolute [4].
• **Variceal size**: larger varices are more likely to bleed but the severity of liver disease should also be taken into account.
Table 15.1 lists the classification of esophageal varices.

Severity of liver disease
Patients with more advanced liver disease (e.g. Child's C) who have small varices are just as likely to bleed as someone with large varices but less severe liver disease (e.g. Child's B). The severity of liver disease also predicts the mortality.

Variceal characteristics
The presence of red signs on varices indicates an increased risk of bleeding. Patients found to have grade II or III (medium or large) varices should receive primary prophylaxis against bleeding with propranolol or variceal band ligation.

For those patients who survive a first variceal bleed, the risk of rebleeding is very high (>60%) and therefore secondary prevention is required. Various options exist for secondary prevention and include pharmacological agents, endoscopic therapy, TIPSS, or surgical shunting.

Pharmacological agents that have been shown to decrease rebleeding rate and bleeding-related mortality, as well as decreasing overall mortality, are nonselective β blockers such as propranolol or nadolol [4]. The mainstay of endoscopic therapy is variceal band ligation, because injection sclerotherapy is now less commonly used due to frequent and severe side effects [5]. TIPSS has been shown to be better than endoscopic therapy in the prevention of variceal rebleeding, but it is not associated with any survival benefit to justify the extra costs involved [6]. There is also an increased risk of encephalopathy after TIPSS insertion. TIPSS remains, however, very valuable to control acute bleeding not responding to endoscopic therapy. Surgical shunts are rarely performed today, because the use of polytetrafluoroethylene (PTFE) stents has significantly decreased TIPSS occlusion rates.

Gastric varices are less common and bleed less frequently than esophageal varices, but when they do bleed they tend to bleed more profusely and are associated with higher transfusion requirements and mortality [7]. The best treatment strategy for bleeding gastric or ectopic varices has not been determined, because most of the available literature consists of small studies with no randomized control studies available. Treatment options for bleeding gastric varices include, injection sclerotherapy with cyanoacrylate, thrombin, and TIPSS. Clinical characteristics of esophageal and gastric varices are very different and this is therefore why the management of each is different. Gastric varices are more deeply seated (submucosa) and are deemed "true veins"; therefore treatment with variceal band ligation is less effective and believed to be associated with rebleeding.

Another simple measure that improves outcome post-variceal hemorrhage and is associated with improved survival is the administration of prophylactic antibiotics for 4–10 days after the initial bleed [8].

In this case of cirrhosis secondary to alcoholic liver disease, it is important to stress to the patient that complete cessation of alcohol is required; abstinence from alcohol has been demonstrated to decrease the incidence of complications in cirrhosis and can result in increased survival [9].

Case 2: abdominal distension in a diabetic patient

Case presentation

A 62-year-old retired mechanic was referred for admission by his general practitioner, after presenting with a 3-week history of increasing abdominal distension and ankle swelling. He also complained of nausea, poor appetite, and dizziness but denied any weight loss or falls. He had no history of liver prob-

lems, but had a background history of poorly controlled type 2 diabetes mellitus, with known retinopathy and mild renal impairment. He also had a history of hypercholesterolemia and hypertension.

With regard to risk factors for liver disease, he denied any previous blood transfusions, tattoos, or high-risk behavior. Alcohol intake was less than 5 units per week and he denied any previous excess. He had had no recent travel and all contacts were well.

Current drug therapy was aspirin 75 mg, metformin 1 g twice daily, gliclazide 80 mg twice daily, simvastatin 40 mg, losartan 50 mg twice daily, and bendrofluazide 5 mg. No documented drug allergy was recorded but he was noted to be previously intolerant of angiotensin-converting enzyme (ACE) inhibitors. He was an ex-smoker for the last 5 years.

On clinical examination he was obese with an estimated BMI of 34, although this was an overestimate due to the presence of ascites.

He was mildly jaundiced with few spider nevi and bilateral Dupuytren's contractures. No flapping tremor.

Temperature 38.5°C

Basal metabolism (BM) 5.2 mmol/L

Cardiovascular: HR 98 beats/min, sinus rhythm; BP 92/48 mmHg; jugular venous pressure not elevated; heart sounds normal; bilateral pitting edema to mid-calf level

Respiratory: O_2 saturation was 94% on room air. Respiratory Rate was 16. Good air entry bilaterally but decreased air entry right base.

Abdomen: moderately distended; soft and non-tender with no masses palpable; bulging flanks. shifting dullness; bowel sounds reduced; rectal examination normal

CNS: alert and oriented: Abbreviated Mental Test score 10/10; no focal limb weakness with bilateral downgoing plantars

Investigations (normal values in brackets)
Bilirubin 52 (3–16) μmol/L
Hb 120 (130–180) g/L
Na$^+$ 127 (135–145) mmol/L
K$^+$ 3.2 (3.5–5.0) mmol/L
ALT 58 (10–50) U/L
MCV 86 (78–98) fL
Bicarbonate 22 (22–30) mmol/L
ALP 125 (40–125) U/L
WCC 17.5 (4–11) × 10^9/L

Urea 8.7 (2.5–6.6) mmol/L
GGT 158 (5–35) U/L
Platelets 58 (150–350) × 10⁹/L
Creatinine 192 (60–120) μmol/L
Albumin 29 (35–50) g/L
PT 16 (10.2–12.7) s
Chest radiograph: elevation of right hemidiaphragm and small right pleural effusion
  Abdominal radiograph: general haziness

Questions

- What is your differential diagnosis?
- How would you investigate this patient further?
- What is your initial management of this patient?
- What complications is he at risk from?

Differential diagnosis

Obvious abdominal distension can be due to fluid, fat, flatus, feces, or fetus! Free fluid is usually relatively easy to identify clinically with shifting dullness and a fluid thrill. The umbilicus is often everted.

Ascites in cirrhosis indicates liver failure and is the most likely diagnosis in this case. The patient was diagnosed with non-alcoholic fatty liver disease (NAFLD)-related cirrhosis in view of the history of type 2 diabetes mellitus and no significant alcohol intake.

The presence of ascites in patients with cirrhosis has important prognostic significance; 50% of patients who develop ascites will die within 2 years so these patients should be referred for consideration for liver transplantation. Classification of ascites is preferably based on serum–albumin ascites gradient (SAAG) which has replaced the older transudate–exudate classification and is linked to the presence of portal hypertension. SAAG is calculated by subtracting the albumin content of the ascitic fluid from the serum albumin level obtained from blood samples taken at approximately the same time. A SAAG result of ≥11g/L is strongly suggestive of portal hypertension, but it should also be remembered that it can be found in ascites due to right heart failure or constrictive pericarditis. Table 15.2 lists other causes of ascites as classified by SAAG gradient.

Ascites occurs in patients with portal hypertension as a result of splanchnic arteriolar vasodilation caused

Table 15.2 Classification of ascites by serum–albumin ascites gradient (SAAG)

SAAG ≥ 11 g/L	SAAG ≤ 11 g/L
Portal hypertension	Hypoalbuminemia
Liver cirrhosis of any cause	nephrotic syndrome (of any cause)
Fulminant liver failure	protein-losing enteropathy
extensive hepatic metastases	severe malnutrition
Budd–Chiari syndrome	
Congestive cardiac failure	Diseased peritoneum:
	(a) infections – bacterial peritonitis, fungal peritonitis, tuberculous peritonitis
	(b) malignancy: – peritoneal carcinomatosis – primary mesothelioma – hepatocellular carcinoma
Constrictive pericarditis	Miscellaneous
	chylous ascites
	pancreatic ascites
	vasculitis
	granulomatous peritonitis
	eosinophilic peritonitis
Tricuspid regurgitation	

by increased production of nitric oxide thus resulting in a reduction in circulating blood volume; this induces compensatory activation of the renin–angiotensin–aldosterone system (RAAS), hypersecretion of antidiuretic hormone (ADH), and increased production of lymph fluid. This mechanism also explains why dilutional hyponatremia is common in these patients. Fluid preferentially collects within the abdomen because of the portal hypertension.

In patients with cirrhosis, examination may reveal the stigmata of chronic liver disease, dilated periumbilical veins, umbilical hernias, and palpable splenomegaly in addition to the presence of ascites. A pleural effusion may also be present which commonly occurs on the right side.

All patients with ascites should have a diagnostic ascitic tap performed not only to assess the SAAG but also to actively exclude the presence of spontaneous bacterial peritonitis (SBP). Approximately 10% of patients with ascites in hospital have SBP (defined as the presence of >250 neutrophils/mL). Many do not complain of pain or tenderness and will be missed without a diagnostic tap. All patients should therefore have fluid sent off for urgent Gram staining, cell count, and culture. If there is any suggestion of malignancy, fluid should be sent for cytology. The presence of ascites is often confirmed with abdominal ultrasonography, which also provides useful diagnostic information such as the overall appearance of the liver parenchyma, the presence or absence of focal lesions, portal vein flow, and degree of splenomegaly.

The patient underwent an ascitic tap and abdominal ultrasonography. A full liver screen was also completed with the results listed below:

ANA negative
ANCA negative
HBsAg negative
HBsAb negative
HCVAb negative
SMA negative
AMA negative
α_1-Antitrypsin 2.12 (1.5–3.5) g/L
Ferritin 379 (20–250) μg/L
Transferrin saturation 26 (22–40)%
Ceruloplasmin 0.24 (<0.35) g/L
AFP 5 (<5) μg/L

Ascitic tap results
RBCs 32
WCC 120×10^9/L, mainly lymphocytes
Gram stain – no organisms seen
MC&S (microscopy, culture, and sensitivity) – no growth
Glucose 5 mmol/L
Albumin 12 g/L

Abdominal ultrasound report
Liver appeared shrunken but echo bright with a coarse irregular outline. No focal abnormality in the liver parenchyma was identified. Spleen size was increased at 14 cm. Moderate amount of ascites present. Hepatic and portal veins appeared patent.

Patient management
He was given dietary advice about his salt intake (i.e. no added salt) and started on spironolactone 100 mg daily. After a week on the ward, only a mild reduction was noted in his weight so his diuretics were titrated up to furosemide 80 mg daily and spironolactone 200 mg daily. This resulted in some improvement and he was therefore mobilized. Unfortunately just before discharge he became pyrexial. A septic screen was performed which included an ascitic tap and confirmed the presence of *Escherichia coli* SBP. He was commenced on intravenous ceftriaxone 2 g daily and after 5 days was changed to oral ciprofloxacin. He was subsequently started on long-term oral co-trimoxazole 960 mg once daily as prophylaxis against SBP. He declined referral for liver transplantation.

Unfortunately this patient was readmitted 3 weeks later after generally feeling unwell and complaining of fevers and diarrhea. Stool cultures grew *Clostridium difficile* and was toxin positive. The co-trimoxazole was stopped and metronidazole started. He was noted to be oligouric with a serum creatinine of 370 μmol/L. Despite appropriate fluid resuscitation he remained oliguric with a serum creatinine of 350 μmol/L.

Discussion

SBP is defined as an infection of the ascitic fluid in patients with underlying cirrhosis with the presence of >250 neutrophils/mL. Its exact pathogenesis is uncertain but increased gut permeability and delayed intestinal transit are thought to be key factors because these factors promote bacterial translocation to mesenteric lymph nodes. The lifetime risk of a cirrhotic patient developing SBP is up to 33% [10] and SBP is especially common in patients with cirrhosis who are in hospital. The long-term prognosis for patients with SBP is poor, with mortality rates in excess of 70% reported at 2 years [11]. Patients who have therefore recovered from an episode of SBP should be considered for liver transplantation.

Risk factors for SBP include severity of liver disease, large-volume ascites (as it is associated with low ascitic fluid albumin levels, and thus low opsonic activity), and a previous episode of SBP. The risk of recurrence of SBP is high and has been reported to be up to 70% in the first year [12].

Treatment of SBP is with intravenous antibiotics, mainly third-generation cephalosporins such as cefotaxime or ceftriaxone. Intravenous albumin has also been shown recently to be very beneficial by reducing the incidence of complications such as hepatorenal syndrome (HRS) and may significantly improve survival [13]. Secondary prophylaxis is indicated in all patients with a documented episode of SBP, with quinolones being the oral antibiotic of choice [14]. However, quinolones have been associated with increase risk of *Cl. difficile* and therefore alternatives include co-trimoxazole 960 mg once daily, but the evidence is not as strong as that with norfloxacin.

The differential diagnosis of this patient's renal dysfunction is acute renal failure secondary to dehydration ± acute tubular necrosis and HRS. Given the history of recent SBP and poor response to rehydration, HRS is more likely.

HRS occurs in patients with portal hypertension and is characterized by renal vasoconstriction and progressive renal failure without any structural kidney abnormalities. The marked renal vasoconstriction is thought to be the end-result of splanchnic vasodilation, activation of the RAAS and sympathetic nervous system, along with local vasoconstrictors.

HRS is subdivided into two groups according to the clinical course and severity:
1 Type 1: defined by a rapid doubling of serum creatinine to >2.5 mg/dL (220 μmol/L) or a reduction in creatinine clearance of >50% within 2 weeks. This is the most severe type with poor prognosis if left untreated. It often develops after a trigger, e.g. SBP, alcoholic hepatitis, large-volume paracentesis without albumin replacement, or following a variceal bleed.
2 Type 2: defined as a slower decline in renal function and usually seen in patients with refractory ascites. It has a better prognosis.

The diagnosis of HRS is based on the exclusion of other causes of renal impairment (e.g. dehydration, hemorrhagic or septic shock, and nephrotoxic drugs) and the presence of major or minor criteria as developed by International Ascites Club [15] as detailed in Box 15.1.

The treatment of HRS involves removal of all nephrotoxic drugs including diuretics and a fluid challenge with human albumin solution (1 mg/kg) to ensure adequate intravascular filling. Central venous pressure (CVP) monitoring is often helpful to avoid fluid overload. If no improvement occurs, splanchnic vaso-

---

Box 15.1 International Ascites Club's diagnostic criteria for hepatorenal syndrome

Major criteria

Chronic or acute liver disease with advanced hepatic failure and portal hypertension

Low glomerular filtration rate as indicated by serum creatinine >1.5 mg/dL or 24-hour creatinine clearance >40 mL/min

Absence of shock, infection, and current or recent nephrotoxic drugs

No sustained improvement in renal function following diuretic withdrawal and expansion of plasma volume with 1.5 L isotonic saline

Proteinuria<500 mg/dL

No ultrasound evidence of parenchymal renal disease or obstructive uropathy

Minor criteria

Low urine volume (<500 mL in 24 h)

Low urinary sodium (<10 mmol/L)

Urine osmolarity > serum osmolarity

Absence of red blood cells in urine (<50 per high power field)

Serum sodium <130 mmol/L

---

constrictors such as terlipressin have been shown to be effective, particularly when used in combination with albumin [16].

Diagnostic paracentesis is important to exclude SBP, but large-volume paracentesis should be avoided because this may precipitate further hypovolemia and deterioration of kidney function.

If, despite the above measures, improvement is not seen, renal replacement therapy, albumin dialysis (molecular adsorbent recirculating system or MARS), TIPSS insertion, or liver transplantation should be considered.

Case 3: confusion in a patient with chronic liver disease

Case presentation

A 54-year-old unemployed secretary was admitted from A&E after falling at home while her son was assisting her to the toilet. Her son reported that she had become increasingly confused over the past 3 days and had been bed bound for the last 48 hours. He noticed that his mother had a fever and had been incontinent of urine. She had not been eating or drinking anything for the last 36 hours. He was unaware of any seizure activity or any recent head injury, but did report that his mother had increasingly poor mobility and a fall 1 week ago. No history was available from the patient.

Her son reported that his mother had a long history of alcohol excess and estimated her current alcohol intake to be half to a full bottle of gin per night. He thought that his mother last had some alcohol 4–5 days ago. He stated that his mother had been admitted 2 years ago with alcohol withdrawal seizures while she was away visiting her sister. He also informed medical staff that his mother had been told by numerous doctors previously to abstain from alcohol and that she had declined to engage in alcohol support services. He was unaware of any other medical problems and reported that she was on no regular medication.

Examination
Mildly jaundiced with multiple spider nevi and marked asterixis. Decreased skin turgor with dry mucous membranes
BM 4.8 mmol/L
Temperature = 38.5°C
Cardiovascular: heart rate 104 beats/min sinus rhythm; BP 94/62 mmHg; heart sounds normal
Respiratory: good air entry bilaterally with no focal signs
Abdomen: soft, mildly tender right upper quadrant with 4 cm smooth liver edge palpable below costal margin. No evidence of ascites. Bowel sounds normal. Rectal examination: hard stool at upper end.
CNS: disoriented to time, place, and person. Glasgow Coma Scale (GCS) E3, V4, M4 = 11. Fundi normal. Neck supple. Difficult to assess cranial nerves as patient non-compliant with examination. No focal deficit but reduced power globally with brisk reflexes. Plantars upgoing bilaterally

Investigations (normal values in brackets)
Bilirubin 98 (3–16) µmol/L
Hb 104 (130–180) g/L

MCV 108 (78–98) fL
Na^+ 130 (135–145) mmol/L
K^+ 2.9 (3.5–5.0) mmol/L
Bicarbonate 24 (22–30) mmol/L
ALT 55 (10–50) U/L
GGT 621 (5–35) U/L
ALP 125 (40–125) U/L
WCC 14.7 (4–11) × 10^9/L
Urea 11.2 (2.5–6.6) mmol/L
Platelets 110 (150–350) × 10^9/L
Creatinine 67 (60–120) µmol/L
Albumin 29 (35–50) g/L
PT 16 (10.2–12.7) s
ECG sinus tachycardia
Chest radiograph normal

Questions

• What is your differential diagnosis?
• How would you initially manage this patient?
• What investigations would you like to perform?
• What is your subsequent management of this patient?

Differential diagnosis

This woman has chronic liver disease with the development of portal hypertension secondary to alcoholic liver disease, as indicated from the history and the demonstration of high MCV and GGT, low platelets and albumin, with a prolonged prothrombin time. In any patient who is confused and possibly could have had a recent head injury, it is important to exclude any intracranial bleeding, especially a subdural hematoma.

In a patient with liver disease it is also important to exclude any reversible metabolic cause such as hypoglycemia (which can also signify liver failure) and hyponatremia.

All patients with pre-existing liver disease are at risk of developing hepatic encephalopathy as the liver disease progresses. Differential diagnoses for hepatic encephalopathy are listed in Table 15.3.

Patients with hepatic encephalopathy can present with a variety of clinical features ranging from minimal confusion and disorientation to life-threatening coma. Its progression can be rapid and in general mirrors liver function or removal of precipitating factors (Table 15.4).

Table 15.3 Differential diagnosis of confusion in pre-existing liver disease

Differential diagnosis	Examples
Metabolic encephalopathies	Hypoglycemia
	Hypoxia or hypercapnia
	Hyponatremia or hypernatremia
Drugs/ toxins	Alcohol (intoxication and withdrawal)
	Sedatives (e.g. benzodiazepines)
Intracranial structural abnormalities	Subdural hematoma
	Subarachnoid hemorrhage
	Space-occupying lesion (including cerebral abscess)
	Cerebrovascular accident
Infection	Encephalitis
	Meningitis
Miscellaneous	Wernicke's encephalopathy
	Seizures
	Head injury

Table 15.4 Precipitating factors for hepatic encephalopathy

Etiology	Precipitating factor
Increased protein load	Upper gastrointestinal hemorrhage
	Ingestion of large protein meal
Decreased ammonia excretion	Constipation
	Renal failure
Infective	Urinary tract infection
	Spontaneous bacterial peritonitis
	Infective diarrhea
	Lower respiratory tract infection
	Skin infections (cellulitis)
Metabolic	Dehydration
	Electrolyte disturbance, e.g. hypokalemia
	Drugs, e.g. sedatives
Other	Large-volume paracentesis without adequate volume replacement
	Creation of portosystemic shunts, e.g. TIPSS

TIPSS, transjugular intrahepatic portosystemic stent.

In patients with chronic liver disease, an episode of acute encephalopathy is often characterized by acute confusion, neuromuscular abnormalities, and fetor hepaticus (a sweet musty smell on the breath which arises due to unmetabolized mercaptans). Asterixis (or liver flap) is often present with brisk tendon reflexes. Neurological signs of variable severity are sometimes present, but do not fit into a unifying focal neurological diagnosis.

Patient management

The patient was initially rehydrated with intravenous fluids and a full septic screen performed. In view of the history of a recent fall and the inability to clarify the history, a CT scan of the head was performed to exclude a subdural hemorrhage. A liver screen (including an abdominal ultrasound scan) was also performed to exclude other causes of cirrhosis.

All outstanding results listed below:
HBV/HCV negative
ANA/AMA/SMA/ANCA negative
α_1-Antitrypsin and ceruloplasmin levels: normal
Ferritin 895 µg/L (normal <150)
CRP 205 mg/L
MSU report: *E. coli* sensitive to ciprofloxacillin
Abdominal ultrasound scan: small shrunken liver with irregular contour consistent with chronic liver disease. Spleen size increased at 14 cm. No ascites demonstrated. Hepatic and portal vessels patent

CT scan of the brain: general atrophy which is advanced for patient's age. No focal lesion demonstrated. No evidence of intracranial hemorrhage

This woman had acute hepatic encephalopathy that was precipitated by an *E. coli* urinary tract infection and dehydration. She made a quick and complete recovery after receiving intravenous fluids and intravenous antibiotics. She was referred to alcohol liaison services and entered into an hepatocelllular carcinoma and variceal surveillance program with regular outpatient review.

Discussion

Hepatic encephalopathy is a reversible neuropsychiatric syndrome, which may complicate acute or chronic liver failure. Its presence signifies liver failure and should prompt consideration for liver transplantation. The diagnosis is essentially clinical but in difficult cases further investigation may be required with the use of electroencephalography (EEG), positron emission tomography (PET), or electrophysiological tests such as visual or brain-stem auditory evoked potentials [17]. Most of these investigations are, however, used largely as research tools.

Hepatic encephalopathy may be subclassified according to onset of symptoms and etiology of liver disease.

Acute encephalopathy secondary to chronic liver disease
This is commonly seen in clinical practice and its features have been described earlier in this case.

Acute encephalopathy in fulminant liver failure
The features of this are essentially the same as for acute encephalopathy secondary to chronic liver disease, but cerebral edema and elevated intracranial pressure (as signified by bradycardia, hypertension, dilated pupils, and decerebrate posturing) are more commonly seen in this patient group.

Subclinical encephalopathy
This term is used to describe the mild brain dysfunction that can be commonly overlooked during routine clinical examination because it results in subtle changes in visuospatial and psychomotor abilities. These abnormalities can be identified from simple psychometric tests such as digit symbol substitution and number connection. Asking the patient to draw a five-pointed star is also useful to identify visuospatial abnormalities.

Chronic persisting encephalopathy
This term is used to describe patients with chronic liver disease who have previously had recurrent episodes of acute encephalopathy and then go on to develop persistent neurological manifestations that range from ataxia and dysarthria to parkinsonism and advanced dementia.

The exact pathogenesis of hepatic encephalopathy remains unclear but it is widely accepted that failure of hepatic detoxification of gut-derived toxins plays a key role. This results from splanchnic venous blood bypassing the liver due to intra- and extrahepatic shunting which occurs in portal hypertension. It has also been suggested that elevated levels of circulating toxins in the central nervous system is the result of a blood–brain barrier with an abnormal or increased permeability [18]. The toxins that have been implicated are ammonia (glutamine–glutamate cycle), manganese, mercaptans, short-chain fatty acids, and aromatic amino acids.

The treatment of hepatic encephalopathy consists of general treatment measures such as adequate hydration and withdrawal of precipitating factors as listed in Table 15.4. A reduction of gut protein/nitrogen load has also been shown to be beneficial and this can be achieved by dietary measures (e.g. low-protein diet), but this unbalanced diet is not advised long term because it will lead to malnutrition. Vegetable protein is beneficial because this is thought to be less ammoniagenic and is associated with high fiber content, which promotes bowel movement and therefore elimination of nitrogenous waste.

Pharmacological measures revolve around non-digestible saccharides such as lactulose, which is the most commonly used and has dual action: metabolism of lactulose by gut bacteria results in lowering of colonic pH, thus enhancing formation of the non-absorbable NH_4^+ from NH_3 and reduction of plasma NH_3 concentration; and it is not absorbed by gut and its action as an osmotic laxative not only reduces the concentration of ammonia-forming gut bacteria, but also results in increased fecal nitrogen elimination.

The evidence base for their use is, however, poor. A reduction in gut flora using poorly absorbed antibiotics such as neomycin has also been shown to be beneficial but long-term use is associated with nephrotoxicity and ototoxicity, so its use is limited.

A newer agent, which is being increasingly used, is high-dose L-ornithine-L-aspartate (LOLA). LOLA has been shown to significantly decrease ammonia levels, and improve mental state parameters and EEG activity [19].

Another new agent is rifaximin, which is a minimally absorbed antibiotic that has been shown to be more effective than lactulose in the treatment of overt hepatic encephalopathy. A large double-blind, placebo-controlled trial has confirmed that rifaximin reduced the risk of an episode of overt hepatic encephalopathy over a 6-month period with no serious adverse events [20].

Conclusion

These three cases highlight the challenges of managing patients with liver cirrhosis and portal hypertension. All patients presenting with ascites, encephalopathy or variceal bleeding have significant portal hypertension associated with advanced liver disease and it is not uncommon that all three manifestations are present in many patients admitted to hospital. Due to the high mortality of portal hypertension-associated complications, specialized management in a critical care setting is recommended. Careful follow-up after the first episode of portal hypertension-related complications is important to address clinical issues such as variceal surveillance, fluid balance, prevention of infection, and nutritional support. Early consideration of liver transplantation, if there are no contraindications, is important to ensure longer-term survival.

References

1 D'Amico G, Luca A. Natural history. Clinical–haemodynamic correlations. Prediction of the risk of bleeding. *Baillière's Clin Gastroenterol* 1997;**11**: 243–56.

2 D'Amico G, Pagliaro L, Bosch J. The treatment of portal hypertension: a meta analytic review. *Hepatology* 1995;**22**:332–54.

3 The North Italian Endoscopic Club for the Study and Treatment of Esophageal Varices. Prediction of the first variceal hemorrhage in patients with cirrhosis of the liver and esophageal varices. A prospective multicenter study. *N Engl J Med* 1988;**319**:983–9.

4 Casado M, Bosch J, Garcia-Pagan JC, et al. Clinical events after transjugular intrahepatic portosystemic shunt: correlation with hemodynamic findings. *Gastroenterology* 1998;**114**:1296–303.

5 Garcia-Pagan JC, Bosch J. Endoscopic band ligation in the treatment of portal hypertension. *Nat Clin Pract Gastroenterol Hepatol* 2005;**2**:526–35.

6 Burroughs AK, Vangeli M. Transjugular intrahepatic portosystemic shunt versus endoscopic therapy: randomized trials for secondary prophylaxis of variceal bleeding: an updated meta-analysis. *Scand J Gastoenterol* 2002;**37**:249–52.

7 Sarin SK, Lahoti D, Saxena SP, et al. Prevalence, classification and natural history of gastric varices: a long-term follow-up study in 568 portal hypertension patients. *Hepatology* 1992;**16**:1343–9.

8 Rolando N, Gimson A, Philpott-Howard J, et al. Infectious sequelae after endoscopic sclerotherapy of oesophageal varices: role of antibiotic prophylaxis. *J Hepatol* 1993;**18**:290–294.

9 Tome S, Lucey MR. Review article: current management of alcoholic liver disease. *Aliment Pharmacol Ther* 2004;**19**:707–14.

10 Sheer TA, Runyon BA. Spontaneous bacterial peritonitis. *Dig Dis* 2005;**23**:39–46.

11 Rimola A, García-Tsao G, Navasa M, et al. Diagnosis, treatment and prophylaxis of spontaneous bacterial peritonitis: a consensus document. International Ascites Club. *J Hepatol* 2000;**32**:142–53.

12 Garcia TG. Identifying new risk factors for spontaneous bacterial peritonitis: how important is it? *Gastroenterology* 1999;**117**:495–9.

13 Sort P, Navasa M, Arroyo V, et al. Effect of intravenous albumin on renal impairment and mortality in patients with cirrhosis and spontaneous bacterial peritonitis. *N Engl J Med* 1999;**341**:403–9.

14 Gentilini P, Casini-Raggi V, Di Fiore G, et al. Albumin improves the response to diuretics in patients with cirrhosis and ascites: results of a randomized control trial. *J Hepatol* 1999;**30**:639–45.

15 Arroyo V, Gines P, Gerbes A, et al. Definition and diagnostic criteria of refractory ascites and hepatorenal syndrome in cirrhosis. International Ascites Club. *Hepatology* 1996;**23**:164–76.

16 Ortega R, Gines P, Uriz J, et al. Terlipressin therapy with and without albumin for patients with hepatorenal syn-

drome: results of a prospective, nonrandomized study. *Hepatology* 2002;**36**:941–8.

17 Davies MG, Rowan MJ, Feely J. Hepatic encephalopathy – a brief review. *Irish J Psychol Med* 1991;**8**:144–6.

18 Mas A. Hepatic encephalopathy: from pathophysiology to treatment. *Digestion* 2006;**73**(suppl 1):86–93.

19 Kircheis G, Wettstein M, Dahl S, et al. Clinical efficacy of L-ornithine-L-aspartate in the management of hepatic encephalopathy. *Metab Brain Dis* 2002;**17**:453–62.

20 Bass NM, Mullen KD, Sanyal, A et al. Rifaximin treatment in hepatic encephalopathy. *N Engl J Med* 2010;**362**:1071–81.

16 Infections in the Liver

Veerendra Sandur and George Therapondos

Multiorgan Transplant Program, Toronto General Hospital, University Health Network, University of Toronto, Ontario, Canada

Case 1: infections in the post-transplantation immunocompromised patient

Case presentation

A 66-year-old Egyptian man with chronic hepatitis C virus (HCV) infection was diagnosed with hepatic encephalopathy and ascites related to cirrhosis. He had not previously been treated with antiviral therapy. His other medical problems were type 2 diabetes mellitus and hypertension. After a careful evaluation, he was placed on the liver transplant waiting list and underwent cadaveric donor split liver transplant, but unfortunately he developed hepatic artery thrombosis and was retransplanted 3 months later. The early postoperative course was uneventful.

Six weeks afterwards, he presented with intermittent, low-grade fever and decreased appetite.

Medications included prednisone, cyclosporine, insulin, metoprolol, and omeprazole.

Examination revealed the following:

Height 170 cm
Weight 63 kg
BMI 21 kg/m²
Temperature 38°C
Mild jaundice
Cardiovascular: pulse 102 beats/min, BP 140/82 mmHg; heart sounds normal with no added sounds
Respiratory: normal examination

Gastrointestinal: abdomen soft, mild hepatomegaly 2 cm firm, non-tender
Splenomegaly 16 cm, small amount of ascites; bowel sounds normal
CNS: conscious, oriented; no flap or tremor

Investigations (normal values in brackets)
Hb 8.8 (13.5–17.5) g/dL
WCC 14.7 (4–11) × 10⁹/L
Platelets 330 (150–400) × 10⁹/L
AST 79 (10–40) IU/L
ALT 119 (5–30) IU/L
Bilirubin 32 (2–17) μmol/L
Albumin 32 (35–55) g/L
ALP 531 (30–130) IU/L
INR 1.4 (0.9–1.2)
Glucose 6.6 (3.5–5.5) mmol/L
Creatinine 97 (50–120) μmol/L
Na⁺ 137 (135–145) mmol/L
K⁺ 3.6 (3.5–5.0) mmol/L
Cyclosporin level: within target limits
Chest radiograph normal

Ultrasound scan report
Liver has a normal appearance with unremarkable Doppler evaluation of the portal veins, hepatic artery and hepatic veins. The bile ducts are not dilated. There are two large peritransplant collections; the first at the epigastrium measuring at 1.7 × 3.8 × 7.4 cm and a second at approximately the midclavicular

Problem-based Approach to Gastroenterology and Hepatology, First Edition. Edited by John N. Plevris, Colin W. Howden.
© 2012 Blackwell Publishing Ltd. Published 2012 by Blackwell Publishing Ltd.

line measuring at $7.9 \times 6.2 \times 5.2$ cm. The spleen is enlarged measuring at 16 cm. A small amount of free fluid is noted within the pelvis. Pancreas and kidneys normal.

Bacterial infection and acute cellular rejection were ruled out and he was found to have CMV infection (positive CMV pp65 antigenemia).

Clinical progress

After successful treatment (see below), his fever recurred 3 months later and on this occasion the ultrasound scan of his abdomen showed multiple small hypodense lesions in the liver parenchyma (largest measuring 2×1.8 cm). The infrahepatic collection was significantly decreased in size and measured 4×3 cm. CT confirmed these lesions and suggested that they were intrahepatic abscesses.

Blood cultures were negative. Ultrasound-guided aspiration of abscesses was performed and a small amount of red-colored material was obtained and sent for culture and sensitivity. A liver biopsy was also performed at the same time and showed granulomatous inflammation with alcohol and acid-fast bacilli typical of tuberculosis. Culture later confirmed *Mycobacterium tuberculosis*. Unfortunately, despite appropriate quadruple treatment for 3 months, he deteriorated further and died.

Questions

- What are the possible causes of fever in this patient on the first and second occasions of this presentation?
- What other investigations are necessary to establish the diagnosis and aid decisions on further management?
- What therapeutic interventions would be necessary in similar cases?

Differential diagnosis

First presentation
The main causes of fever in a patient in the early post-liver transplantation period that need to be excluded are:
- Postoperative sepsis – bacteremia from a variety of sources, e.g. urinary tract, skin, lungs, and biliary tract (especially in biliary structuring). Intra-abdominal infection (especially if ascites is present) must also be excluded (abdominal collections are common postoperatively and are not *necessarily* a cause of sepsis).
- Opportunistic infections:
  - viral: cytomegalovirus virus (CMV) infection, Epstein–Barr virus (EBV) infection, herpes virus infection
  - fungal: *Pneumocystic jiroveci (carinii)* pneumonia, aspergillosis
- Post-transplantation lymphoproliferative disorder (PTLD)
- Reactivation of previous dormant chronic infections (tuberculosis, herpes zoster)
- Acute cellular rejection
- Drug-related fever (uncommon).

Second presentation
In this situation, all of the above diagnoses are possible, although the presence of intrahepatic small abscesses is unlikely to be due to viral infection, rejection, or PTLD. Although these conditions may coexist, bacterial or fungal infections must be considered as the most likely.

Diagnosis

This case illustrates the unusual types of infection that can affect the liver in immunosuppressed hosts such as transplant recipients.

First presentation
The diagnosis on this occasion was CMV infection which was made by the detection of CMV antigenemia in the blood. The liver biopsy added confirmatory evidence by showing the typical changes of CMV infection, although the absence of these changes does not exclude the disease (Figure 16.1).

Blood and urine cultures for bacteremia and fungemia were consistently negative and the CT scan also identified the intra-abdominal collections seen on ultrasound, which are a common finding post-surgery. Ultrasound-guided aspiration of these perihepatic collections yielded no growth. Acute cellular rejection was a possibility, given the slight increase in aminotransferases but was ruled out with the liver biopsy. There was no other evidence of local infection focus to support an alternative diagnosis at this stage, and he was therefore treated with intravenous ganciclovir

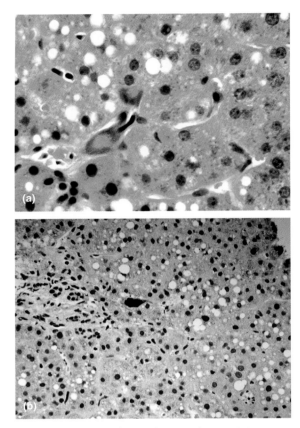

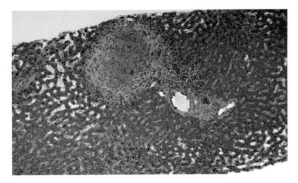

Figure 16.2 Typical liver tuberculosis granuloma. (Image courtesy of Dr Oyedele Adeyi.)

Figure 16.1 (a) Liver biopsy showing characteristic cytomegalovirus (CMV) inclusion body; (b) immunohistochemistry of the same biopsy. (Images courtesy of Dr Oyedele Adeyi.)

which cleared his CMV antigenemia and resolved his fever and other symptoms within 4 days.

CMV infection in immunocompetent individuals is common but is generally asymptomatic. Occasional organ-specific complications such as hepatitis have been reported and elevated aminotransferases are a common finding although rarely severe [1]. In immunocompetent hosts, CMV infection is generally self-limited with complete recovery over a period of days to weeks.

In immunosuppressed hosts, and specifically in the case of liver transplant (LT) recipients, CMV infection is a relatively common complication as well as the single most important viral pathogen. CMV has been shown to predispose to acute and chronic rejection, HCV recurrence, and susceptibility to other opportunistic infections. In addition, it is known that delayed-onset CMV disease after liver transplantation is associated with increased mortality [2].

CMV can present with fever, myelosuppression, and malaise as well as with tissue-invasive disease such as gastrointestinal problems, hepatitis, pneumonitis, CNS disease, and retinitis.

The most common predisposing factor for CMV disease after liver transplantation is lack of immunity and therefore the patients most at risk are the donor-positive/recipient-negative combinations (D+ve/R−ve).

The ease of diagnosis has recently been greatly enhanced by the availability of polymerase chain reaction (PCR) assays which can be used in most clinical scenarios [3], although not in the presented case. Strategies currently used against CMV infection include preemptive therapy as well as antiviral prophylaxis with ganciclovir or valganciclovir in high-risk patients (those who are D+ve/R−ve or those who received induction therapy with anti-thymocyte globulin).

Second presentation
The history and ethnic or travel background of the patient may be relevant in cases such as this one. The diagnosis of tuberculosis (TB) can be difficult in cases that do not show the typical chest radiograph findings. This patient showed the liver biopsy changes of TB (Figure 16.2) and the diagnosis was indeed confirmed by culture of the material aspirated form the hepatic abscesses. TB infection attacks various tissues

or organs, including the lung, lymph nodes, vertebral column, pancreas, and liver. Making a diagnosis of TB can be difficult because of the atypical clinical presentation, especially among those with other bacterial or fungal infections. TB is an important although relatively uncommon cause of morbidity and mortality among solid organ transplant recipients.

Patient management

This patient had HCV chronic infection which ultimately led to decompensated cirrhosis, transplantation, retransplantation, and subsequent opportunistic infections that caused his death.

Hepatitis C infection continues to be a major disease burden worldwide and is estimated to affect approximately 170 million people. There is a difference in prevalence between countries. In Europe, the general prevalence is about 1%, although it is more common in southern Europe (approximately 4.6%). In North America, the prevalence rate is 1.7%, in south-east Asia 2.15%, and in Africa 5.3%, although there are some very wide variations in some countries (e.g. Egypt 28%) [4].

HCV is divided into six genotypes with numerous subtypes. Genotype 1 is the most dominant genotype in North America and Europe, whereas genotype 3 is the most common genotype on the Indian subcontinent. Genotype 4 is most commonly found in Africa and the Middle East [4].

HCV infection is diagnosed by the presence of anti-HCV antibody but the presence of active ongoing infection needs to be documented by the finding of HCV RNA (PCR technique), which enables genotyping and measurement of viral load. It is recommended that all patients with chronic HCV be assessed to determine whether they may benefit from therapy [5].

The decision to treat with antiviral therapy can be complex and is guided by the risk:benefit ratio for each individual patient. Response depends mostly on genotype and viral load and is adversely affected by the presence of significant fibrosis and especially cirrhosis. The patient's ability to tolerate antiviral therapy and compliance are also important [5].

Treatment consists of pegylated interferon (weekly injections) and ribavirin (oral daily) for a period that again depends on genotype (genotypes 1 and 4 need longer treatment than genotypes 2 and 3). Successful treatment is achieved in approximately 45–50% in genotype 1 patients and in 85% in patients with genotype 2/3 disease. Treatment regimes continuously evolve (e.g. triple schemes using protease inhibitors) and this can significantly impact response rates.

Hepatitis C infection is the most common indication for liver transplantation in the developed world but invariably recurs after liver transplantation.

Liver transplant recipients are predisposed to opportunistic infections due to their immunocompromised status. As the symptoms are often masked by immunosuppression, the diagnosis may be delayed.

The most common clinical manifestation of TB is pleuropulmonary disease, accounting for approximately 60% of the infected cases among solid organ transplant recipients [6,7]. Tuberculous liver abscesses are rare. When present they are usually associated with a focus of infection in the lung or gastrointestinal tract, and bacteria probably reach the subcapsular region of liver through hematogenous dissemination from occult lesions.

History and physical examination are important. The diagnostic methods for TB infection include PPD (purified protein derivative) test, chest radiograph, bronchioalveolar lavage, and biopsy of possible infected organs. However, a negative PPD test in an immunocompromised patient does not exclude TB infection [8]. Patients with a history of TB have a higher risk of reactivation during the first month after transplantation, independent of the type of immunosuppression [8], and all post-transplantation patients with pyrexia of unknown origin should be investigated aggressively to exclude TB infection, especially among those with a history of TB infection. Tentative antituberculous treatment may be applied to patients with clinical presentations that were highly suspicious of TB infection.

The treatment of TB in liver transplant recipients is difficult. Hepatotoxicity of antituberculous agents and drug interactions with immunosuppressants may render the graft more susceptible to injury. Rifampin and isoniazid are microsomal enzyme inducers with a particular affinity for liver cytochrome P450 IIIa [9], which can augment the catabolism of immunosuppressants, increasing rejection risk [10]. Ofloxacin is a second-line drug for anti-TB therapy, with a high efficacy and weaker hepatotoxicity and interactions with immunosuppressants. For the reasons mentioned above, less hepatotoxic yet effective antituberculous drugs should be chosen for patients and immunosuppressant levels should be monitored frequently. Organ rejection may manifest with the same clinical and laboratory findings, including elevated bilirubin levels, and liver enzymes including alanine aminotransferase and aspartate aminotransferase, as seen in drug-induced toxicity. If liver damage occurs, liver biopsy should be used to confirm the diagnosis.

In conclusion, TB is a rare but severe and difficult-to-treat infection after liver transplantation. TB infection should be suspected in liver transplant recipients with fever of unknown cause. Careful monitoring of liver function and immunosuppressant levels is essential.

Case 2: chronic hepatitis B infection in the post-transplantation patient

Case presentation

A 54-year-old Iraqi man with a history of chronic hepatitis B viral (HBV) infection and lamivudine treatment for 3 years was found to have hepatocellular carcinoma. He was listed for transplantation and at the time of his operation he was HBsAg positive with a detectable but low HBV DNA level. Lamivudine was continued postoperatively, and he was started on monthly hepatitis B immunoglobulin (HBIg) prophylaxis. Serum HBsAg and HBV DNA levels became undetectable post-transplantation.

His medications included tacrolimus, mycophenolate mofetil, and lamivudine.

Three months after transplantation, he complained of jaundice, generalized weakness, and loss of appetite.

Examination revealed the following:

Jaundice

Cardiovascular: pulse 88/min, regular; BP 130/80 mmHg; normal

Respiratory: normal examination

Gastrointestinal: mild tenderness in the right hypochondrium. No hepatosplenomegaly or ascites

CNS: conscious, oriented

Investigations (normal values in brackets)
Hb 13.7 (13.5–17.5) g/dL
WCC 6.9 (4–11) × 10^9/L
Platelets 104 (150–400) × 10^9/L

MCV 74 (76–98) fL
INR 2.47 (0.9–1.2)
AST 1649 (10–40) IU/L
ALT 1394 (5–30) IU/L
ALP 204 (30–130) IU/L
Albumin 32 (35–55) g/L
Bilirubin 120 (2–17) µmol/L
Urea 9.1 (2.5–6.5) mmol/L
Creatinine 188 (50–120) µmol/L
Na^+ 137 (135–145) mmol/L
K^+ 4.6 (3.5–5.0) mmol/L
Glucose 8.2 (3.5–5.5) mmol/L
HBsAg positive
HBsAb negative
HBeAg negative
Antibody to HBeAg positive
HCVAb negative
HBV DNA 1.31 × 10^5 IU/mL
(HBV DNA conversion: 1 copy/mL = 0.19 IU/mL or 1 IU = 5.26 copies/mL)

Ultrasound scan report
The hepatic morphology is normal. There is no dilation of the intrahepatic biliary tree. The hepatic and portal veins are patent. Within the liver, good arterial flow was identified with normal acceleration times. No focal hepatic lesion was noted. No other abnormality.

Liver biopsy (transjugular route)
Microscopic description:
Portal inflammation: minimal, lymphoid
No portal phlebitis or duct injury or hepatic vein inflammation
No lobular necroinflammation
Steatosis: mild, some small fat droplets present
Cholestasis
Shikata/orcein stain: positive in the cytoplasm of many hepatocytes

Questions

• How would you interpret the AST, ALT, and INR levels in this patient?
• What other virological studies would be important?
• What is the likely cause of the elevated liver enzymes in this patient?

• What methods could be used to assess the prognosis and aid decisions on further management?
• What are the options for the management of antiviral drug resistance emerging during treatment of chronic HBV?

Differential diagnosis

The main causes of acute hepatitis in this case which need to be excluded are:
• Viral:
  – reactivation of HBV due to emergence of HBV resistance to lamivudine
  – acute hepatitis A, E infection or CMV/herpes/EBV
• Acute cellular rejection
• Hepatic artery thrombosis
• Portal vein or hepatic vein occlusion
• Drug reaction.

In many cases the clinical history will point to the diagnosis but it is still essential to exclude many of the above pathologies. In all cases Doppler ultrasonography of the portal vein and hepatic vessels is essential to exclude occlusion of vessels and, if patency of these vessels cannot be easily demonstrated by this method, CT or MR angiography should be considered.

Acute cellular rejection is possible although such high aminotransferases are rarely seen. A liver biopsy is usually indicated especially if the diagnosis cannot be determined from the appropriate serological or radiological investigations.

Diagnosis

The diagnosis in this case was acute HBV flare due to the emergence of lamivudine resistance. This diagnosis was supported by the finding of a positive HBsAg as well as a high HBV DNA level. In addition, the histology and special stains were supportive of this diagnosis and did not in fact show any evidence of ischemic damage or acute cellular rejection. Other causes of infectious hepatitis were excluded by the investigations presented above.

Tenofovir therapy was added to lamivudine and there was a slow normalization of bilirubin, AST, ALT, and INR. Serum HBV DNA titer declined by more than $4\log_{10}$, and treatment with both drugs is ongoing.

Patient management

Chronic hepatitis B infection affects an estimated 350 million people worldwide [11]. HBV carriers have an increased risk of developing cirrhosis and hepatocellular cancer. Screening of people from high-prevalence areas (south Asia, Middle East, southern Europe, and Africa), as well as other high-risk groups (e.g. intravenous drug users, men who have sex with men, prison inmates) is recommended [12].

HBV immunization is effective and there are a number of strategies used worldwide in terms of target populations depending on local factors.

The evaluation of patients with chronic HBV infection should include assessment of markers of HBV replication (HBeAg and HBV DNA) as well as markers for coinfection with HCV, hepatitis δ, and HIV. Patients should also be screened for hepatocellular cancer by ultrasonography. Treatment with antiviral therapy is generally guided by HBeAg status, ALT level, and liver biopsy findings. An excellent approach to the treatment of chronic HBV is published by Lok and McMahon [13].

The aims of treatment are to achieve sustained suppression of HBV replication and ultimately prevent cirrhosis and hepatocellular cancer. Treatment modalities may include interferon-α or nucleoside/nucleotide analogues.

The emergence of lamivudine-resistant HBV after liver transplantation is a potentially deadly complication often promoting a state of panic that culminates in treatment based largely on anecdotal evidence. Successful long-term outcome after liver transplantation for HBV requires an effective strategy to prevent graft reinfection. Until effective anitviral treatments became available, the results of liver transplantation for HBV-infected individuals were poor.

The first effective strategy required the administration of HBIg. Passive immunoprophylaxis usually prevented graft reinfection when transplantation was performed for patients with low levels of viral replication. However, passive immunoprophylaxis was often unsuccessful when transplantation was undertaken for patients with high levels of replication [14]. Thus, although serum HBsAg negativity could be sustained for a variable period after transplantation, graft reinfection and recurrent HBs antigenemia typically ensued during the first post-transplantation year.

Lamivudine is a potent inhibitor of HBV replication and now has an established role for the prevention of graft reinfection after liver transplantation. Published experience confirms that lamivudine monotherapy, given before and after liver transplantation, can prevent significant graft reinfection for selected patients [15]. Unfortunately, however, graft reinfection can occur despite lamivudine prophylaxis, and is associated with selection and then emergence of viral species with specific mutations in the polymerase gene. These changes comprise a methionine for valine (M552V) or methionine for isoleucine (M552I) substitution at amino acid residue 552, with other changes including methionine for leucine at position 528 (L528M) of the polymerase. Indeed, these lamivudine-resistant species were first described in the context of failed prophylaxis after liver transplantation [16]. As observed for HBIg prophylaxis, failure of lamivudine prophylaxis may be predicted for patients with high pretreatment serum HBV titer [17].

Currently, prophylaxis protocols employing both HBIg and lamivudine have been adopted by most centers and HBV relapse in this context is rare. However, our patient relapsed despite the use of lamivudine before, and lamivudine and HBIg after transplantation. We believe that failure of prophylaxis is a consequence of the emergence of lamivudine-resistant virus before transplantation. The patient commenced lamivudine 3 years before transplantation and, although not confirmed by genetic sequencing, reappearance of serum HBV DNA after 2 years of suppression is strongly suggestive of the emergence of a resistant species. It is recognized that resistant species emerge in most patients during long-term therapy [18]. Thus, in the absence of ongoing suppression by lamivudine, HBIg constituted the mainstay of post-transplantation prophylaxis for the patient. Simultaneous detection of both HBsAg and high-titer anti-HBs in his serum during HBIg therapy suggests selection of an "escape mutant" at the time of HBIg failure. Subsequently, despite ongoing administration of HBIg, the serum titer of anti-HBs declined, and then biochemical liver dysfunction ensued.

In the context of immunosuppression, HBV infection can cause aggressive hepatitis and subacute liver failure. The histological appearance associated with this type of liver failure can be distinctive, frequently referred to as fibrosing cholestatic hepatitis (FCH) [19,20]. Early reports of this condition highlighted the almost universal fatal outcome. It has been suggested that liver failure associated with FCH may be due to massive viral antigen expression associated with extremely high levels of viral replication. Our patient developed liver failure associated with very high levels of viral replication (reflected by the high serum HBV DNA titer and by immunohistology). Adefovir dipivoxil is the oral prodrug of an acyclic nucleotide monophosphate analogue. It has a broad spectrum of antiviral activity against retroviruses, hepadnaviruses, and herpesviruses. Treatment with adefovir of wild-type HBV in non-immunosuppressed patients effects potent inhibition of replication and rapid decline of serum HBV titers [21]. A potential role of adefovir for the treatment of lamivudine-resistant virus has been suggested by in vitro studies [22,23]. In vitro, adefovir retains activity against HBV polymerase containing lamivudine resistance mutations.

Tenofovir, a novel nucleotide analog that belongs to the class of acyclic nucleoside phosphonates, may offer an option for this group of patients. The site of tenofovir action against HBV is at the reverse transcriptase (D domain), which acts as a nucleotide analogue in the acyclic nucleoside phosphonates class [23], and it appears to be safe and effective for lowering HBV DNA in liver transplant recipients with HBV lamivudine resistance. Recent work in non-transplant recipients with lamivudine-resistant HBV revealed a promising effect in a short-term study [24].

Importantly, tenofovir has a long intracellular half-life (12–50 h), allowing for infrequent dosing in any patient with renal insufficiency. Dose adjustment is necessary with both adefovir and tenofovir when patients are diagnosed with renal insufficiency.

Tenofovir can decrease the replication of lamivudine-resistant HBV variants in liver transplant recipients. Normalization of aminotransferase levels tended to occur in most of the authors' patients. These results demonstrate another potential option for treatment of lamivudine-resistant HBV after liver transplantation.

Case 3: parasitic liver infections

Case presentation

A 73-year-old Greek man was referred because of an abnormal mass lesion found on ultrasonography and

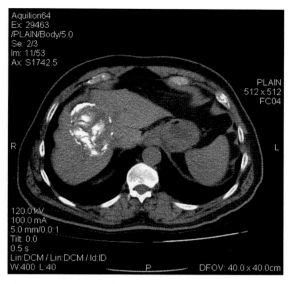

Figure 16.3 CT scan showing hydatid cyst.

subsequently a CT scan (Figure 16.3) which was performed after he mentioned at his routine yearly check-up that he had a previous liver mass found in his liver about 30 years earlier. He had no symptoms.

Examination was unremarkable.

He had type 2 diabetes mellitus, hypertension, hyperlipidemia, and hypothyroidism.

He was on standard medications for the above conditions and had no relevant family history.

He had been a factory worker for most of his adult life in Canada but was a farmer in Greece before that.

Investigations (normal values in brackets)
Hb 13.7 (13.5–17.5) g/dL
MCV 65 (76–98) fL
Platelets 202 (150–400) × 10^9/L
INR 1 (0.9–1.2)
Microcytic blood film
LFTs normal
AFP <5 μg/L (normal)

CT scan of the abdomen
Calcified right lobe cyst at the dome of the liver measured 8.6 × 6.6 cm with a second component measuring 4.5 × 3.5 cm. There are multiple other cysts without calcification. There is a hemangioma in the right lobe. There is also a lower pole renal cyst.

Overall the liver appearances are consistent with a calcified hydatid cyst.

Questions

• What is the likely diagnosis?
• How should this be managed?

Differential diagnosis

The differential diagnosis of a calcified liver mass or cyst includes the following:
Inflammatory conditions: granulomatous conditions such as TB
Echinococcus cyst (hydatid cyst)
Large hemangiomas
Hepatocellular adenoma
Fibrolamellar carcinoma
Intrahepatic cholangiocarcinoma
Mucin-producing metastases (usually colon or ovary)

Diagnosis

This calcified cyst has the typical appearance of a hydatid cyst.

Patient management

Hydatid disease is a parasitic infestation by a tapeworm of the genus *Echinococcus*. *E. granulosus* causes cystic echinococcosis whereas *E. multilocularis* causes alveolar echinococcosis. Echinococcosis is endemic in Mediterranean countries, the Middle East, South America, Australia, and New Zealand, as well as southern parts of Africa. Alveolar echinococosis is the rarer form of the disease [25].

This patient had the cystic form of the disease which is associated with morbidity due to rupture or infection of the cyst as well as dysfunction of the affected organs. Mortality is usually caused by anaphylaxis secondary to rupture.

Many cysts remain asymptomatic into advanced age when their expanding size may cause space-occupying symptoms. A history of living or visiting an endemic area must be established. Although *Echinococcus* may involve any organ, it is most commonly found in the liver (65%) and the lungs (25%). Symptoms may be due to mass effect or cyst complications such as infection. Patients who become symptomatic often present with abdominal pain, mass, or symptoms mimicking cholelithiasis or biliary obstruction. Rupture or episodic leakage from a hydatid cyst may produce fever, pruritis, urticaria, or anaphylaxis. Pulmonary symptoms may include cough, dyspnea, chest pain, or hemoptysis. Rupture of a hydatid cyst or at surgery may lead to dissemination, which can form additional cysts.

Physical examination findings are non-specific. Laboratory studies in patients with liver involvement yield non-specific findings such as elevated bilirubin or ALP as well as esinophilia (25% of patients). Serological testing has variable results. CT scanning shows a high degree of accuracy in diagnosis and MRI offers no real advantage. The most pathognomonic feature of these cysts on imaging is the finding of daughter cysts within the larger cyst. In addition, eggshell or mural calcification on CT is often seen [26].

Therapy is based on considerations of size, location, and manifestations of cysts. Surgery has traditionally been the principal definitive method of treatment but, for most cysts nowadays, PAIR (percutaneous aspiration, infusion of scolicidal agents, and reaspiration) is now recommended, with the concomitant administration of albendazole before the procedure and for 4 weeks afterwards. For complicated cysts, especially for those communicating with the biliary tree, surgery is still the treatment of choice. Certain cysts are regarded as inactive (those with a thick calcified wall or heterogeneous contents) and do not cause discomfort or organ dysfunction and can be left untreated [26]. This was considered to be the case in this patient who appears to have an inactive cyst that has not progressed in size for a number of years.

Discussion

These cases demonstrate the various types of infection that can affect the liver. The first two cases discuss patients with chronic liver disease secondary to viral hepatitis (HBV, HCV), and their clinical course after the onset of liver decompensation and subsequent liver transplantation. They illustrate that, although huge strides have been made in the treatment of these conditions with antiviral agents, both these infections continue to present with the complications of long-term untreated disease and remain extremely common and important causes of morbidity and mortality worldwide.

The last case illustrates some of the important issues in managing a disease that is infrequently seen in the developed world and for which solid evidence to support treatment options is not established.

References

1 Horwitz CA, Henle W, Henle G, et al. Clinical and laboratory evaluation of cytomegalovirus-induced mononucleosis in previously healthy individuals. Report of 82 cases. *Medicine (Baltimore)* 1986;**65**:124–34.

2 Razonable RR. Cytomegalovirus infection after liver transplantation: current concepts and challenges. *World J Gastroenterol* 2008;**14**:4849–60.

3 Razonable RR, Brown RA, Espy MJ, et al. Comparative quantitation of cytomegalovirus (CMV) DNA in solid organ transplant recipients with CMV infection by using two high-throughput automated systems. *J Clin Microbiol* 2001;**39**:4472–6.

4 Sy T, Jamal MM. Epidemiology of hepatitis C virus (HCV) infection. *Int J Med Sci* 2006;**3**:41–6.

5 Sherman M, Shafran S, Burak K, et al. Management of chronic hepatitis C: consensus guidelines. *Can J Gastroenterol* 2007;**21**(suppl C):25C–34C.

6 Singh N, Paterson DL. *Mycobacterium tuberculosis* infection in solid-organ transplant recipients: impact and implications for management. *Clin Infect Dis* 1998;**27**:1266–77.

7 Meyers BR, Halpern M, Sheiner P, Mendelson MH, Neibart E, Miller C. Tuberculosis in liver transplant patients. *Transplantation* 1994;**58**:301–6.

8 Aguado JM, Herrero JA, Gavalda J, et al. Clinical presentation and outcome of tuberculosis in kidney, liver, and heart transplant recipients in Spain. Spanish Transplantation Infection Study Group, GESITRA. *Transplantation* 1997;**63**:1278–86.

9 O'Brien RJ, Long MW, Cross FS, Lyle MA, Snider DE, Jr. Hepatotoxicity from isoniazid and rifampin among children treated for tuberculosis. *Pediatrics* 1983;**72**: 491–9.

10 Sinnott JT, Emmanuel PJ. Mycobacterial infections in the transplant patient. *Semin Respir Infect* 1990;**5**: 65–73.

11 Lavanchy D. Hepatitis B virus epidemiology, disease burden, treatment, and current and emerging prevention and control measures. *J Viral Hepat* 2004;**11**:97–107.

12 Mast EE, Weinbaum CM, Fiore AE, et al. A comprehensive immunization strategy to eliminate transmission of

hepatitis B virus infection in the United States: recommendations of the Advisory Committee on Immunization Practices (ACIP) Part II: immunization of adults. *MMWR Recomm Rep* 2006;**55**:1–33.

13 Lok AS, McMahon BJ. Chronic hepatitis B. *Hepatology* 2007;**45**:507–39.

14 Samuel D, Muller R, Alexander G, et al. Liver transplantation in European patients with the hepatitis B surface antigen. *N Engl J Med* 1993;**329**:1842–7.

15 Grellier L, Mutimer D, Ahmed M, et al. Lamivudine prophylaxis against reinfection in liver transplantation for hepatitis B cirrhosis. *Lancet* 1996;**348**:1212–15.

16 Ling R, Mutimer D, Ahmed M, et al. Selection of mutations in the hepatitis B virus polymerase during therapy of transplant recipients with lamivudine. *Hepatology* 1996;**24**:711–13.

17 Mutimer D, Pillay D, Dragon E, et al. High pre-treatment serum hepatitis B virus titre predicts failure of lamivudine prophylaxis and graft re-infection after liver transplantation. *J Hepatol* 1999;**30**:715–21.

18 Benhamou Y, Bochet M, Thibault V, et al. Long-term incidence of hepatitis B virus resistance to lamivudine in human immunodeficiency virus-infected patients. *Hepatology* 1999;**30**:1302–6.

19 Davies SE, Portmann BC, O'Grady JG, et al. Hepatic histological findings after transplantation for chronic hepatitis B virus infection, including a unique pattern of fibrosing cholestatic hepatitis. *Hepatology* 1991;**13**:150–7.

20 Harrison RF, Davies MH, Goldin RD, Hubscher SG. Recurrent hepatitis B in liver allografts: a distinctive form of rapidly developing cirrhosis. *Histopathology* 1993;**23**:21–8.

21 Gilson RJ, Chopra KB, Newell AM, et al. A placebo-controlled phase I/II study of adefovir dipivoxil in patients with chronic hepatitis B virus infection. *J Viral Hepat* 1999;**6**:387–95.

22 Xiong X, Flores C, Yang H, Toole JJ, Gibbs CS. Mutations in hepatitis B DNA polymerase associated with resistance to lamivudine do not confer resistance to adefovir in vitro. *Hepatology* 1998;**28**:1669–73.

23 Ying C, De CE, Nicholson W, Furman P, Neyts J. Inhibition of the replication of the DNA polymerase M550V mutation variant of human hepatitis B virus by adefovir, tenofovir, L-FMAU, DAPD, penciclovir and lobucavir. *J Viral Hepat* 2000;**7**:161–5.

24 van BF, Zollner B, Sarrazin C, et al. Tenofovir for patients with lamivudine-resistant hepatitis B virus (HBV) infection and high HBV DNA level during adefovir therapy. *Hepatology* 2006;**44**:318–25.

25 Craig PS, McManus DP, Lightowlers MW, et al. Prevention and control of cystic echinococcosis. *Lancet Infect Dis* 2007;**7**:385–94.

26 Junghanss T, da Silva AM, Horton J, Chiodini PL, Brunetti E. Clinical management of cystic echinococcosis: state of the art, problems, and perspectives. *Am J Trop Med Hyg* 2008;**79**:301–11.

17 The Liver Transplant Recipient

Prakash Ramachandran and Andrew J. Bathgate
Centre for Liver & Digestive Disorders and Scottish Liver Transplant Unit, The Royal Infirmary of Edinburgh, Edinburgh, UK

Case 1: abnormal LFTs in the liver transplant recipient

Case presentation

A 61-year-old retired nursing assistant was referred for consideration of liver transplantation. She had primary biliary cirrhosis (PBC) diagnosed 17 years previously after a wedge liver biopsy at the time of a laparoscopic cholecystectomy for right upper quadrant (RUQ) pain and jaundice. Anti-mitchondrial antibodies were positive with a titer of 1 in 80. She subsequently developed intractable pruritus, refractory to medical therapies including cholestyramine, ursodeoxycholic acid, rifampicin, cimetidine, ultraviolet B light, and subcutaneous naloxone. She was listed for a liver transplantation and underwent orthotopic liver transplantation 12 years ago. Her initial postoperative course was complicated by early acute cellular rejection (Figure 17.1), treated with intravenous methylprednisolone first, and subsequently requiring OKT3 (muromonab-CD3). She was eventually discharged with good graft function on the unit's standard immunosuppression in the form of tacrolimus, azathioprine, and a reducing course of prednisolone.

At follow-up clinic, 4 years after her transplantation, she was noted to have developed abnormal liver function tests, with an elevated alkaline phosphatase (ALP) and γ-glutamyltransferase (GGT). These remained elevated persistently. An abdominal ultrasound scan was unremarkable, in particular confirming adequate vascular flow. A magnetic resonance cholangiopancreatography (MRCP) was performed to exclude biliary obstruction. This suggested a possible biliary anastomotic stricture. An endoscopic retrograde cholangiopancreatography (ERCP) did not, however, demonstrate a significant stricture. A liver biopsy was thus undertaken; 12 months later, she once again developed pruritus, which was once more refractory to standard medical therapies and she underwent a trial on plasma exchange. This initially showed some benefit but has become less effective, requiring more frequent treatments, and vascular access has become problematic. Thus, she was referred to consider retransplantation.

Other medical history
- Polyarticular rheumatoid arthritis for 28 years (steroid dependent for 25 years)
- Two previous deep vein thromboses (one postoperatively and one after thrombophlebitis)
- Cholecystectomy and appendectomy.

Current medications
Prednisolone 10 mg once daily, azathioprine 100 mg once daily, tacrolimus, Adcal D3, alendronate 70 mg weekly, ursodeoxycholic acid 500 mg twice daily.

Social history
Non-smoker, no alcohol consumption, quality of Life rated 2/10 – unable to sleep at night due to pruritus.

Problem-based Approach to Gastroenterology and Hepatology, First Edition. Edited by John N. Plevris, Colin W. Howden.
© 2012 Blackwell Publishing Ltd. Published 2012 by Blackwell Publishing Ltd.

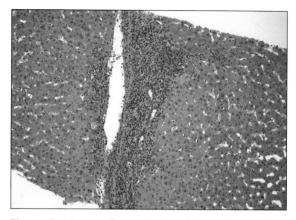

Figure 17.1 Acute cellular rejection with portal expansion, biliary ductulitis, and venous endothelialitis (image courtesy of Dr Chris Bellamy).

Examination findings
Pigmented skin, anicteric, xanthelasma, multiple skin excoriations from scratching, visible spider nevi, and palmar erythema. Left subclavian Hickman line *in situ*.

Gastrointestinal: abdomen non-distended, with no palpable organomegaly; no tremor

Cardiovascular: Pulse 90 beats/min regular, BP 110/60 mmHg, heart sounds normal, no peripheral edema

Respiratory: normal examination

Investigations (normal values in brackets)
Hb 113 (115–165) g/dL
MCV 85 (78–98) fL
WCC 8.0 (4–11) × 10^9/L
Platelets 160 (150–350) × 10^9/L
GGT 250 (5–35) IU/L
ALP 809 (40–125) IU/L
ALT 103 (10–50) IU/L
Albumin 38 (35–50) g/L
Bilirubin 44 (3–16) μmol/L
INR = 1.0
Urea 13.0 (2.5–6.6) mmol/L
Creatinine 149 (60–120) μmol/L
Na^+ 135 (135–145) mmol/L
K^+ 3.8 (3.5–5.0) mmol/L
Anti-mitochondrial antibody positive 1 in 640
AFP 3 (1–5) kU/L
Remaining liver screen normal
CT of the abdomen

Normal liver, splenomegaly, no ascites
Pulmonary function tests normal
Echocardiogram normal
Upper GI endoscopy grade 2 esophageal varices – in banding program

Questions

• What are the most commonly used scoring systems to assess severity of chronic liver disease in patients awaiting liver transplantation?
• What are the common causes of cholestasis after liver transplantation?

Severity of liver disease

There are a number of scoring systems to assess the severity of chronic liver disease. The Childs–Pugh score has been used for many years but requires a subjective assessment of ascites and encephalopathy in addition to bilirubin, albumin, and prothrombin time. The model for end-stage liver disease (MELD) has no subjective assessments and incorporates the international normalized ratio (INR), bilirubin, and creatinine. It is a reasonable predictor of death from chronic liver disease. A score of >15 is generally regarded as the cut-off at which listing should be seriously considered. Attempts to improve predicting outcome have included sodium and the UKELD (UK model for end-stage liver disease) incorporates this value in addition to the above three values and is used in the minimal listing criteria for transplantation (UKELD > 49) in the UK [1]. This patient has a MELD score of 15 and a UKELD score of 50.

Differential diagnosis

The differential diagnosis in this case is that of severe cholestasis related to graft dysfunction. This can be due to either cholestasis related to the extrahepatic biliary tree, in particular anastomotic biliary stricturing, or intrahepatic cholestasis.

An ERCP suggesting no significant bile hold-up at the anastomosis or other larger ducts makes the diagnosis more likely to be intrahepatic cholestasis. The main differential diagnosis lies between chronic rejection and recurrent PBC. Severe or steroid-resistant rejection is a risk factor for chronic rejection. Liver biopsy is required to establish the diagnosis because

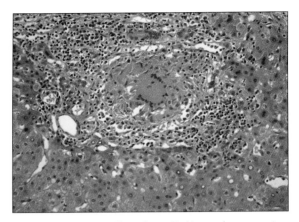

Figure 17.2 Hepatic allograft needle biopsy demonstrating focal bile duct damage and granuloma typical of recurrent primary biliary cirrhosis (image courtesy of Dr Chris Bellamy).

chronic rejection leads to bile duct loss and foamy arteriopathy, although the latter is seldom seen on a graft needle biopsy.

Diagnosis

Recurrent primary biliary cirrhosis as evidenced by focal bile duct inflammation and graft damage on needle biopsy (Figure 17.2).

Discussion

Acute cellular rejection requiring treatment after liver transplantation occurs in around 20% of patients. It is termed "early acute rejection" if it occurs within the first 30 days after liver transplantation and "late" if beyond this time. It is a T-cell-mediated liver injury, which is very responsive to treatment with high-dose methylprednisolone. A single episode of early acute cellular rejection does not deleteriously influence graft or patient survival. Steroid-resistant acute rejection and late acute rejection do influence graft outcome but both are relatively rare events in the present era of immunosuppression. This case is therefore unusual in that antibody therapy was required to treat steroid-resistant rejection. There are various antibody therapies available including anti-thymyocyte globulin, OKT3, and interleukin 2 receptor antagonists. Recipients transplanted for cholestatic liver disease with reasonably preserved liver function, as in this

case, are at a higher risk of acute rejection [2]. Tacrolimus is now the most commonly used calcineurin inhibitor and was used in this case before licensing.

The subsequent developments in this case highlight a common issue in transplantation for primary biliary cirrhosis, namely disease recurrence. Recurrent disease occurs in around 50% of recipients within 8 years [3], although many will be asymptomatic and only have histological changes and minimally abnormal cholestatic liver enzymes. There is much discussion about the possibility of an increase in recurrence with the use of tacrolimus compared with cyclosporine (ciclosporin), although this remains unproven at present. Most units start ursodeoxycholic acid although again this remains unproven.

Severe recurrent symptomatic disease, as in this case, is not common. The common stepwise approach to cholestatic pruritus in native PBC is often used in the post-transplantation setting as in this case. The initial trial of cholestyramine in increasing doses rarely works and an antihistamine may lead to a slight improvement in symptoms. The other medications used include rifampicin, which can increase metabolism of tacrolimus significantly, naltrexone (an opiate antagonist), and sertraline. In extreme cases plasmapheresis may be of benefit. Ultimately retransplantation may be required for severe symptomatology or graft failure.

Case 2: hepatopulmonary syndrome in alcoholic cirrhosis

Case presentation

A 49-year-old woman was referred for liver transplantation assessment. She had a long history of alcohol excess, consuming 1 liter of vodka per day for a number of years. She was diagnosed with alcoholic liver disease 3 years previously and was known to be cirrhotic with portal hypertension and esophageal varices. She presented 12 months ago with shortness of breath and significant hypoxia. Echocardiography showed a normal left ventricle, trivial mitral regurgitation, and a normal right ventricular size and function. Peak systolic pulmonary artery pressure was estimated at 25 mmHg. Pulmonary artery catheterization showed normal pulmonary artery pressures and no ventilation–perfusion

($\dot{V}/\dot{Q}$) mismatch. She was diagnosed with hepatopulmonary syndrome and commenced on home oxygen therapy. She had been abstinent from alcohol since the diagnosis of liver disease. She continued on home oxygen therapy and had significantly impaired exercise tolerance.

Past medical history
Hysterectomy.

Drug history
Spironolactone 300 mg once daily, furosemide 40 mg once daily, omeprazole 20 mg once daily.

Social history
Ex-smoker. Now abstinent from alcohol. Not currently employed. Has a supportive family, living with her husband.

Examination findings
Short of breath on minimal exertion; finger clubbing; spider nevi and palmar erythema

Respiratory: oxygen saturations 83% on air at rest, 69% on air after exertion; chest clear

Cardiovascular: jugular venous pressure elevated; bilateral pitting ankle edema; audible pansystolic murmur loudest over lower left sternal edge

Gastrointestinal: no jaundice/flapping tremor; abdomen soft, non-tender; no ascites clinically

Investigations (normal values in brackets)
Hb 150 (115–165) g/dL
MCV 90 (78–98) fL
WCC 10.5 (4–11) × 10^9/L
Platelets 120 (150–350) × 10^9/L
Bilirubin 29 (3–16) μmol/L
ALT 20 (10–50) IU/L
ALP 155 (40–125) IU/L
GGT 354 (5–35) IU/L
Albumin 33 g/L
PT 10 s (control 9 s)
INR 1.1
Urea 4.7 (2.5–6.6) mmol/L
Creatinine 75 (60–120) μmol/L
Na^+ 138 (135–145) mmol/L
K^+ 3.9 (3.5–5.0) mmol/L
MELD 9
UKELD 47
Child–Pugh grade A
Remaining liver screen normal

Ultrasound scan of abdomen – cirrhotic liver, vessels patent, splenomegaly, no ascites

Upper GI endoscopy – grade 3 esophageal varices – in banding program

Pulmonary function tests: normal ventilatory capacity, gas transfer reduced with TCO 3.37 (43% predicted) and KCO 0.82 (54% predicted)

Arterial blood gas on air: PO_2 5.8 kPa, PCO_2 4.8 kPa, H^+ 34 nmol/L, HCO_3^- 20.4 mmol/L

Contrast echocardiography to further assess: normal left ventricular function, Right heart normal, microbubbles identified in left atrium three to six cycles after right atrium, right heart pressure estimated at 23 mmHg, thus excluding pulmonary hypertension.

Questions

• What are the two main respiratory syndromes associated with chronic liver disease?
• What clinical signs and investigations help differentiate between them?
• What is the role and risk of liver transplantation in managing these syndromes?
• What are the key alcohol-related contraindications to liver transplantation?

Differential diagnosis

Dyspnea associated with cirrhosis can be related to anemia, primary cardiorespiratory disease, or a respiratory complication of cirrhosis and portal hypertension.

The differential diagnosis is therefore broad in this case. Simple blood tests, routine imaging, pulmonary function tests, and conventional echocardiography narrow the differential diagnosis rapidly to one of the two respiratory syndromes associated with chronic liver disease – hepatopulmonary syndrome or portopulmonary hypertension. Further investigation often requires contrast-enhanced echocardiography, technetium-99-labeled albumin, macroaggregate perfusion scan, and right heart catheterization with measurement of oxygen saturations and pressures.

Clinical examination can assist in making the diagnosis, because patients with hepatopulmonary syndrome are often cyanosed with finger clubbing whereas patients with portopulmonary hypertension are not.

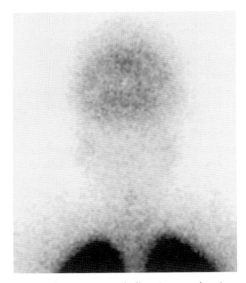

Figure 17.3 Macroaggregated albumin scan showing uptake in the brain consistent with a diagnosis of hepatopulmonary syndrome.

Diagnosis

The diagnosis in this case is hepatopulmonary syndrome associated with alcoholic cirrhosis and portal hypertension (Figure 17.3). The level of hypoxaemia is very marked and a positive contrast-enhanced echocardiogram with no elevation of pulmonary artery pressure clinches the diagnosis.

Management

A TIPSS (transjugular intrahepatic portosystemic stent) was performed initially in an attempt to reduce the perioperative risk. Despite achieving a portal pressure gradient of 3 mmHg, the improvement in the patient's symptoms was minimal and she remained very short of breath on minimal exertion.

She had a further deterioration in her symptoms 6 months later. She thus underwent an orthotopic liver transplantation. Her postoperative course was protracted due to hypoxia on mobilization, meaning a hospital stay of 6 weeks. However, graft function was good. She was discharged on high-flow oxygen at home.

She had continued good graft function in subsequent follow-up. However, respiratory symptoms persisted and at 3 months post-transplantation she was still requiring continuous home oxygen with exercise tolerance limited to walking 5 meters.

A slow improvement was first noted 6 months after surgery, when she was requiring oxygen non-continuously and was able to mobilize around the house. Progress continued over the next 2 years before cessation of home oxygen therapy. She is currently feeling well with no significant restrictions on her daily activities.

Discussion

Assessment of patients with alcoholic liver disease remains a controversial issue. There have been many attempts to identify robust criteria that will predict a return to drinking. However, this has proved very difficult and most units will utilize the assessment of a specialist in alcohol and substance misuse in making their decision about suitability. A period of abstinence allows liver improvement and is important to ascertain the necessity of liver transplantation, but has not been shown as a consistent predictor of relapse. In the UK previous non-compliance with medical therapy, a return to drinking after full professional assessment, concomitant illicit drug misuse, and alcoholic hepatitis are regarded as absolute contraindications to listing for transplantation [4]. None of these applied in this case and a favorable report from an alcohol specialist meant that she was deemed suitable for listing from the alcohol point of view.

This case also illustrates the issue of the pulmonary vascular problems associated with portal hypertension. This is a fascinating area because the two extremes of pulmonary vasculature tension are seen. First, portopulmonary hypertension where there is constriction of the pulmonary arteries and does not improve after liver transplantation. The second entity demonstrated in this case is the hepatopulmonary syndrome, which results in dilation of the pulmonary arteries and does improve after liver transplantation. Clinically, patients with hepatopulmonary syndrome tend to be cyanosed with clubbing and do not show signs of right heart failure. There is no doubt that both conditions contribute significantly to the operative risk of liver transplantation. The degree of hypoxia associated with hepatopulmonary syndrome is associated with increased mortality in the non-transplant setting as well as affecting outcome at the time of transplantation [5]. This case highlights that very acceptable levels of synthetic liver function can be present in patients with incapacitating hepatopulmonary syndrome.

TIPSS was attempted in this case because liver function was good and there were case reports of significant improvement in hepatopulmonary syndrome after the reduction in portal hypertension that occurs with TIPSS placement. There was, however, no significant improvement, leaving the only therapeutic option as liver transplantation.

If patients survive the early postoperative period there is usually, as in this case, a slow improvement in oxygenation. This can take months or years. The mechanisms involved in this syndrome are not as yet clearly defined but both reversal of portal hypertension and a functioning liver appear to be required suggesting that the presumed imbalance of vasoactive mediators responsible are in some way modulated by the liver.

Case 3: immunosuppression complications post-liver liver transplant

Case presentation

A 45-year-old man underwent orthotopic liver transplantation for fulminant hepatic failure of uncertain etiology, having presented with a 3-week history of jaundice and 1-day history of encephalopathy. He had no other significant medical or family history, with no regular medications. The initial postoperative course was complicated by blood loss, requiring a second laparotomy, and sepsis and renal failure necessitating a period of continuous venovenous hemofiltration. However, subsequent recovery was excellent, with good graft function and renal function back to normal, with urea 5.0 mmol/L and creatinine 100 μmol/L at discharge. Medications on discharge incorporated an immunosuppression regimen of prednisolone 20 mg once daily, cyclosporine, and azathioprine, as well as antibiotic prophylaxis with co-trimoxazole and amphotericin lozenges.

Questions

• What are the common side effects of post-transplantation immunosuppression regimens and how they are managed?
• What are the management options once this juncture of management has been reached?

Post-transplantation management

At follow-up 2 months post-transplantation the patient was noted to be hypertensive with a blood pressure of 150/90 mmHg. In addition he had a degree of renal impairment, with a urea of 11.3 (2.5–6.6) mmol/L and creatinine of 144 (60–120) μmol/L. His hepatic allograft was functioning well. He was started on nifedipine and continued on azathioprine and cyclosporine with a reducing dose of prednisolone.

Further deterioration in his renal function was detected over the subsequent year, with urea of 10 mmol/L and creatinine of 208 μmol/L 1 year post-transplantation. His BP was now well controlled and his cyclosporine dose had been reduced.

His condition remained stable at follow-up appointments over the next 4 years. An elevated BP had necessitated an increase in his nifedipine dose. Three years post-transplantation he had noticed an abnormal skin lesion on his finger. This was excised by dermatology and found to be a squamous carcinoma in situ of Bowen's type.

He continued to be stable over the next 18 months, although he required an increase in his nifedipine dose. However, at follow-up 6 years post-transplantation his renal function had deteriorated significantly with urea 20 mmol/L, creatinine 400 μmol/L (Figure 17.4). His cyclosporine dose was reduced and he was admitted for investigation and review by the nephrologists. A formal 24-hour urinary protein and creatinine clearance were 4.5 g/day and 17.5 mL/min respectively. A renal biopsy was then performed which showed sclerosed glomeruli and severe interstitial fibrosis with tubular atrophy, consistent with severe end-stage irreversible parenchymal scarring due to vascular disease related to calcineurin inhibitors and/or hypertension.

Further management

More aggressive BP control was instituted with the addition of metoprolol. An attempt was made to convert his cyclosporine to mycophenolate mofetil (MMF). However, 1 month after the transition he presented with jaundice and abnormal liver function. A liver biopsy confirmed acute cellular rejection, which was treated with intravenous methylprednisolone. His liver function improved and he was kept on tacrolimus, MMF and reducing dose prednisolone.

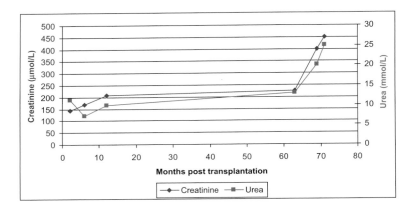

Figure 17.4 Renal function following liver transplantation in case 3.

At this juncture he was also commenced on peritoneal dialysis.

He was listed for a cadaveric renal transplant 8 years following his liver transplant and underwent this 6 months later. His liver and kidney grafts both functioned well following this and he was maintained on tacrolimus and MMF. He subsequently developed type 2 diabetes mellitus and hyperlipidemia, requiring drug treatment. Unfortunately he was admitted to his local hospital with a short history of dyspnea and investigations revealed disseminated malignancy from which he died soon after.

Diagnosis

Renal biopsy confirmed the diagnosis of calcineurin inhibitor (CNI)-induced nephrotoxicity.

Differential diagnosis

Renal dysfunction after orthotopic liver transplantation is a common occurrence. There are not many liver conditions that affect both organs. Polycystic disease affecting both liver and kidney and Caroli's disease with medullary sponge kidney are two such conditions but both are relatively uncommon. Hepatitis B and C, and alcoholic cirrhosis may be associated with glomerular lesions, although again these are not common. In the setting of acute liver failure there is often acute renal impairment and a return to pre-morbid renal function can occur, but one of the main predictors of ongoing renal dysfunction is the need for renal replacement therapy at the time of transplantation.

The main differential in this case lies between CNI-induced nephrotoxicity and hypertensive nephropathy.

Discussion

The principal lessons from this case are in the post-transplantation follow-up rather than the transplantation episode. Liver transplantation for acute liver failure is dealt with in Chapter 13.

Immunosuppression strategies have evolved from the early years with an emphasis now on a more tailored approach. In this case the recipient received the standard triple therapy used around 15 years ago – cyclosporine, azathioprine, and corticosteroids in the form of prednisolone.

Renal impairment is a common problem after liver transplantation and appears to have significant impact on survival [6]. There are multiple insults to the kidneys around the time of transplantation and it is well established that renal replacement therapy at the time of transplantation is a predictor of long-term renal impairment. The other modifiable renal insults, in the longer term, are hypertension and calcineurin nephrotoxicity. Hypertension often occurs within the first year after liver transplantation as in this case. Corticosteroids and CNIs contribute significantly to blood pressure.

This case illustrates that the CNIs are problematic in terms of adverse affects but are also very effective in preventing rejection. Weaning of the cyclosporine dose was performed but complete withdrawal led to a severe acute rejection episode even after 7 years. This has very much been the experience of several liver transplant units that have employed withdrawal strategies, with only the minority of patients able to remain off immunosuppression.

End-stage renal disease occurs in around 5% of patients receiving a liver transplant and this case indicates the need for vigilance in follow-up of transplant recipients with early intervention if possible. Strategies employed now include replacing CNIs with other less nephrotoxic agents such as mycophenolate mofetil and prednisolone. Control of hypertension is more aggressive with targets of 120 mmHg systolic and 80 mmHg diastolic. Often a combination of agents is required to achieve this and all the commonly used antihypertensive agents can be used, although nifedipine, in particular, may increase the levels of the CNIs. There may also be problems with hyperkalemia with the combination of CNIs and blockade of the angiotensin system.

Another teaching point of this case is that overall immunosuppressive load has a significant effect on mortality. The major causes of death with a functioning graft are cardiovascular and malignancy. Skin malignancies are common but rarely affect survival; however, solid-organ and hematological malignancies are the principal non-hepatic cause of death after 3 years [7].

Case 4: Hepatitis C post-liver transplant

Case presentation

A 45-year-old man was referred for liver transplant assessment for advanced chronic liver disease and possible hepatocellular carcinoma (HCC). He had been diagnosed with chronic hepatitis C some 6 months earlier. The likely route of transmission was plasma infusion 18 years previously after significant burns. There was also a significant alcohol history with excess in the previous 7 years of around 50–100 units per week. He had been abstinent for 2 months at the time of initial assessment.

Past medical history
Burns 1984, bilateral mastectomy for gynecomastia 1998, acute pancreatitis 1999 (? alcohol related).

Examination
Cardiovascular and respiratory examination: unremarkable

Mildly icteric; spider nevi and palmar erythema present
Small amount of ascites detectable clinically
No evidence of hepatic encephalopathy

Investigations (normal values in brackets)
Hb 113 (125–170) g/dL
MCV 87 (78–98) fL
WCC 9.5 (4–11) × 10^9/L
Platelets 101 (150–350) × 10^9/L
PT 17 s (control 10 s)
Bilirubin 71 (3–16) μmol/L
ALT 143 (10–50) IU/L
ALP 209 (40–125) IU/L
GGT 107 (5–35) IU/L
Albumin 22 (35–50) g/L
INR 1.7
Urea 3.9 (2.5–6.6) mmol/L
Creatinine 84 (60–120) μmol/L
Na^+ 137 (135–145) mmol/L
K^+ 4.1 (3.5–5.0) mmol/L
AFP 359 (1–5) kU/L
Hepatitis C antibody positive
Hepatitis C PCR-positive genotype 1
MELD 18
UKELD 53.6
Child–Pugh grade C
Extensive imaging including ultrasonography, CT, MRI, and hepatic angiography showed no evidence of HCC.

Two liver biopsies performed at 6-monthly intervals showed micronodular cirrhosis with chronic hepatitis C (mild activity), no evidence of alcohol-induced liver disease, and no evidence of dysplasia or HCC.

Ongoing management
Listed for transplantation; last hepatitis C PCR 40 000 copies/mL

Eight weeks later he was admitted with worsening jaundice, dehydration, spontaneous bacterial peritonitis, and renal failure. Liver transplantation was performed.

Liver function tests (LFTs) remained abnormal during inpatient recovery post transplantation:
Bilirubin 29 μmol/L
ALT 96 IU/L
ALP 722 IU/L
GGT 639 IU/L
PT 9 s

Further investigations included a CT scan that showed two collections adjacent to that graft which were drained under ultrasound guidance. This raised the suspicion of bile leak, which was confirmed on ERCP demonstrating a leak from duct anastomosis. This was treated with a biliary stent across the leak.

After this he made a good clinical recovery and was discharged from hospital on immunosuppression consisting of prednisolone, tacrolimus, and azathioprine. The biliary stent was removed and the leak had resolved.

However, his LFTs remained abnormal being:
bilirubin 29 µmol/L
ALT 89 IU/L
ALP 682 IU/L
GGT 1428 IU/L
5 months after transplantation. At clinic 6 months post-transplantation his LFTs had deteriorated with: bilirubin 373 µmol/L
ALT 112 IU/L
ALP 314 IU/L
GGT 227 IU/L
urea 6.9 mmol/L
creatinine 92 µmol/L
Na^+ 136 mmol/L
albumin 37 g/L
PT 11 s

Questions

- What are the common causes of abnormal LFTs post-transplantation?
- How would you investigate abnormal LFTs post-transplantation?
- What is the risk of recurrent hepatitis C post-transplantation?
- How effective is hepatitis C treatment in the post-transplantation setting?

Differential diagnosis

Liver enzyme abnormalities occur commonly after liver transplantation. Early graft dysfunction, however, with an increasing bilirubin and PT, is usually related to a problem with the vascular supply to the graft or acute rejection.

Liver enzyme abnormalities, as in this case, without graft dysfunction can reflect several pathologies including drug hepatotoxicity, systemic infection, and biliary anastomotic problems. Investigation often, therefore, involves cross-sectional imaging followed by ERCP if there is a suspicion of a biliary problem. Liver biopsy is often performed if imaging does not suggest a problem.

The main differential diagnosis in this case as follow-up continued was between ongoing biliary anastomotic problems and recurrent hepatitis C infection. The latter is universal although severity is very variable and histology is required to make the diagnosis because HCV RNA is positive in virtually all cases.

Management

He was readmitted for further investigation of deterioration. An abdominal ultrasound scan showed a dilated common bile duct at 17 mm. A repeat ERCP showed a tight stricture across the biliary anastomosis, which was stented, with improvement in LFTs (Figure 17.5).

LFTs were noted to deteriorate again 13 months after the initial transplantation, with
bilirubin 106 µmol/L
ALT 273 IU/L,

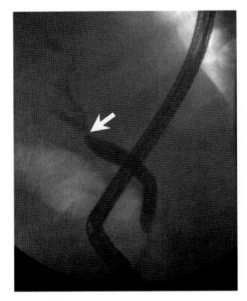

Figure 17.5 Biliary anastomotic stricture (white arrow identifies anastomosis between donor and recipient duct).

ALP 170 IU/L,
GGT 152 IU/L,
albumin 27 g/L,
urea 5.1 mmol/L
creatinine 76 μmol/L,
Na$^+$ 138 mmol/L
Hb 131 g/dL
platelets 119 × 10^9/L
PT 14 s

He was once again admitted for investigation. An abdominal ultrasound scan showed no biliary dilation and patent hepatic artery and portal vein. An MRI/MRCP was then performed, which suggested a caliber change at the site of the biliary anastomosis but a non-dilated duct system. The patency of the hepatic artery was confirmed. As no explanation for the blood abnormalities was demonstrated on imaging, a liver biopsy was then performed. Surprisingly, this demonstrated micronodular cirrhosis in the graft with recently formed fibrous septa. Chronic portal interface and lobular hepatitis with moderate activity were seen, suggesting recurrent hepatitis C to be a strong contributor to the cirrhosis.

Hepatitis C PCR at this time was 424 000 IU/mL.

Diagnosis

The liver biopsy at month 13 after the first transplantation diagnosed severe recurrent hepatitis C infection as the principal diagnosis.

Hepatitis C recurrence

Recurrent hepatitis C is universal with a very variable rate of progression. Severe recurrence resulting in rapid graft failure occurs in less than 5% of cases. The treatment of recurrent hepatitis C with pegylated interferon and ribavirin is, in general, poorly tolerated and requires dose modification in most patients. This results in a sustained virological response rate of around 30% overall, compared with around 50% in the non-transplantation setting.

Progress

He was subsequently readmitted to hospital 15 months after his initial transplantation with decompensated liver disease in the form of jaundice, sepsis, ascites, and renal failure. Imaging demonstrated portal vein thrombosis. Liver function showed minimal improvement despite treatment and thus he was re-listed for transplantation.

The patient underwent a second transplantation 16 months after the initial graft. He made steady progress postoperatively and was discharged 3 weeks later on the same immunosuppression regimen as after his first graft. Bloods on discharge were:
bilirubin 27 μmol/L
ALT 74 IU/L
ALP 553 IU/L
GGT 399 IU/L
urea 8.3 mmol/L
creatinine 90 μmol/L
Na$^+$ 136 mmol/L
PT 11 s

A hepatitis C PCR assay 2 weeks after discharge was 850 000 IU/mL with an estimated value of 1750 000 IU/mL of HCV RNA.

One month after the transplantation he was again noticed to develop abnormal LFTs with:
bilirubin 38 μmol/L
ALT 313 IU/L
ALP 325 IU/L
GGT 731 IU/L
albumin 32 g/L
PT 12 s

An abdominal ultrasound scan was normal.

A liver biopsy was performed, which showed inflammation and lobulitis with significant collapse around terminal venules. Whether this represented atypical acute cellular rejection or reactivation of HCV infection was not definitive from the pathology.

However, given the HCV PCR levels, he was treated for hepatitis C recurrence with pegylated interferon and ribavirin, in addition to continuing his immunosuppression regimen of tacrolimus, azathioprine, and prednisolone. He also required erythropoietin injections for treatment-induced anemia.

Despite hepatitis C therapy, his liver function tests remained abnormal 2 months later:
bilirubin 65 μmol/L
ALT 139 IU/L
ALP 183 IU/L
GGT 538 IU/L
albumin 26 g/L
PT 11 s

Hepatitis C PCR showed a viral load >850 000 IU/mL with an estimated value 2 150 000 IU/mL.

A surveillance biopsy showed fibrosing cholestatic hepatitis with extensive collapse, parenchymal injury, and cholestasis. This was significantly worse than the previous biopsy and consistent with aggressive recurrent hepatitis C infection. He continued on hepatitis C treatment, but his viral load remained high. A further surveillance biopsy was performed 3 months later, which showed similar histological changes. Unfortunately, he was then admitted with decompensated liver disease with jaundice, ascites, and encephalopathy, and died 8 months after his second transplantation.

Discussion

This case highlights two significant problems that can complicate liver transplantation. The first problem is that of a bile leak. These occur either at the site of the anastomosis between donor common bile duct and recipient donor common bile duct (or roux-en-Y anastomosis if this anastomosis is formed as in PSC patients) or from the cut surface of a split liver graft. A bile leak occurs early in the postoperative period and may give very few symptoms as in this case. The derangement in liver function leads to imaging, usually a CT scan, which shows a collection around the liver graft. Percutaneous drainage of the collection reveals bile-stained fluid. It is then important to improve biliary drainage either internally into the duodenum, as was achieved in this case by stenting the common bile duct at ERCP, or occasionally externally with a percutaneous approach. This allows the leak to heal but may lead to future problems at the anastomosis as happened in this case.

Biliary anastomotic strictures occur in around 10% of cases and are more likely to occur in the setting of bile leaks and arterial compromise, e.g. hepatic artery stenosis [8]. In this case biliary dilation was seen on ultrasonography, but MRCP is often being used for diagnosis of strictures at the anastomosis where the recipient has cholestatic liver enzymes but no significant dilation of the biliary system on ultrasonography.

The two approaches to treatment of biliary strictures are either endoscopic, with balloon dilation of the stricture and the placement of an increasing number of stents to widen the anastomosis, or surgical, with the formation of a hepaticojejunostomy. The

improvement of liver enzymes, as occurred in this case, is a sign of improved biliary drainage. This may not have been the case because it detracted attention from any other potential graft problem.

This case also highlights the significant problem of recurrent hepatitis C infection. Most units will perform protocol biopsies on an annual basis and consider treatment if there is progression of disease in terms of fibrosis. This case highlights that even at 12 months there can be significant fibrosis or even cirrhosis from recurrent disease. This patient's biliary problems may have contributed to the liver injury but the biopsy suggested recurrent hepatitis C as the principal problem. Graft failure from recurrent disease leads to the difficult decision about considering retransplantation. In this case no attempts had been made to intervene in the process of recurrent disease progression and therefore a decision was made to retransplant.

Further aggressive hepatitis C re-infection occurred with therapy started very early after transplantation. Unfortunately this had no impact on disease progression. Treatment of hepatitis C in the context of liver transplantation is very challenging due to adverse affects of treatment in terms of both symptoms and reduced cell counts. Many units use growth factors to support both red cell and white cells, although hard evidence is lacking. Response to treatment, as highlighted in this case, is often poor with substantially reduced efficacy compared with the native situation.

Unified discussion

There are four main reasons to consider liver transplantation as a therapeutic option. The first is acute liver failure, which has been dealt with in Chapter 13. The second is for end-stage chronic liver disease where the risk of dying is such that liver transplantation is required to improve survival. The third is for HCC where the prospect of long-term survival is increased with transplantation despite well-preserved liver function. The last, and most contentious, is transplantation for "quality of life," where chronic liver disease-associated symptoms are considered to be so debilitating that liver transplantation is considered despite no obvious survival benefit. Most of the transplantations that fall into this category are for either troublesome encephalopathy or severe pruritus associated with PBC.

The point at which the risk of dying without a transplantation exceeds the risk with one is based on scoring systems for chronic liver disease such as the MELD and the UKELD score.

The listing of patients for transplantation with HCC has principally been based on the Milan criteria established many years ago, which are:
• a single lesion <5 cm in maximum diameter
• no more than three lesions all <3 cm in maximum diameter
• no evidence of extrahepatic spread or vascular invasion.

There is much debate about extending these criteria as imaging techniques have improved considerably, and the biology of the tumor may also influence outcome after transplantation. In the UK we have recently extended the criteria to include up to five lesions all <3 cm and a single lesion between 5 and 8 cm that does not increase in size over 6 months with or without locoregional therapy.

As well as the medical issues involved in determining whether liver transplantation is an appropriate mode of therapy, there are other factors that are taken into consideration. Alcoholic liver disease is an extremely common condition in the west and liver transplantation as a therapy in this condition has been controversial. The outcome of liver transplantation for this condition is in general very good, with relatively few individuals returning to harmful drinking. The selection criteria for suitable candidates are based on relatively scanty evidence but often include a period of abstinence when relatively well and out of hospital, compliance with medical therapy and no other form of substance misuse [9]. The most common indication for liver transplantation worldwide is chronic hepatitis C infection where intravenous drug use has often been a significant issue. Again firm evidence-based criteria for transplantation in this setting have been difficult to establish and many centers have specialists in substance misuse as part of the team to help in making decisions about suitability for listing.

Early follow-up

Renal dysfunction in the early postoperative period is a common occurrence and a significant predictor of late renal dysfunction. Attempts to minimize early exposure to the nephrotoxic CNIs, cyclosporine and tacrolimus, with interleukin-2 receptor antagonists have some effect but lack long-term outcome data at present.

Infection can occur at any time after liver transplantation but the early period is when patients are at their most immunocompromised and require prophylaxis against certain specific infections such as with *Candida* spp., *Pneumocystis jiroveci*, and cytomegalovirus (particularly if the donor is CMV positive and the recipient negative).

Immunosuppressive regimens differ between centers and countries. The mainstays of therapy are the CNIs, with tacrolimus being the most commonly used. At least in the first few months most centers will use additional immunosuppression in the form of azathioprine or mycophenolate mofetil and a reducing dose of prednisolone.

Acute rejection occurs most commonly in the first 30 days when the recipient's immune system encounters the donor antigen in both direct and indirect recognition. It is T-cell mediated and is a histological diagnosis with the main targets of attack being the biliary ductules and venous endothelium. Late acute cellular rejection most often occurs in the context of reduced calcineurin levels or viral infection and is more detrimental to the graft, particularly if recurrent.

With improvements in immunosuppressive therapy, chronic rejection has become very uncommon, accounting for less than 5% of late graft loss. Recurrent acute rejection and poor compliance with CNIs are the most common precipitants of chronic rejection, where there is loss of bile ducts and an arteriopathy resulting in ischaemic injury to the graft, which often results in the need for retransplantation.

Viral hepatitis

Liver transplantation for liver disease where hepatitis C has contributed to the requirement for transplantation is very common and is the principal indication in most centers throughout the world. The outcome for transplantation for hepatitis C is worse than for other causes of cirrhosis and recurrent disease contributes to this poorer outcome. Hepatitis B recurrence can be prevented by the administration of hepatitis immunoglobulin and lamivudine. In cases where lamivudine resistance is present either before or after transplantation, newer nucleoside analogues can control the infection. It is now extremely rare to lose a graft to recurrent hepatitis B infection because there are such effective therapies available [10]. This, however, is not the case for hepatitis C infection.

Trials of preemptive therapy with pegylated interferon and ribavirin have failed to show any benefit in reducing the risk of significant re-infection, and most units adopt a wait-and-see approach with protocol biopsies every year and commencement of therapy when there is histological progression. The rate of progression is variable between centers with immunosuppressive regimens and donor age probably being the most significant modifiable factors concerned [11]. The response to therapy in the transplant situation is significantly less than in the naive setting, with sustained virological responses in the order of 30% overall commonplace. The dose reduction required is commonly required in the post-transplantation setting despite the use of growth factors and erythropoeitin. Significant fibrosis causing graft dysfunction occurs in the region of 20% of HCV-related transplantations at 5 years.

Disease recurrence

The other common indications for transplantation in the western world are PBC, primary sclerosing cholangitis (PSC), and alcoholic and non-alcoholic fatty liver disease (NAFLD). All of these conditions can recur with alcoholic liver disease being the most modifiable. In most series the relapse rate is around 10–15% [9]. The cholestatic liver diseases, however, recur in a significant proportion as follow-up increases. Recurrent PBC has been discussed previously and there is controversy about the importance of the contribution of inflammatory bowel disease to the recurrence of PSC. In the UK, at least, it does appear that having an intact colon at the time of transplantation is significant in terms of the risk of recurrent PSC [12]. At present there is very little information about recurrent NAFLD although there are cases of graft failure related to recurrent disease [13].

Recurrent disease does occur in some patients transplanted for autoimmune hepatitis, but for other conditions such as hemochromatosis and Wilson's disease there is no recurrence.

Long-term issues

Liver transplant recipients have a survival of around 75% at 5 years and 60% at 10 years. The common causes of death in this population are graft failure, malignancy, and cardiovascular death [14]. The long-term use of immunosuppression increases the risk of malignancy of all types with the specific PTLD occurring usually in the first 3 years. This is driven by the Epstein–Barr virus and may respond to reduction in immunosuppression, cytotoxic T-cell therapy, or conventional chemotherapy.

Surveillance colonoscopy is performed annually in patients transplanted for PSC and regular mammography and cervical smears are recommended for female patients. Sunscreen is advised because the incidence of all skin tumors is significantly increased. One group that appears particularly susceptible are patients transplanted for alcoholic liver disease with an increase in esophageal and laryngeal tumors [15].

Allocation of allografts

Allocation systems for liver transplantation vary between countries, although most systems have a "super-urgent" category that permits transplantation of individuals with acute liver failure or early graft failure due to hepatic artery thrombosis or primary non-function. The USA now allocates grafts according to the MELD score with additional points given for patients with HCC, because these patients often have a very low MELD score. The death rate on the waiting list for liver transplantation is around 25% and therefore other alternatives have been sought with living-related liver transplantation being the most radical. This involves, in most cases, the removal of the right lobe from a healthy individual and transplanting this into the related recipient. Careful work-up of the donor is required in terms of liver size as well as general physical and mental health. Biliary complications occur in around 20% of donors and there is a reported mortality rate of around 0.4% [16].

References

1 Neuberger J, Gimson A, Davies M, for the Liver Advisory Group, and UK Blood and Transplant. Selection of patients for liver transplantation and allocation of donated livers in the UK. *Gut* 2008;57:252–7.

2 Bathgate AJ, Hynd P, Sommerville D, Hayes PC. The prediction of acute cellular rejection in orthotopic liver transplantation. *Liver Transpl* 1999;**5**:475–9.

3 Sylvestre PB, Batts KP, Burgart LJ, Poterucha JJ, Wiesner RH. Recurrence of primary biliary cirrhosis after liver transplantation: Histologic estimate of incidence and natural history. *Liver Transpl* 2003;**9**:1086–93.

4 Bathgate AJ, UK Liver Transplant Units. Recommendations for alcohol-related liver disease. *Lancet* 2006;**367**:2045–6.

5 Rodriguez-Roisin R, Krowka MJ. Hepatopulmonary syndrome – a liver-induced lung vascular disorder. *N Engl J Med* 2008;**358**:2378–87.

6 Ojo AO, Held PJ, Port FK, et al. Chronic renal failure after transplantation of a nonrenal organ. *N Engl J Med* 2003;**349**:931–40.

7 Pruthi J, Medkiff KA, Esrason KT, et al. Analysis of causes of death in liver transplant recipients who survived more than 3 years. *Liver Transpl* 2001;**7**: 811–15.

8 Sharma S, Gurakar A, Jabbour N. Biliary strictures following liver transplantation: Past, present and preventive strategies. *Liver Transpl* 2008;**14**:759–69.

9 McCallum S, Masterton G. Liver transplantation for alcoholic liver disease: a systematic review of psychosocial selection criteria. *Alcohol* 2006;**41**:358–63.

10 Mutimer D. Review article: hepatitis B and liver transplantation. *Aliment Pharmacol Ther* 2006;**23**:1031–41.

11 Berenguer M, Aguilera V, Prieto M, et al. Effect of calcineurin inhibitors on survival and histologic disease severity in HCV-infected liver transplant recipients. *Liver Transpl* 2006;**12**:762–7.

12 Vera A, Moledina S, Gunson B, et al. Risk factors for recurrence of primary sclerosing cholangitis of liver allograft. *Lancet* 2002;**360**:1943–4.

13 Contos MJ, Cales W, Sterling RK, et al. Development of nonalcoholic fatty liver disease after orthotopic liver transplantation for cryptogenic cirrhosis. *Liver Transpl* 2001;**7**:363–73.

14 Jain A, Reyes J, Kashyap R, et al. Long-term survival after liver transplantation in 4,000 consecutive patients at a single center. *Ann Surg* 2000;**232**:490–500.

15 Lake JR, David KM, Steffen BJ, Chu AH, Gordon RD, Wiesner RH. Addition of MMF to dual immunosuppression does not increase the risk of malignant short-term death after liver transplantation. *Am J Transplant* 2005;**5**:2961–7.

16 Middleton PF, Duffield M, Lynch SV, et al. Living donor liver transplantation – adult donor outcomes: a systematic review. *Liver Transpl* 2006;**12**:24–30.

18 Incidental Radiological Findings in the Asymptomatic Patient

Tiffany J. Campbell[1] *and Dilip Patel*[2]

[1]Forth Valley Royal Hospital, Larbert, UK
[2]Department of Radiology, The Royal Infirmary of Edinburgh, Edinburgh, UK

Case 1: echogenic lesion in the right lobe of the liver

Case presentation

A previously well 35-year-old woman with a family history of colorectal carcinoma presented with vague abdominal pain. Physical examination was unremarkable. Routine blood results including FBC, urea and electrolytes, liver function tests, ESR, CRP, and CEA (carcinoembryonic antigen) were all normal. The fecal occult blood test was also negative.

An abdominal ultrasound scan was requested and was reported as follows:

32-mm well-circumscribed echogenic lesion peripherally within the right lobe of the liver. The liver is otherwise normal. No significant abnormality in relation to the gallbladder, biliary tree, kidneys, spleen, pancreas, or aorta. No evidence of free fluid or lymph node enlargement.

Questions

- What is the most likely diagnosis?
- What is the differential diagnosis?
- What further imaging modalities can be utilized to investigate this lesion further?

Discussion

The ultrasound appearances are typical of a hepatic hemangioma. Hepatic hemangiomas are a common incidental finding at imaging and are the most common benign liver tumor with a frequency of 7.3% at autopsy [1]. Hepatic hemangiomas are more common in women, with a female:male ratio of up to 5:1 [2], and associated with an increased incidence in postmenopausal, multiparous women. They tend to be solitary, are typically <4 cm in size, and are found most commonly in the posterior right lobe of liver peripherally or in a subcapsular location.

Up to 70% of hemangiomas have a typical ultrasonic appearance (Figure 18.1), being well defined, uniformly echogenic lesions <4 cm, which demonstrate posterior acoustic enhancement [1]. Microscopically they are made up of large vascular channels lined by a thin layer of endothelial cells, separated by thin, fibrous septa. It is these vascular channels and the multiple interfaces that are thought to cause its appearance on an ultrasound scan.

The classic ultrasonic appearance of a hemangioma detected as an incidental finding in a patient who is otherwise entirely well requires no further investigation. The principal ultrasonic differential diagnosis is metastasis, particularly from neuroendocrine tumors and adenocarcinomas.

When there is a concern that the lesion could represent a neoplastic lesion such as a metastasis CT or MRI is the next investigation of choice. CT until recently has been the cross-sectional imaging modality most frequently used for further characterization of a lesion identified on ultrasonography. Non-contrast scans of the upper abdomen are initially

Problem-based Approach to Gastroenterology and Hepatology, First Edition. Edited by John N. Plevris, Colin W. Howden.
© 2012 Blackwell Publishing Ltd. Published 2012 by Blackwell Publishing Ltd.

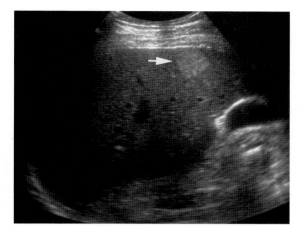

Figure 18.1 Ultrasound scan showing well-defined subcapsular echogenic lesion within the right lobe of the liver, typical of a hemangioma.

obtained and the patient is subsequently scanned after the administration of intravenous iodinated contrast in the arterial, portal venous, and late venous phases.

Up to 70% demonstrate the classic appearance of a low attenuation lesion on the pre-contrast images, with globular peripheral enhancement on arterial phase imaging and then gradual centripetal in-filling on the portal and late venous phases. The enhancement of the lesion is identical to the blood pool in each phase. Classically, hemangiomas demonstrate complete "in-filling" and, depending on the size of the lesion, this can take up to 20 min or longer. The sensitivity and specificity of CT for diagnosing hemangioma have been reported as 88% and 84–100% respectively [3,4].

Since the development of faster sequences and liver-specific contrast agents, hepatic MRI is now an established imaging tool for the liver. MRI also has the added advantage of not using ionizing radiation, which is a relevant consideration because many of the patients investigated are young and repeated scans are often required to demonstrate the typical enhancement pattern, thus increasing radiation exposure.

On MRI, hemangiomas have variable degrees of T1- and T2-lengthening values but typically have longer T2-weighted values than any other tumor. Lesions are typically well circumscribed and are of increased signal on T2-weighted imaging, with signal intensity similar to cerebrospinal fluid (CSF) [5,6]. On

T1-weighted pre-contrast images, hemangiomas are usually of lower signal-to-background intensity than liver but can be of variable intensity and may be of higher signal-to-background intensity due to the presence of hepatocytes containing fat and hemorrhage. The contrast enhancement characteristics with gadolinium-based contrast agents are identical to those of iodinated contrast with CT (Figure 18.2). MRI is considered the most accurate imaging technique for characterizing hemangiomas with accuracy rates approaching 100% [7].

The enhancement characteristics of hemangiomas using intravenous ultrasound contrast agents are similar to those for CT and MRI [8]. However, this technique is not as widely available as CT and MRI, and its success depends on both the skill of the operator and the suitability of the patient, particularly with respect to body habitus.

Unfortunately not all hemangiomas present typically or have classic imaging appearances. Most hemangiomas remain stable in size or demonstrate very slow growth over time. Some can be seen to grow rapidly, and this has been seen during pregnancy or in cases of estrogen use. If the lesion exceeds 4 cm in diameter the term "giant hemangioma" is used. The mechanism of enlargement is thought to be vascular ectasia, and the role of estrogens has been postulated. Complications for hemangiomas are rare and vary from 4.5% to 19.7% [5]. Complication rates increase with the size of the lesion and include pain, upper abdominal mass, inflammation, intratumoral hemorrhage, and even hemoperitoneum secondary to spontaneous rupture. The Kasabach–Merritt syndrome is a rare complication of hemangioma in adults which involves the presence of multiple liver lesions and a coagulopathy consisting of intravascular coagulation, clotting, and fibrinolysis within the hemangioma. The initially localized coagulopathy may progress to secondary increased systemic fibrinolysis and thrombocytopenia, leading to a fatal outcome in 20–30% of patients [5].

The most frequent atypical appearance on ultrasonography, with reports up to 40% [1], is of a hypoechoic lesion with an echogenic rim. This appearance is thought to be due to central hemorrhage, necrosis, or scarring within the lesion. Other rarer atypical appearances include: calcification, hyalinization, cystic or multilocular, pedunculated, and containing fluid–fluid levels.

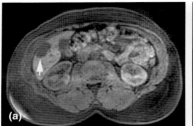
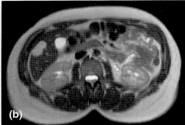
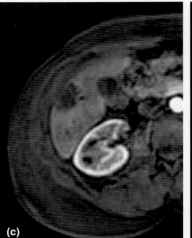
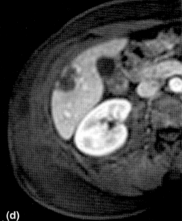
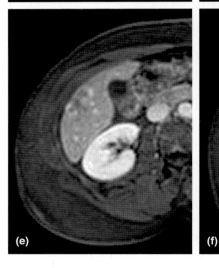

Figure 18.2 (a) T1-weighted image (a) demonstrating well-circumscribed low signal characteristics of a hemangioma. (b) The T2-weighted image shows the corresponding high signal appearances. Sequential post-contrast MR images acquired in the (c) arterial, (d) portal, (e) 3-min, and (f) 10-min phases, demonstrating the typical enhancement characteristics of a hemangioma with progressive centripetal enhancement. By 10 min the lesion has completely "filled-in."

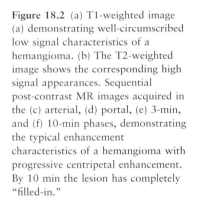

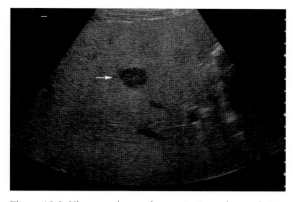

Figure 18.3 Ultrasound scan demonstrating a hypoechoic hemangioma with background increased liver echotexture in keeping with fatty infiltration.

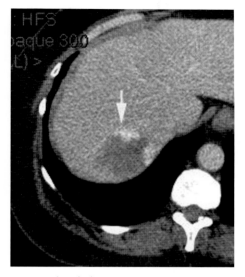

Figure 18.4 Delayed phase post-contrast CT scan showing non enhancement of the central portion of the hemangioma. This can be seen in large lesions and can be due to fibrosis or necrosis.

With background fatty infiltration of the liver hemangiomas may appear iso- or hypoechoic on ultrasound scan compared with the rest of the liver (Figure 18.3) and can mimic other lesions such as metastases. In these situations the lesion still tends to show posterior acoustic enhancement. Contrast-enhanced CT or MRI is usually indicated to demonstrate the typical enhancement characteristics. Giant hemangiomas can be hypoattenuating and heterogeneous, and on contrast administration demonstrate a central scar or area that does not enhance even on delayed phase imaging (Figure 18.4). Sixteen percent of hemangiomas may also demonstrate rapid flash filling [5] in the arterial phase (Figure 18.5), which is a pattern that can be seen particularly with background fatty infiltration and can make them difficult to distinguish from other hypervascular lesions, particularly hypervascular metastases. The diagnosis can generally be made, however, on the delayed phase imaging where hemangiomas tend to retain their enhancement, whereas hypervascular metastases tend to wash out contrast and are hypoattenuating/hypointense compared with normal background liver.

With advances in imaging techniques, a confident imaging diagnosis of hemangioma can be made in over 95% of cases based on the imaging appearances alone. Biopsy is indicated only when the appearances are atypical and a malignancy in particular needs to be excluded. Despite the vascular nature of these lesions, percutaneous biopsy is a proven safe

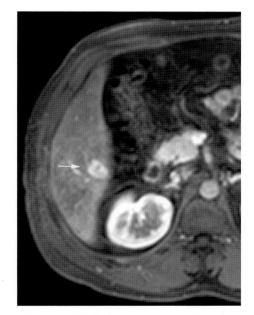

Figure 18.5 Arterial phase post-contrast MR scan showing atypical enhancement pattern with flash filling and uniform contrast enhancement.

229

procedure using an 18 G needle [9]. With subcapsular lesions, where it is not possible to access the lesion by traversing normal hepatic parenchyma, laparoscopic biopsy is indicated to reduce the risk of bleeding-related complications.

Case 2: incidental adrenal lesion

Case presentation

A 51-year-old man presents with dysphagia and weight loss. Endoscopy demonstrates a 3-cm malignant stricture of the distal esophagus, with biopsy confirming squamous cell carcinoma.

The patient undergoes a staging CT scan of the thorax and upper abdomen with oral water and intravenous contrast, with the thoracic and abdominal phases acquired at 25 s and 60 s respectively.

The following report is obtained:

Concentric thickening of the distal esophagus over a length of 3 cm with preservation of the periesophageal fat planes. Several peritumoral nodes are identified measuring up to 6 mm in short axis diameter. No other significant findings within the mediastinum or lung fields.

22 mm well-circumscribed nodule (Figure 18.6) within the right adrenal gland. The upper abdominal viscera are otherwise normal. No evidence of upper abdominal lymph node enlargement or free fluid.

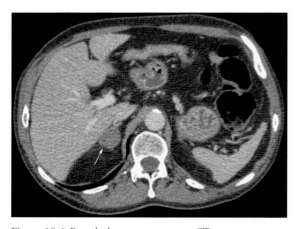

Figure 18.6 Portal phase post contrast CT scan demonstrating 22-mm right adrenal mass.

Conclusion: distal esophageal carcinoma with local staging T3N1 by CT criteria. Right adrenal nodule.

Questions

• What is the most likely diagnosis of the adrenal nodule?
• What differential diagnoses should be considered?
• How should the patient be investigated further?

Diagnosis and differential diagnosis

The right adrenal lesion is typically termed an adrenal "incidentaloma" which is defined as a lesion detected on imaging performed in patients not suspected of having adrenal disease. The principal differential diagnoses are a benign adrenal adenoma and metastasis.

Several other benign mass lesions can occur in the adrenal glands which can be characterized accurately by their morphological appearances on CT and MRI, including adrenal cysts and myelolipomas, with the identification of fat in an adrenal mass – virtually pathognomonic of the latter. Other benign lesions include hemangioma, hematoma, and granulomatous disease.

Adrenal carcinoma is usually >5 cm at presentation and appears as a heterogeneous soft-tissue mass which may have areas of necrosis and show features of local invasion of adjacent organs such as the liver and also of vascular structures particularly the adrenal veins and inferior vena cava (IVC). Therefore, adrenal carcinoma is rarely mistaken for an incidentaloma.

Discussion

Incidental adrenal lesions are common, with a prevalence of 9% within the general population at autopsy [10,11]. With the increasing use of cross-sectional imaging in the assessment of the abdomen, incidental adrenal lesions are being identified with a frequency of up to 5%, with the incidence increasing in patients with diabetes and hypertension [11].

Most incidental adrenal lesions are benign in those patients who do not have a history of malignancy [12,13]. Adrenal cortical adenoma is the most common benign tumor, with recent studies demonstrating that 75% of benign adrenal lesions are adenomas, with myelolipomas and hematomas being the next most common [4]. The vast majority of adrenal adenomas are hormonally non-functional and, once correctly characterized, do not require further intervention. However, the differential diagnosis includes functioning lesions resulting in conditions such as Cushing's disease, Conn's syndrome, virilization syndromes, and pheochromocytoma.

The chance of an incidental adrenal lesion being malignant increases if there is an underlying history of extra-adrenal malignancy, with up to 50% of such lesions representing metastases [12,13].

Accordingly, the accurate characterization of these lesions is essential, especially in the oncology setting where the characterization of an adrenal incidentaloma as malignant classifies the patient as having stage IV disease, effectively ending the option of treatment with curative intent.

Consequently, intensive hormonal and imaging work-up is required before these lesions can be ignored and non-invasive adrenal imaging techniques can usually determine if a lesion is benign or malignant.

The follow-up of lesions characterized as benign is not universally agreed, with some guidelines suggesting follow-up for 2 years despite no supporting evidence base [12]. More recent work has demonstrated that these lesions do not require follow-up in low-risk population groups where there is no history of malignancy [14].

Functional assessment

Functional assessment of adrenal nodules includes measurement of 24-hour urinary catecholamines and urinary free cortisol, overnight dexamethasone suppression tests, and measurement of plasma renin activity, and aldosterone and adrenal androgens [15].

Functional assessment

Ultrasonography can be a useful imaging tool for adrenal glands in children but has virtually no role in characterizing adrenal lesions in adults.

CT and MRI are the mainstay of non-invasive imaging assessment of adrenal lesions. Positron emission tomography (PET)/CT is also being increasingly utilized for lesion characterization in the oncology population.

Image-guided biopsy is usually reserved for those cases where imaging has failed to characterize a lesion

and immediate patient management depends on knowing the nature of the lesion.

Benign adrenal adenomas are usually small, measuring 2–4 cm in diameter, well-defined round or ovoid lesions, and of uniform appearance. More than 70% of all adrenal adenomas will have high intracytoplasmic lipid content, a feature very rarely seen in malignant lesions, and has a very high correlation with benign disease.

This can be demonstrated non-invasively on both CT and MRI with sensitivities and specificities in excess of 90%.

CT scan

Formal CT of the adrenal gland involves acquiring both pre- and delayed post-contrast (10–15 min after administration) scans. However, most incidental adrenal lesions are detected on post-contrast portal phase scans, during routine reporting after the patient has left the CT department! It is very difficult to classify a lesion as benign on this single phase alone, particularly in the oncology setting.

On non-contrast CT, benign adenomas with a high intracytoplasmic lipid content have a mean Hounsfield unit (HU) of ≤10. Using this threshold a benign adenoma can be diagnosed with a specificity of 98% and a sensitivity of 71% [16].

However, 30% of benign adenomas are "lipid poor" and therefore have a mean HU >10, as do most malignant lesions. Patients with atypical lesions with a HU >10 on non-contrast CT are further assessed with contrast-enhanced scans and delayed imaging. Although both benign adenomas and malignant lesions enhance early after intravenous contrast, it has been shown that benign adenomas "wash out" contrast faster than their malignant counterparts.

Contrast washout is calculated by measuring the mean HU of the lesion at 60s and 10–15 min after intravenous iodinated contrast administration. Percentage washout is calculated as either absolute (if non-contrast HU values are available) or relative if based on post-contrast measurements using only the formulae outlined below. Using absolute (APW) and relative (RPW) percentage washout thresholds of >60% and >40%, respectively, lesions can be characterized as benign adenomas with sensitivities and specificities approaching 100% [16]. Lesions with washout thresholds less than these or with mean HU

>43 on non-contrast CT should be considered malignant [16].

$$RPW = 100 \times$$
$$\text{(enhanced HU - delayed HU)/enhanced HU}$$
$$APW = 100 \times$$
$$\text{(enhanced HU - delayed HU)/enhanced HU -}$$
$$\text{non-contrast HU.}$$

MRI scan

This can be used to characterize benign adenomas utilizing chemical shift imaging (CSI) to demonstrate intracytoplasmic lipid. CSI exploits the differing resonance frequency rates of protons in water and fat molecules, and images of the adrenal glands are obtained with the water and fat protons "in" and "out" of phase.

In lesions that contain high content of both water and fat, "in-phase" MR images will combine the two factors to give a high signal lesion. In the "out-of-phase" imaging, the water and fat signals will cancel each other out and produce very low signal intensity, which can usually be appreciated by visual assessment of the images (Figure 18.7). CSI signal loss can also be measured quantitatively by calculating the adrenal:spleen CSI ratio with a CSI ratio of 0.71 indicating a benign lipid-rich adenoma.

The sensitivity and specificity of CSI for characterizing an adrenal lesion as benign are reported at 78–100% and 87–100% respectively [17]. Although there is no significant difference between CT and MRI in characterizing lipid-rich lesions, the evidence suggests that CSI may be superior to CT for evaluating lesions with a CT HU value of 10–30. Contrast washout has also been evaluated using MRI but is not a robust technique suitable for routine clinical practice.

MR diffusion-weighted imaging and MR spectroscopy have recently been shown to have promising applications for adrenal lesion characterization but are not currently used in routine clinical practice.

PET/CT scan

[18F]Fluorodeoxyglucose (FDG) PET/CT is now a pivotal part of the imaging assessment of some cancers including lung and colorectal carcinoma and lymphoma. FDG is a glucose analogue and the basic imaging principle is based on most malignant tumors preferentially using glucose as an energy source. Tumor cells take up FDG preferentially to glucose and compete with glucose for enzymatic phosphorylation by hexokinase. Once FDG is phosphorylated into FDG-6-phosphate it is trapped inside the cell and does not undergo further metabolism. The 18F decays to emit a positron which collides with an electron to emit gamma rays; these are detected by scintillation counters from which the images are formed. The patient also undergoes a CT scan that is used to accurately localize the abnormal activity, therefore providing both functional and anatomical information.

Normal adrenal glands and 95% of benign adenomas do not take up FDG, whereas malignant lesions do and can be detected by FDG PET scanning, with sensitivities and specificities approaching 100% in lesions >10 mm [18]. Metastases are also increasingly being identified in adrenal glands showing minimal thickening of the limb architecture and even in morphologically normal looking glands (Figure 18.8).

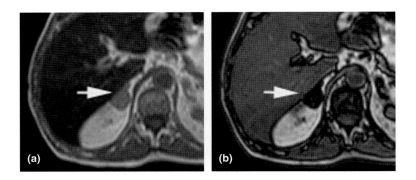

Figure 18.7 (a) In- and (b) out-of-phase MR scans. The out-of-phase image demonstrates signal loss within the right adrenal gland which appears almost black, indicating a lipid-rich benign adenoma.

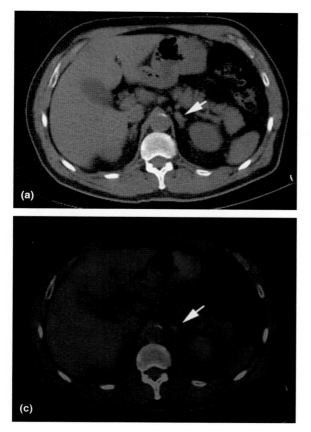

Figure 18.8 Positron emission tomography (PET/CT) series in a patient with esophageal carcinoma with resectable disease demonstrated on conventional CT and endoscopic ultrasonography. (a) The CT scan demonstrates minimally thickened left adrenal gland. (b) The PET image shows corresponding [^{18}F] fluorodeoxyglucose uptake confirmed by the fusion image (c). Metastasis was confirmed at laparoscopic adrenalectomy.

PET/CT is being increasingly used to characterize lesions classed as indeterminate using CT and MRI and too small to biopsy percutaneously.

Biopsy

Adrenal biopsy is reserved for those patients in whom non-invasive imaging has failed to characterize a lesion and a diagnosis is required, and management will be altered particularly if there is a history of malignancy. The procedure is usually performed under CT guidance using a coaxial technique that allows a number of passes to be made through a single outer needle. The adrenal gland can usually be accessed directly with the patient prone or in a lateral decubitus position. Difficult right-sided lesions can also be accessed by a transhepatic approach. Image guide adrenal biopsy is a safe procedure with a high degree of accuracy (83–96%) and a low complication rate (3%) usually related to hemorrhage or pneumothorax [14].

Case 3: pancreatic cystic mass

Case presentation

A 32-year-old woman presents to the emergency department with a 12-hour history of right-sided loin pain. She has no significant past medical history other than occasional RUQ pain. On examination she is overweight, apyrexial, and mildly tender to palpation in the right flank. Routine blood tests including CBC, U&Es, liver function tests, blood glucose, and CRP are normal. Dipstick urinalysis reveals 1+ hematuria.

A clinical diagnosis of right renal colic is made and a non-contrast CT of the kidneys, ureter, and bladder

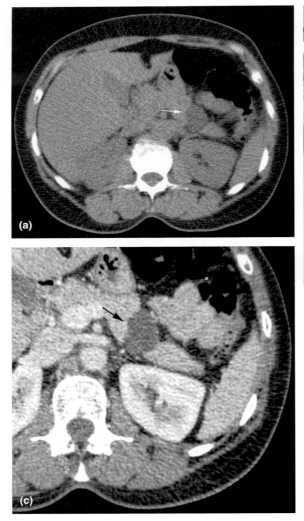

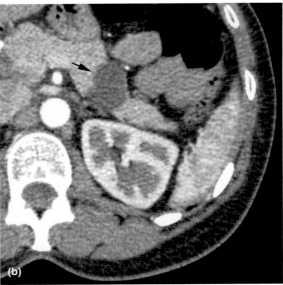

Figure 18.9 (a) Non-contrast CT demonstrating well-circumscribed, non-calcified, cystic attenuation pancreatic tail mass. (b,c) Arterial and portal phase post-contrast CT scans; both demonstrate no evidence of enhancement of the cystic mass shown in (a) compared with the adjacent normal pancreatic parenchyma.

is requested. This demonstrates a normal renal tract with no evidence of radio-opaque renal stone disease. However, a well-circumscribed, non-calcified, 3-cm cystic attenuation mass is noted in relation to the pancreatic tail (Figure 9a). No other significant findings are noted.

Questions

• What differential diagnoses should be considered for the pancreatic mass?
• How should the patient be investigated further?

Differential diagnosis

The differential diagnosis for a cystic pancreatic mass is wide and is detailed in Table 18.1. With the greater use of high-resolution cross-sectional imaging, these lesions are diagnosed in increasing numbers as an incidental finding in patients investigated for non-pancreatic-related conditions.

They are often small, usually asymptomatic, and in some studies can occur in up to 20% of the imaged population [19]. They are usually identified in the older patient in whom the surgical risk is higher due to associated co morbidities.

Table 18.1 Differential diagnosis of pancreatic cystic masses

Congenital	Multiple:
	adult polycystic kidney disease
	von Hippel–Lindau disease
	Single: epithelial, lymphoepithelial cysts
Inflammatory	Pseudocyst, abscess
Exocrine pancreatic lesions	Mucinous adenocarcinoma
	Microcystic adenoma
	Macrocystic adenoma
	Intraductal papillary mucinous neoplasm
Endocrine lesions	Insulinoma, glucagonoma
Non-epithelial lesions	Sarcoma, metastases

Many cystic lesions are known to be benign and after proper imaging workup can be either ignored or safely followed up with serial scanning. It is important to accurately characterize cystic neoplasms and to distinguish cystic neoplasms of the pancreas from pancreatic pseudocysts which are the commonest pancreatic cystic masses detected in symptomatic patients. Serous cystadenomas, mucinous cystic neoplasms, and intraductal papillary mucinous neoplasms (IPMNs) account for 90% of all primary cystic pancreatic neoplasms [20]. Serous cystadenomas are benign tumors and in asymptomatic patients can be safely followed up obviating the need for surgery, whereas mucin-producing lesions such as IPMNs and mucinous cystic neoplasms have malignant potential that warrants surgery [21]. Solid tumors of the pancreas such as islet cell tumors and adenocarcinomas can occasionally present as cystic masses. It is also important to differentiate cystic neoplasms from pancreatic adenocarcinomas because the prognosis for malignant cystic neoplasms is better than that for ductal adenocarcinomas [21,22].

Discussion

Imaging plays a crucial role in the non-invasive characterization of pancreatic cystic lesions and those lesions detected incidentally either on ultrasonography or on "routine" CT/MRI should be re-evaluated by CT or MRI with dedicated pancreatic imaging protocols.

Multidetector CT is still currently the modality of choice for imaging the pancreas because it is possible to obtain very-high-resolution images as a result of the thin slices from which the images are acquired. This allows reconstruction of the images in multiple planes without loss of resolution, which is essential to evaluate the relationship of any mass identified to adjacent structures and vessels; this is an important part in assessing for operability.

Pre-contrast images are useful to identify calcifications that may help in lesion characterization. The pancreas is subsequently imaged in the arterial and portal phases after giving intravenous contrast for vascular and parenchymal assessment (Figure 18.9b,c).

With the development of faster pulse sequences, MRI is increasingly used for pancreatic imaging. The superior soft-tissue resolution compared with CT often allows more accurate characterization of the internal architecture of cystic lesions by demonstrating internal septa, debris, and microcysts not appreciated on CT (Figure 18.10). MRI can also be used to

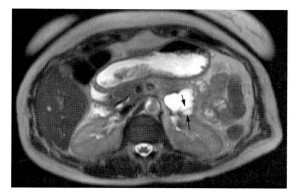

Figure 18.10 T2-weighted MR scan demonstrating the cystic mass in Figure 18.9 as a high signal lesion. An internal septum is noted that is not seen on the CT, demonstrating the superiority of MRI in depicting internal cyst architecture.

characterize hemorrhagic and proteinaceous cysts based on cyst signal characteristics. MR cholangio-pancreatography (MRCP) is also an accurate non-invasive technique for demonstrating the relationship of the cyst to the pancreatic duct, which can help to characterize lesions such as pancreatic pseudocysts and IPMNs.

Endoscopic ultrasonography (EUS) can be used to characterize small lesions when CT/MRI is indeterminate and can also be used for image-guided fine needle aspiration (FNA)/biopsy, particularly for those lesions that are inaccessible for percutaneous CT- or ultrasound-guided biopsy. However, access outside major centers is still limited. It is an operator-dependent technique requiring a high level of expertise and, although generally well tolerated, is still relative invasive compared with CT or MRI.

Several groups have attempted to classify cystic pancreatic lesions to help stratify the further management of these lesions [23,24] and can be grouped as follows.

Unilocular cysts

Pancreatic pseudocysts are the most common cause of unilocular cysts [25]. Most patients are symptomatic and the diagnosis is usually confirmed by clinical evidence of a preceding history of pancreatitis and appropriate risk factors. Imaging usually provides further support, demonstrating other features of pancreatitis such as peripancreatic inflammatory changes and free fluid. Gallstones may also be identified as the precipitating cause, particularly if they are intraductal stones. Features of chronic pancreatitis may be present such as pancreatic calcification, parenchymal atrophy, and pancreatic duct dilation.

Pseudocysts are typically well-circumscribed, uniformly thin-walled, oval or round masses measuring up to 20 cm (Figure 18.11). Uncomplicated pseudocysts are of uniform fluid attenuation/signal on CT and MRI respectively. Hemorrhagic or infected pseudocysts are of high attenuation on CT and the presence of gas can be seen with enteric communication or infection.

When a pseudocyst is detected incidentally and there is diagnostic doubt, cyst puncture can be a useful procedure to obtain fluid for amylase measurement.

Multiple unilocular cysts are usually due to pseudocysts but can also be seen in von Hippel–Lindau

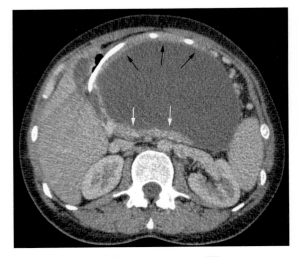

Figure 18.11 Portal phase post-contrast CT scan demonstrating a large pseudocyst compressing the stomach anteriorly (black arrows), which contains a nasogastric tube. The pseudocyst lies immediately anterior to the pancreas which is also compressed (white arrows).

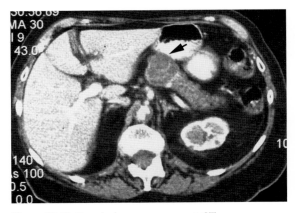

Figure 18.12 Portal phase post-contrast CT scan demonstrating the typical appearance of a serous cystadenoma with multiple tiny cysts. (Image courtesy of Dr Stephen Glancy, The Royal Infirmary of Edinburgh.)

disease in which there may also be cysts in the liver and kidneys.

Microcystic lesions

Serous cystadenomas are benign lesions that usually measure between 2 and 20 cm [26]. The majority demonstrate a polycystic pattern consisting of cysts measuring between 2 and 20 mm (Figure 18.12). The presence of a central scar with or without stellate calcification is a highly specific feature seen in approximately 30% of patients and is virtually pathognomonic. Pancreatic duct dilation is rarely seen. MRI and EUS are useful modalities to demonstrate the microcystic nature of the lesion when CT is indeterminate. If a confident imaging diagnosis of serous cystadenoma can be made, imaging surveillance in asymptomatic patients is a recognized imaging strategy obviating the need for surgery.

A macrocystic variant is also recognized and seen in less than 10% of cases, in which the lesion consists of a unilocular cyst or multiple cysts >2 cm (which was the diagnosis in this particular case). This variant can be difficult to differentiate on imaging grounds from mucinous cystic tumors [27].

Macrocystic lesions

Macrocystic lesions These are characterized by fewer compartments and individual loculations >2 cm. This category includes mucinous cystic tumors and IPMNs.

Mucinous cystadenomas These can be asymptomatic in 75% of cases and are typically located in the body and tail of pancreas [28]. The complex internal architecture is best seen on MRI or EUS (Figure 18.13) which helps to differentiate from serous cystadenoma. Peripheral eggshell calcification is an uncommon feature but is associated with malignancy. These lesions can sometimes be difficult to distinguish from complex pseudocysts. Surgical resection is indicated for mucinous cystadenoma because of the propensity for malignancy.

IPMNs These are classified as main duct, side branch, or mixed based on the site and extent of involvement. Side-branch and mixed lesions can present as cystic masses.

These lesions are multiseptated and typically communicate with the pancreatic duct, which helps to differentiate them from mucinous cystadenomas [29]. Both multidetector CT and MRI can demonstrate the relationship of the lesion to the duct. MRCP is the investigation of choice, obviating the need for endoscopic retrograde cholangiopancreatography (ERCP) and its associated risks. These lesions do have malignant potential and surgery is therefore usually recommended.

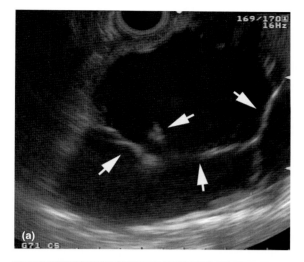
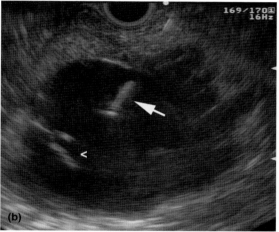

Figure 18.13 (a) Endoscopic ultrasonography (EUS) image showing mucinous cystadenoma with the typical internal septations. (b) The cyst was aspirated under EUS guidance (needle arrowed) and biochemical analysis confirmed an elevated carcinoembryonic antigen (CEA) which is an accurate predictive feature of a mucinous neoplasm. (Image courtesy of Dr Ian Penman.)

Other cystic lesions

Some solid tumors may have a cystic component or undergo cystic degeneration; this group includes islet cell tumors, solid pseudopapillary tumors, pancreatic adenocarcinomas, and metastases. These are rarely identified as incidental findings in asymptomatic patients and therefore require intervention appropriate for the clinical circumstances.

Conclusion

The increasing use of cross-sectional imaging including ultrasonography, CT, and MRI has resulted in a significant increase in the detection of incidental lesions often unrelated to the patient's presenting complaint.

These cases outline three lesions frequently encountered as incidental findings in the course of imaging patients with suspected gastrointestinal (GI) or hepatic disease.

Hepatic hemangiomas are a common incidental imaging finding, usually identified on an abdominal ultrasound scan. Although hepatic hemangiomas have a typical ultrasonic appearance, CT or MRI is increasingly being used for further confirmation, particularly when the patient is being investigated for possible malignant disease to exclude metastasis. Percutaneous biopsy is a safe technique reserved in a minority of cases when the imaging appearances are atypical and malignancy in particular needs to be excluded.

Likewise, adrenal adenoma, although not strictly a "gastrointestinal incidentaloma," is an important lesion for the GI physician to be familiar with because these lesions are frequently encountered both during the routine investigation of patients with abdominal symptoms and during the staging of patients with proven GI malignancy. The vast majority of these are benign in the general population and even in the oncology population the proportion of benign lesions is 50%. The correct characterization of these lesions is crucial to patient management, particularly in the oncology setting, and may determine whether the patient will be offered treatment with curative intent if benign or palliative treatment in those patients upstaged to stage IV disease, where the lesion has been shown to be a metastasis.

Pancreatic cystic lesions are encountered with increasing frequency as an incidental finding and again accurate imaging assessment is crucial to ensure appropriate clinical management, particularly to avoid major surgery for those lesions <2 cm and with no complex features, where there is increasing evidence that these can be safely followed up after careful workup.

As illustrated, incidental lesions often require further clinical, laboratory, and imaging investigations to assess their significance and consequently are labor and resource intensive. Some patients are left with a sense of bewilderment and anxiety as they are faced with a barrage of investigations often unrelated to their presenting complaint.

Although imaging assessment forms the core basis of further investigation of these lesions, a multidisciplinary team approach is crucial to ensure that these patients are investigated and managed in a cost-effective manner.

References

1 Moody AR, Wilson SR. Atypical hepatic haemangioma: a suggestive sonographic morphology. *Radiology* 1993;**188**:413–17.

2 Semelka RC, Sofka CM. Hepatic hemangiomas. *Magn Reson Imaging Clin North Am* 1997;**5**:241–53.

3 Leslie DF, Johnson CD, Johnson CM, Ilstrup DM, Harmsen WS. Distinction between cavernous hemangiomas of the liver and hepatic metastases on CT: value of contrast enhancement patterns. *AJR Am J Roentgenol* 1995;**164**:625–9.

4 Quinn SF, Benjamin GG. Hepatic cavernous hemangiomas: simple diagnostic sign with dynamic bolus CT. *Radiology* 1992;**182**:545–8.

5 Vilgrain V, Boulos L, Vullierme MP, et al, Imaging of atypical haemangiomas of the liver with pathological correlation. *RadioGraphics* 2000;**20**:379–97.

6 Nelson RC, Chezmar JL, Diagnostic approach to hepatic haemangiomas. *Radiology* 1990;**176**:11–13.

7 Soyer P, Gueye C, Somveille E, et al. MR diagnosis of hepatic metastases from neuroendocrine tumors versus hemangiomas: relative merits of dynamic gadolinium chelate–enhanced gradient-recalled echo and unenhanced spin-echo images. *AJR Am J Roentgenol* 1995;**165**:1407–13.

8 Brannigan M, Burns PN, Wilson SR. Blood flow patterns in focal liver lesions at microbubble-enhanced US. *RadioGraphics* 2004;**24**:921–35.

9 Cronan JJ, Esparza AR, Dorfman GS, Ridlen MS, Paolella LP. Cavernous hemangioma of the liver: role of percutaneous biopsy. *Radiology* 1988;**166**:135–8.

10 Abrams HL, Spiro R, Goldstein N. Metastases in carcinoma; analysis of 1000 autopsied cases. *Cancer* 1950;**3**:74–85.

11 Copeland PM. The incidentally discovered adrenal mass. *Ann Intern Med* 1983;**98**:940–5.

12 Young WF Jr. The incidentally discovered adrenal mass. *N Engl J Med* 2007;**356**:601–10.

13 Song JH, Fakhra S, Chaudhry FS, Mayo-Smith WW. The incidental adrenal mass on CT: Prevalence of adrenal disease in 1,049 consecutive adrenal masses in patients with no known malignancy. *Am J Roentgenol* 2008;**190**:1163–8.

14 Welch TJ, Sheedy PF II, Stephens DH, Johnson CM, Swensen SJ, Percutaneous adrenal biopsy review of 10-year experience. *Radiology* 1994;**193**:341–4.

15 Grumbach MM, Biller BM, Braunstein GD et al. Management of the clinically inapparent adrenal mass ("Incidentaloma"). *Ann Intern Med* 2003;**138**:424–30.

16 Boland GW, Lee MJ, Gazelle GS, et al. Characterization of adrenal masses using unenhanced CT: an analysis of the CT literature. *Am J Roentgenol* 1998;**171**:201–4.

17 Li J, Kalra MK, Small WC. Adrenal mass: differentiation by attenuation characteristics using dual-energy MDCT. *Am J Roentgenol* 2007;**188**(suppl 5):A59–62.

18 Chong S, Lee KS, Kim HY, et al. Integrated PET-CT for the characterization of adrenal gland lesions in cancer patients: diagnostic efficacy and interpretation pitfalls. *RadioGraphics* 2006;**26**:1811–24.

19 Zhang XM, Mitchell DG, Dohke M, et al. Pancreatic cysts: depiction on single-shot fast spin-echo MR images. *Radiology* 2002;**223**:547–53.

20 Fernandez-del Castillo C, Warshaw AL. Cystic tumors of the pancreas. *Surg Clin North Am* 1995;**75**:1001–16.

21 Compagno J, Oertel JE. Mucinous cystic neoplasms of the pancreas with overt and latent malignancy (cysta-denocarcinoma and cystadenoma): clinicopathologic study of 41 cases. *Am J Clin Pathol* 1978;**69**:573–80.

22 Madura JA, Wiebke EA, Howard TJ, et al. Mucin hyper-secreting intraductal neoplasms of the pancreas: a precursor to cystic pancreatic malignancies. *Surgery* 1997;**122**:786–93.

23 Sahani DV, Kadavigere R, Saokar A, et al. Cystic pancreatic lesions: a simple imaging-based classification system for guiding management. *RadioGraphics* 2005;**25**:1471–84.

24 Planner AC, Anderson EM, Slater A et al. An evidence-based review for the management of cystic pancreatic lesions. *Clin Radiol* 2007;**62**:930–7.

25 Balthazar EJ, Ranson JH, Naidich DP, Megibow AJ, Caccavale R, Cooper MM. Acute pancreatitis: prognostic value of CT. *Radiology* 1985;**156**:767–72.

26 Bounds BC, Brugge WR. EUS diagnosis of cystic lesions of the pancreas. *Int J Gastrointest Cancer* 2001;**30**:27–31.

27 Khurana B, Mortele KJ, Glickman J, Silverman SG, Ros PR. Macrocystic serous adenoma of the pancreas: radiologic–pathologic correlation. *AJR Am J Roentgenol* 2003;**181**:119–23.

28 Buetow PC, Rao P, Thompson LD. Mucinous cystic neoplasms of the pancreas: radiologic–pathologic correlation. *RadioGraphics* 1998;**18**:433–49.

29 Chiua SS, Lima JH, Leea WJ et al. Intraductal papillary mucinous tumour of the pancreas: differentiation of malignancy and benignancy by CT. *Clin Radiol* 2006;**61**:776–83.

Index

Problem-based Approach to Gastroenterology and Hepatology, First Edition. Edited by John N. Plevris, Colin W. Howden.
© 2012 Blackwell Publishing Ltd. Published 2012 by Blackwell Publishing Ltd.